IOM ROUNDTABLE ON EVIDENCE-BASED MEDICINE

THE LEARNING HEALTHCARE SYSTEM

Workshop Summary

LeighAnne Olsen, Dara Aisner, and J. Michael McGinnis

Roundtable on Evidence-Based Medicine

INSTITUTE OF MEDICINE
OF THE NATIONAL ACADEMIES

THE NATIONAL ACADEMIES PRESS
Washington, D.C.
www.nap.edu

THE NATIONAL ACADEMIES PRESS   500 Fifth Street, N.W.   Washington, DC 20001

NOTICE: The project that is the subject of this report was approved by the Governing Board of the National Research Council, whose members are drawn from the councils of the National Academy of Sciences, the National Academy of Engineering, and the Institute of Medicine.

This project was supported by the contracts between the National Academy of Sciences and Agency for Healthcare Research and Quality, America's Health Insurance Plans, AstraZeneca, Blue Shield of California Foundation, Burroughs Wellcome Fund, California Health Care Foundation, Centers for Medicare and Medicaid Services, Department of Veterans Affairs, Food and Drug Administration, Johnson & Johnson, sanofi-aventis, and Stryker. Any opinions, findings, conclusions, or recommendations expressed in this publication are those of the author(s) and do not necessarily reflect the view of the organizations or agencies that provided support for this project.

Library of Congress Cataloging-in-Publication Data

The learning healthcare system : workshop summary / [edited by] LeighAnne Olsen, Dara Aisner, and J. Michael McGinnis ; Roundtable on Evidence-Based Medicine.
      p. ; cm.
   Includes bibliographical references.
   ISBN-13: 978-0-309-10300-8 (pbk. : alk. paper)
   ISBN-10: 0-309-10300-2 (pbk. : alk. paper) 1. Evidence-based medicine. 2. Medical care—Research—Methodology. 3. Health education. I. Olsen, LeighAnne. II. Aisner, Dara. III. McGinnis, J. Michael. IV. Institute of Medicine (U.S.). Roundtable on Evidence-Based Medicine.
   [DNLM: 1. Delivery of Health Care—organization & administration. 2. Biomedical Research. 3. Evidence-Based Medicine. 4. Learning. 5. Quality of Health Care. W 84.1 L438 2007]
   R723.7.L43 2007
   616—dc22
                                                      2007015074

Additional copies of this report are available from the National Academies Press, 500 Fifth Street, N.W., Lockbox 285, Washington, DC 20055; (800) 624-6242 or (202) 334-3313 (in the Washington metropolitan area); Internet, http://www.nap.edu.

For more information about the Institute of Medicine, visit the IOM home page at: **www.iom.edu.**

The serpent has been a symbol of long life, healing, and knowledge among almost all cultures and religions since the beginning of recorded history. The serpent adopted as a logotype by the Institute of Medicine is a relief carving from ancient Greece, now held by the Staatliche Museen in Berlin.

Suggested citation: Institute of Medicine (IOM). 2007. *The Learning Healthcare System: Workshop Summary.* Washington, DC: The National Academies Press.

"Knowing is not enough; we must apply.
Willing is not enough; we must do."
—Goethe

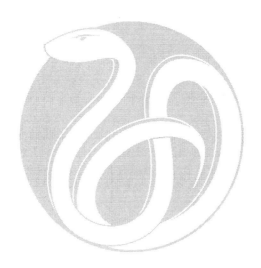

INSTITUTE OF MEDICINE
OF THE NATIONAL ACADEMIES

Advising the Nation. Improving Health.

THE NATIONAL ACADEMIES
Advisers to the Nation on Science, Engineering, and Medicine

The **National Academy of Sciences** is a private, nonprofit, self-perpetuating society of distinguished scholars engaged in scientific and engineering research, dedicated to the furtherance of science and technology and to their use for the general welfare. Upon the authority of the charter granted to it by the Congress in 1863, the Academy has a mandate that requires it to advise the federal government on scientific and technical matters. Dr. Ralph J. Cicerone is president of the National Academy of Sciences.

The **National Academy of Engineering** was established in 1964, under the charter of the National Academy of Sciences, as a parallel organization of outstanding engineers. It is autonomous in its administration and in the selection of its members, sharing with the National Academy of Sciences the responsibility for advising the federal government. The National Academy of Engineering also sponsors engineering programs aimed at meeting national needs, encourages education and research, and recognizes the superior achievements of engineers. Dr. Wm. A. Wulf is president of the National Academy of Engineering.

The **Institute of Medicine** was established in 1970 by the National Academy of Sciences to secure the services of eminent members of appropriate professions in the examination of policy matters pertaining to the health of the public. The Institute acts under the responsibility given to the National Academy of Sciences by its congressional charter to be an adviser to the federal government and, upon its own initiative, to identify issues of medical care, research, and education. Dr. Harvey V. Fineberg is president of the Institute of Medicine.

The **National Research Council** was organized by the National Academy of Sciences in 1916 to associate the broad community of science and technology with the Academy's purposes of furthering knowledge and advising the federal government. Functioning in accordance with general policies determined by the Academy, the Council has become the principal operating agency of both the National Academy of Sciences and the National Academy of Engineering in providing services to the government, the public, and the scientific and engineering communities. The Council is administered jointly by both Academies and the Institute of Medicine. Dr. Ralph J. Cicerone and Dr. Wm. A. Wulf are chair and vice chair, respectively, of the National Research Council.

www.national-academies.org

I. Steven Udvarhelyi, Senior Vice President and Chief Medical Officer, Independence Blue Cross
Frances M. Visco, President, National Breast Cancer Coalition
William C. Weldon, Chairman and Chief Executive Officer, Johnson & Johnson
Janet Woodcock, Deputy Commissioner and Chief Medical Officer, Food and Drug Administration

Roundtable Staff

Dara L. Aisner, Program Officer
Pamela Bradley, Science and Technology Policy Fellow
Katharine Bothner, Senior Program Assistant
J. Michael McGinnis, Senior Scholar
LeighAnne Olsen, Program Officer
Julie Wiltshire, Financial Associate

Reviewers

This report has been reviewed in draft form by individuals chosen for their diverse perspectives and technical expertise, in accordance with procedures approved by the National Research Council's Report Review Committee. The purpose of this independent review is to provide candid and critical comments that will assist the institution in making its published report as sound as possible and to ensure that the report meets institutional standards for objectivity, evidence, and responsiveness to the study charge. The review comments and draft manuscript remain confidential to protect the integrity of the deliberative process. We wish to thank the following individuals for their review of this report:

Carmella Bocchino, America's Health Insurance Plans
Kathy Buto, Johnson & Johnson
Don Goldmann, Institute for Healthcare Improvement
Paul Wallace, The Care Management Institute and KP-Health Solutions, Permanente Federation, Kasier Permanente

Although the reviewers listed above have provided many constructive comments and suggestions, they were not asked to endorse the final draft of the report before its release. The review of this report was overseen by **Dr. Elaine L. Larson,** School of Nursing, Columbia University. Appointed by the National Research Council and the Institute of Medicine, she was responsible for making certain that an independent examination of this report was carried out in accordance with institutional procedures and that all review comments were carefully considered. Responsibility for the final content of this report rests entirely with the authors and the institution.

Institute of Medicine
Roundtable on Evidence-Based Medicine
Charter and Vision Statement

The Institute of Medicine's Roundtable on Evidence-Based Medicine has been convened to help transform the way evidence on clinical effectiveness is generated and used to improve health and health care. Participants have set a goal that, by the year 2020, ninety percent of clinical decisions will be supported by accurate, timely, and up-to-date clinical information, and will reflect the best available evidence. Roundtable members will work with their colleagues to identify the issues not being adequately addressed, the nature of the barriers and possible solutions, and the priorities for action, and will marshal the resources of the sectors represented on the Roundtable to work for sustained public-private cooperation for change.

* *

The Institute of Medicine's Roundtable on Evidence-Based Medicine has been convened to help transform the way evidence on clinical effectiveness is generated and used to improve health and health care. We seek the development of a *learning healthcare system* that is designed to generate and apply the best evidence for the collaborative healthcare choices of each patient and provider; to drive the process of discovery as a natural outgrowth of patient care; and to ensure innovation, quality, safety, and value in health care.

Vision: Our vision is for a healthcare system that draws on the best evidence to provide the care most appropriate to each patient, emphasizes prevention and health promotion, delivers the most value, adds to learning throughout the delivery of care, and leads to improvements in the nation's health.

Goal: By the year 2020, 90 percent of clinical decisions will be supported by accurate, timely, and up-to-date clinical information, and will reflect the best available evidence. We feel that this presents a tangible focus for progress toward our vision, that Americans ought to expect at least this level of performance, that it should be feasible with existing resources and emerging tools, and that measures can be developed to track and stimulate progress.

Context: As unprecedented developments in the diagnosis, treatment, and long-term management of disease bring Americans closer than ever to the promise of personalized health care, we are faced with similarly unprecedented challenges to identify and deliver the care most appropriate for individual needs and conditions. Care that is important is often not delivered. Care that is delivered is often not important. In part, this is due to our failure to apply the evidence we have about the medical care that is most effective—a failure related to shortfalls in provider knowledge and accountability, inadequate care coordination and support, lack of insurance, poorly aligned payment incentives, and misplaced patient expectations. Increasingly, it is also a result of our limited capacity for timely generation of evidence on the relative effectiveness, efficiency, and safety of available and emerging interventions. Improving the value of the return on our healthcare investment is a vital imperative that will require much greater capacity to evaluate high priority clinical interventions, stronger links between clinical research and practice, and reorientation of the incentives to apply new insights. We must quicken our efforts to position evidence development and application as natural outgrowths of clinical care—to foster health care that learns.

Approach: The IOM Roundtable on Evidence-Based Medicine serves as a forum to facilitate the collaborative assessment and action around issues central to achieving the vision and goal stated. The challenges are myriad and include issues that must be addressed to improve evidence development, evidence application, and the capacity to advance progress on both dimensions. To address these challenges, as leaders in their fields, Roundtable members will work with their colleagues to identify the issues not being adequately addressed, the nature of the barriers and possible solutions, and the priorities for action, and will marshal the resources of the sectors represented on the Roundtable to work for sustained public–private cooperation for change.

Activities include collaborative exploration of new and expedited approaches to assessing the effectiveness of diagnostic and treatment interventions, better use of the patient care experience to generate evidence on effectiveness, identification of assessment priorities, and communication strategies to enhance provider and patient understanding and support for interventions proven to work best and deliver value in health care.

Core concepts and principles: For the purpose of the Roundtable activities, we define evidence-based medicine broadly to mean that, *to the greatest extent possible, the decisions that shape the health and health care of Americans—by patients, providers, payers, and policy makers alike—will be grounded on a reliable evidence base, will account appropriately for individual variation in patient needs, and will support the generation of new insights on clinical effectiveness.* Evidence is generally considered to be information from clinical experience that has met some established test of validity, and the appropriate standard is determined according to the requirements of the intervention and clinical circumstance. Processes that involve the development and use of evidence should be accessible and transparent to all stakeholders.

A common commitment to certain principles and priorities guides the activities of the Roundtable and its members, including the commitment to the right health care for each person; putting the best evidence into practice; establishing the effectiveness, efficiency, and safety of medical care delivered; building constant measurement into our healthcare investments; the establishment of healthcare data as a public good; shared responsibility distributed equitably across stakeholders, both public and private; collaborative stakeholder involvement in priority setting; transparency in the execution of activities and reporting of results; and subjugation of individual political or stakeholder perspectives in favor of the common good.

Foreword

One of the important functions of the Institute of Medicine is use of its convening capacity to draw together key stakeholders in a neutral venue, one that allows them to discuss issues and foster collaborative activities around issues in which they have a strong common interest. No issue better demonstrates the importance of such convening than that of evidence-based medicine. We all want to ensure that, as a society, we are doing everything we can to marshal the best evidence in support of the best care for Americans. Yet, we too often fall far short of that ideal. As the Roundtable members have noted in their vision statement, too much care that is important is often not delivered, and too much care that is delivered is often not important.

Part of the problem is due to our inability to provide the evidence we have, and part is due to the inadequacy of the evidence base to keep pace with new tools and approaches for diagnosis and treatment. Both are of central importance to meeting our potential. The latter challenge, in particular, is soon to become much more acute, as new pharmaceuticals, medical devices, biologics, and procedures are introduced into the marketplace—and as advances in genetics give us a better sense of individual differences in response to various interventions. We clearly need a very different approach to the way we develop evidence. Fortunately, the tools are developing to refashion our approaches. The emerging era of individualized medicine and widespread utilization of health information technology presents a dramatically different terrain for clinical research, practice, and healthcare delivery. We can see rich opportunities for improving health through the creation of new knowledge about what works best for whom under what circumstance, and to apply it more expeditiously. Still, ongoing systemic issues pose significant barriers to our ability to generate and translate such knowledge to improved patient care. Improvements in health care are increasingly to be determined by our capacity to manage information and our ability to develop accurate, timely, and reliable information and expedite the application of evidence in clinical decision making. The IOM Roundtable on Evidence-Based Medicine was created in 2006 to bring together leaders from multiple sectors—patients, health providers, payers, employees, health product manufacturers, information technology companies, policy makers, and researchers—to identify and discuss the issues and approaches to help transform how evidence on clinical effectiveness is generated and used to improve health and health care. As part of the charge, the Roundtable has developed a vision for a healthcare system that has the capacity to draw on the best evidence to provide the care most appropriate to each patient as well as the ability to add to knowledge throughout the delivery of care—a healthcare system that learns.

This publication, *The Learning Healthcare System*, presents a summary of a workshop held in July 2006 to identify and discuss the broad range of issues that must be engaged if we are to meet the ever-growing demand for evidence that will help bring better health and economic value for our sizable investment in health care. In that workshop, experts from a variety of fields came together to discuss the current approach to evidence development, the standards that are used in drawing conclusions, new research methodologies, some promising initiatives that are under way, and what is needed to enhance the cooperative roles of patients and providers in this work. This volume is rich with insights and sets a solid stage for follow-on activities and discussions on the issues identified.

I would like to offer my personal thanks to the Roundtable members for the important service they are performing on behalf of better health for Americans, to the Roundtable staff for their excellent contributions in coordinating the activities, and importantly, to the sponsors who support this vital activity: the Agency for Healthcare Research and Quality, America's Health Insurance Plans, AstraZeneca, Blue Shield of California Foundation, Burroughs Wellcome Fund, California Health Care Foundation, Centers for Medicare and Medicaid Services, Department of Veterans Affairs, Food and Drug Administration, Johnson & Johnson, sanofi-aventis, and Stryker. It is this sort of commitment and leadership that give us confidence in our healthcare future.

Harvey V. Fineberg, M.D., Ph.D.
President, Institute of Medicine

Preface

The Learning Healthcare System is the first formal product of the Institute of Medicine (IOM) Roundtable on Evidence-Based Medicine. It is a summary of a two-day workshop held in July 2006, convened to consider the broad range of issues important to reengineering clinical research and healthcare delivery so that evidence is available when it is needed, and applied in health care that is both more effective and more efficient than we have today. Embedded in these pages can be found discussions of the myriad issues that must be engaged if we are to transform the way evidence is generated and used to improve health and health care—issues such as the potential for new research methods to enhance the speed and reliability with which evidence is developed, the standards of evidence to be used in making clinical recommendations and decisions, overcoming the technical and regulatory barriers to broader use of clinical data for research insights, and effective communication to providers and the public about the dynamic nature of evidence and how it can be used. Ultimately, our hope and expectation are that the process of generating and applying the best evidence will be natural and seamless components of the process of care itself, as part of a learning healthcare system.

The aim of the IOM Roundtable on Evidence-Based Medicine is to help accelerate our progress toward this vision. Formed last year, and comprised of some of the nation's most senior leadership from key sectors—consumers and patients, health providers, payers, employees, health product manufacturers, information technology companies, policy makers, and researchers—the work of the Roundtable is anchored in a focus on three dimensions of the challenge:

1. Fostering progress toward the long-term vision of a learning health-care system, in which evidence is both applied and developed as a natural product of the care process.
2. Advancing the discussion and activities necessary to meet the near-term need for expanded capacity to generate the evidence to support medical care that is maximally effective and produces the greatest value.
3. Improving public understanding of the nature of evidence-based medicine, the dynamic nature of the evidence development process, and the importance of supporting progress toward medical care that reflects the best evidence.

The workshop summarized here was intentionally designed to cast the net broadly across the key topics, to identify issues and commonalties in the perspectives of the various participants. As indicated in the Summary, in the course of workshop discussions, a number of fundamental challenges to effective health care in this country were heard, as were a number of uncertainties, and a number of compelling needs for change.

Among the many challenges heard from participants were that missed opportunity, preventable illness, and injury are too often features in health care, and inefficiency and waste are too familiar characteristics. Insufficient attention to the evidence—both its application and its development—is at the core of these problems. Without a stronger focus on getting and using the right evidence, the pattern is likely to be accentuated as intervention options become more complex and greater insight is gained into patient heterogeneity. In the face of this change, the prevailing approach to generating clinical evidence is impractical today, and may be irrelevant tomorrow. Current approaches to interpreting the evidence and producing guidelines and recommendations often yield inconsistencies and confusion. Meeting these challenges may be facilitated by promising developments in information technology, but those developments must be matched by broader commitments to make culture and practice changes that will allow us to move clinical practice and research into closer alignment.

Among the uncertainties participants underscored were some key questions: Should we continue to call the randomized controlled clinical trial (RCT) the "gold standard"? Although clearly useful and necessary in some circumstances, does this designation over-promise? What do we need to do to better characterize the range of alternatives to RCTs, and the applications and implications for each? What constitutes evidence, and how does it vary by circumstance? How much of evidence development and evidence application will ultimately fall outside of even a fully interoperable and universally adopted electronic health record (EHR)? What are the boundaries of a technical approach? What is the best strategy to get to the right standards and interoperability for a clinical record system that can be a fully functioning part of evidence development and application? How much can some of the problems of post-marketing surveillance be obviated by the emergence of linked clinical information systems that might allow information about safety and effectiveness to emerge naturally in the course of care?

Engaging the challenges and uncertainties, participants identified a number of pressing needs: adapting to the pace of change, through continuous learning and a much more dynamic approach to evidence development and application; a culture of shared responsibility among patients, providers, and researchers; a new clinical research paradigm that draws clinical research more closely to the experience of clinical practice; clinical decision support systems that accommodate the pace of information growth; full and effective application of electronic health records as an essential prerequisite for the evolution of the learning healthcare system; advancing the notion of clinical data as a public good and a central common resource for advancing knowledge and evidence for effective care; database linkage, mining, and use; stronger incentives to draw research and practice closer together, forging interoperable patient record platforms to foster more rapid learning; better consistency and coordination in efforts to generate, assess, and advise on the results of new knowledge; and the importance of strong and trusted leadership to provide the guidance, shape the priorities, and marshal the vision and actions necessary to create a learning healthcare system.

The workshop then laid out a number challenges requiring the attention and action of stakeholders such as those represented on the Roundtable. We will be following up with deeper consideration of many of these issues through other workshops, commissioned papers, collaborative activities, and public communication efforts. The challenges are large but the Roundtable is populated by committed members who will also reach out to involve their colleagues more widely in the work, assisted by what has been heard and reported through this initial contribution.

We would like to acknowledge all the individuals and organizations that donated their valuable time toward the development of this workshop summary. In particular, we acknowledge the contributors to this volume for their presence at the workshop as well as their efforts to further develop their presentations into the manuscripts contained in this summary. In this respect, we should emphasize that the workshop summary is a collection of individually authored papers and is intended to convey only the views and opinions of individuals participating in the workshop—not the deliberations of the Roundtable on Evidence-Based Medicine, its sponsors, or the Institute of Medicine. We would also like to acknowledge those that provided counsel during the planning stages of this workshop, including Carol Diamond (Markle Foundation), Steve Downs (Robert Wood Johnson

Foundation), Lynn Etheredge (George Washington University), Joe Francis (Department of Veterans Affairs), Brent James (Intermountain Healthcare), Missy Krasner (Google), Nancy Nielsen (American Medical Association), Richard Platt (Harvard), Jeff Shuren (Food and Drug Administration), Susan Shurin (National Institutes of Health), Steven Udverheyli (Independence Blue Cross), and Paul Wallace (Kaiser Permanente). A number of IOM staff were instrumental in the preparation and conduct of the two-day workshop in July, including Shenan Carroll, Amy Grossman, Leon James, Paul Lee, and David Tollerud. Roundtable staff, in particular LeighAnne Olsen along with Dara Aisner and Katharine Bothner helped translate the workshop proceedings and discussion into this workshop summary. We would also like to thank Lara Andersen, Michele de la Menardiere, Bronwyn Schrecker, and Tyjen Tsai for helping to coordinate the various aspects of review, production, and publication.

Encouraging signs exist in our quest toward a learning healthcare system. Progress has been accelerating and we need to sustain this momentum. We look forward to building on this workshop's insights, and the vision of *The Learning Healthcare System* is a welcome first step along the path.

Denis A. Cortese, M.D.
Chair, Roundtable on Evidence-Based Medicine

J. Michael McGinnis, M.D., M.P.P.
Senior Scholar, Institute of Medicine

Contents

Summary   1

**1 Hints of a Different Way—Case Studies in Practice-Based
   Evidence**   37
   Overview, 37
   Coverage with Evidence Development, 39
      Peter B. Bach
   Use of Large System Databases, 46
      Jed Weissberg
   Quasi-Experimental Designs for Policy Assessment, 50
      Stephen Soumerai
   Practical Clinical Trials, 57
      Sean Tunis
   Computerized Protocols to Assist Clinical Research, 61
      Alan H. Morris
   References, 71

**2 The Evolving Evidence Base—Methodologic and Policy
   Challenges**   81
   Overview, 81
   Evolving Methods: Alternatives to Large Randomized
   Controlled Trials, 84
      Robert M. Califf

Evolving Methods: Evaluating Medical Device Interventions in a
Rapid State of Flux, 93
   Telba Irony
Evolving Methods: Mathematical Models to Help Fill the
Gaps in Evidence, 99
   David M. Eddy and David C. Kendrick
Heterogeneity of Treatment Effects: Subgroup Analysis, 113
   Sheldon Greenfield and Richard L. Kravitz
Heterogeneity of Treatment Effects: Pharmacogenetics, 123
   David Goldstein
Broader Post-Marketing Surveillance for Insights on Risk and
Effectiveness, 128
   *Harlan Weisman, Christina Farup, Adrian Thomas,
   Peter Juhn, and Kathy Buto*
Adjusting Evidence Generation to the Scale of Effects, 134
   Steve M. Teutsch and Marc L. Berger
HIPAA and Clinical Research: Protecting Privacy, 138
Protecting Privacy While Linking Patient Records, 140
   Janlori Goldman and Beth Tossell
References, 144

3   **Narrowing the Research-Practice Divide—Systems
   Considerations**   151
Overview, 151
Feedback Loops to Expedite Study Timeliness and Relevance, 152
   Brent James
Electronic Health Records and Evidence-Based Practice, 163
   Walter F. Stewart and Nirav R. Shah
Standards of Evidence, 171
   Steven Pearson
Implications for Accelerating Innovation, 174
   Robert Galvin
References, 181

4   **New Approaches—Learning Systems in Progress**   185
Overview, 185
Implementation of Evidence-Based Practice in the VA, 187
   Joel Kupersmith
Practice-Based Research Networks, 198
   Robert L. Phillips, Jr., James Mold, and Kevin Peterson
National Quality Improvement Process and Architecture, 203
   George Isham

Envisioning a Rapid Learning Healthcare System, 210
  Lynn Etheredge
References, 213

5   Developing the Test Bed—Linking Integrated Service
    Delivery Systems   217
    Overview, 217
    NIH and Reengineering Clinical Research, 218
      Stephen I. Katz
    AHRQ and the Use of Integrated Service Delivery Systems, 221
      Cynthia Palmer
    The HMO Research Network as a Test Bed, 223
      Eric B. Larson
    Council of Accountable Physician Practices, 233
      Michael A. Mustille
    References, 239

6   The Patient as a Catalyst for Change   243
    Overview, 243
    The Internet, eHealth, and Patient Empowerment, 244
      Janet M. Marchibroda
    Joint Patient-Provider Management of the Electronic Health
    Record, 250
      Andrew Barbash
    Evidence and Shared Decision Making, 254
      James N. Weinstein and Kate Clay
    References, 264

7   Training the Learning Health Professional   267
    Overview, 267
    Clinicians and the Electronic Health Record as a
    Learning Tool, 268
      William W. Stead
    Embedding an Evidence Perspective in Health Professions
    Education, 275
      Mary Mundinger
    Knowledge Translation: Redefining Continuing Education
    Around Evolving Evidence, 281
      Mark V. Williams
    References, 285

8 Structuring the Incentives for Change 289
Overview, 289
Opportunities for Private Insurers, 290
  Alan Rosenberg
Opportunities for CMS, 295
  Steve Phurrough
Opportunities for Pharmaceutical Companies, 300
  *Wayne A. Rosenkrans, Jr., Catherine Bonuccelli, and
  Nancy Featherstone*
Opportunities for Standards Organizations, 304
  Margaret E. O'Kane
References, 313

APPENDIXES
A Workshop Agenda   315
B Biographical Sketches of Participants   321
C Workshop Attendee List   345
D IOM Roundtable on Evidence-Based Medicine   353

Summary

Seven years ago, the Institute of Medicine (IOM) Committee on the Quality of Health Care in America released its first report, *To Err Is Human*, finding that an estimated 44,000 to 98,000 Americans may die annually due to medical errors. If mortality tables routinely included medical errors as a formal cause of death, they would rank well within the ten leading killers (IOM 2000). Two years later, the Committee released its final report, *Crossing the Quality Chasm*, underscoring the need for redesigning health care to address the key dimensions on which improvement was most needed: safety, effectiveness, patient centeredness, timeliness, efficiency, and equity (IOM 2001). Although these reports sounded appropriate alerts and have triggered important discussion, as well as a certain level of action, the performance of the healthcare system remains far short of where it should be.

Evidence on what is effective, and under what circumstances, is often lacking, poorly communicated to decision makers, or inadequately applied, and despite significant expenditures on health care for Americans, these investments have not translated to better health. Studies of current practice patterns have consistently shown failures to deliver recommended services, wide geographic variation in the intensity of services without demonstrated advantage (and some degree of risk at the more intensive levels), and

---

The planning committee's role was limited to planning the workshop, and the workshop summary has been prepared by Roundtable staff as a factual summary of what occured at the workshop.

waste levels that may approach a third or more of the nation's $2 trillion in healthcare expenditures (Fisher et al. 2003; McGlynn 2003). In performance on the key vital statistics, the United States ranks below at least two dozen other nations, all of which spend far less for health care.

In part, these problems are related to fragmentation of the delivery system, misplaced patient demand, and responsiveness to legal and economic incentives unrelated to health outcomes. However, to a growing extent, they relate to a structural inability of evidence to keep pace with the need for better information to guide clinical decision making. Also, if current approaches are inadequate, future developments are likely to accentuate the problem. These issues take on added urgency in view of the rapidly shifting landscape of available interventions and scientific knowledge, including the increasing complexity of disease management, the development of new medical technologies, the promise of regenerative medicine, and the growing utility of genomics and proteomics in tailoring disease detection and treatment to each individual. Yet, currently, for example, the share of health expenses devoted to determining what works best is about one-tenth of 1 percent (AcademyHealth September 2005; Moses et al. 2005).

In the face of this changing terrain, the IOM Roundtable on Evidence-Based Medicine ("the Roundtable") has been convened to marshal senior national leadership from key sectors to explore a wholly different approach to the development and application of evidence for health care. Evidence-based medicine (EBM) emerged in the twentieth century as a methodology for improving care by emphasizing the integration of individual clinical expertise with the best available external evidence (Sackett et al. 1996) and serves as a necessary and valuable foundation for future progress. EBM has resulted in many advances in health care by highlighting the importance of a rigorous scientific base for practice and the important role of physician judgment in delivering individual patient care. However, the increased complexity of health care requires a deepened commitment by all stakeholders to develop a healthcare system engaged in producing the kinds of evidence needed at the point of care for the treatment of individual patients.

Many have asserted that beyond determinations of basic efficacy and safety, the dependence on individually designed, serially constructed, prospective studies to establish relative effectiveness and individual variation in efficacy and safety is simply impractical for most interventions (Rosser 1999; Wilson et al. 2000; Kupersmith et al. 2005; Devereaux et al. 2005; Tunis 2005; McCulloch et al. 2002). Information technology will provide valuable tools to confront these issues by expanding the capability to collect and manage data, but more is needed. A reevaluation of how health care is structured to develop and apply evidence—from health professions training, to infrastructure development, patient engagement, payments, and measurement—will be necessary to orient and direct these tools toward the creation of a sustainable system that gets the right care to people when they need it and then captures the results for improvement. The nation needs a healthcare system that learns.

About the Workshop

To explore the central issues in bringing about the changes needed, in July 2006 the IOM Roundtable convened a workshop entitled "The Learning Healthcare System." This workshop was the first in a series that will focus on various issues important for improving the development and application of evidence in healthcare decision making. During this initial workshop, a broad range of topics and perspectives was considered. The aim was to identify and discuss those issues most central to drawing research closer to clinical practice by building knowledge development and application into each stage of the healthcare delivery process, in a fashion that will not only improve today's care but improve the prospects of addressing the growing demands in the future. Day 1 was devoted to an overview of the methodologic and institutional issues. Day 2 focused on examples of some approaches by different organizations to foster a stronger learning environment. The workshop agenda can be found in Appendix A, speaker biosketches in Appendix B, and a listing of workshop participants in Appendix C. Synopses follow of the key points from each of the sessions in the two-day workshop.

THE LEARNING HEALTHCARE SYSTEM WORKSHOP

Common Themes

In the course of the workshop discussions, several common themes and issues were identified by participants. A number of current challenges to improving health care were raised, as were a number of uncertainties, and a number of compelling needs for change.

Among challenges heard from participants were the following:

- Missed opportunities, preventable illness, and injury are too often features in health care.
- Inefficiency and waste are too familiar characteristics in much of health care.
- Deficiencies in the quantity, quality, and application of evidence are important contributors to these problems, and improvement requires a stronger system-wide focus on the evidence.
- These challenges are likely to be accentuated by the increasing com-

plexity of intervention options and increasing insights into patient heterogeneity.
- The prevailing approach to generating clinical evidence is inadequate today and may be irrelevant tomorrow, given the pace and complexity of change. The current dependence on the randomized controlled clinical trial (RCT), as useful as it is under the right circumstances, takes too much time, is too expensive, and is fraught with questions of generalizability.
- The current approaches to interpreting the evidence and producing guidelines and recommendations often yield inconsistencies and confusion.
- Promising developments in information technology offer prospects for improvement that will be necessary to deploy, but not sufficient to effect, the broad change needed.

Among the uncertainties participants underscored were some key questions:

- Should we continue to call the RCT the "gold standard"? Although clearly useful and necessary in some circumstances, does this designation overpromise?
- What do we need to do to better characterize the range of alternatives to RCTs and the applications and implications for each?
- What constitutes evidence, and how does it vary by circumstance?
- How much of evidence development and evidence application will ultimately fall outside of even a fully interoperable and universally adopted electronic health record (EHR)? What are the boundaries of a technical approach to improving care?
- What is the best strategy to get to the right standards and interoperability for a clinical record system that can be a fully functioning part of evidence development and application?
- How much can some of the problems of post-marketing surveillance be obviated by the emergence of linked clinical information systems that might allow information about safety and effectiveness to emerge naturally in the course of care?

Among the most pressing needs for change (Box S-1) identified by participants were those related to:

- *Adaptation to the pace of change:* continuous learning and a much more dynamic approach to evidence development and application, taking full advantage of developing information technology to

---

BOX S-1
Needs for the Learning Healthcare System

- Adaptation to the pace of change
- Stronger synchrony of efforts
- Culture of shared responsibility
- New clinical research paradigm
- Clinical decision support systems
- Universal electronic health records
- Tools for database linkage, mining, and use
- Notion of clinical data as a public good
- Incentives aligned for practice-based evidence
- Public engagement
- Trusted scientific broker
- Leadership

---

match the rate at which new interventions are developed and new insights emerge about individual variation in response to those interventions;

- *Stronger synchrony of efforts:* better consistency and coordination of efforts to generate, assess, and advise on the results of new knowledge in a way that does not produce conflict or confusion;

- *Culture of shared responsibility:* to enable the evolution of the learning environment as a common cause of patients, providers, and researchers and better engage all in improved communication about the importance of the nature of evidence and its evolution;

- *New clinical research paradigm:* drawing clinical research closer to the experience of clinical practice, including the development of new study methodologies adapted to the practice environment and a better understanding of when RCTs are most practical and desirable;

- *Clinical decision support systems:* to accommodate the reality that although professional judgment will always be vital to shaping care, the amount of information required for any given decision is moving beyond unassisted human capacity;

- *Universal electronic health records:* comprehensive deployment and effective application of the full capabilities available in EHRs as an essential prerequisite for the evolution of the learning healthcare system;

- *Tools for database linkage, mining, and use:* advancing the potential for structured, large databases as new sources of evidence, including issues in fostering interoperable platforms and in developing new means of ongoing searching of those databases for patterns and clinical insights;

- *Notion of clinical data as a public good:* advancement of the notion of the use of clinical data as a central common resource for advancing knowledge and evidence for effective care—including directly addressing current challenges related to the treatment of data as a proprietary good and interpretations of the Health Insurance Portability and Accountability Act (HIPAA) and other patient privacy issues that currently present barriers to knowledge development;
- *Incentives aligned for practice-based evidence:* encouraging the development and use of evidence by drawing research and practice closer together, and developing the patient records and interoperable platforms necessary to foster more rapid learning and improve care;
- *Public engagement:* improved communication about the nature of evidence and its development, and the active roles of both patients and healthcare professionals in evidence development and dissemination;
- *Trusted scientific broker:* an agent or entity with the public and scientific confidence to provide guidance, shape priorities, and foster the shift in the clinical research paradigm; and
- *Leadership:* to marshal the vision, strategy, and actions necessary to create a learning healthcare system.

PRESENTATION SUMMARIES

Hints of a Different Way—Case Studies in Practice-Based Evidence

Devising innovative methods to generate and apply evidence for healthcare decision making is central to improving the effectiveness of medical care. This workshop took the analysis further by asking how we might create a healthcare system that "learns"—one in which knowledge generation is so embedded into the core of the practice of medicine that it is a natural outgrowth and product of the healthcare delivery process and leads to continual improvement in care. This has been termed by some "practice-based evidence" (Green and Geiger 2006). By emphasizing effectiveness research over efficacy research (see Table S-1) practice-based evidence focuses on the needs of decision makers and on narrowing the research-practice divide. Research questions identified are relevant to clinical practice, and effectiveness research is conducted in typical clinical practice environments with unselected populations to increase generalizability (Clancy 2006 [July 20-21]).

TABLE S-1 Characteristics of Efficacy and Effectiveness Research

Efficacy	Effectiveness
Clinical trials—idealized setting	Clinical practice—everyday setting
Treatment vs. placebo	Multiple treatment choices, comparisons
Patients with a single diagnosis	Patients with multiple conditions (often excluded from efficacy trials)
Exclusions of user groups (e.g., elderly)	Use is generally unlimited
Short-term effects measured through surrogate endpoints, biomarkers	Longer-term outcomes measured through clinical improvement, quality of life, disability, death

SOURCE: Clancy 2006 (July 20-21).

The first panel session of the workshop was devoted to several examples of efforts that illustrate ways to use the healthcare experience as a practical means of both generating and applying evidence for health care. Presentations highlighted approaches that take advantage of current resources through innovative incentives, study methodologies, and study design and demonstrated their impact on decision making.

Coverage with Evidence Development

Provision of Medicare payments for carefully selected interventions in specified groups, in return for their participation in data collection, is beginning to generate information on effectiveness. Peter B. Bach of the Centers for Medicare and Medicaid Services (CMS) discussed Coverage with Evidence Development (CED), a form of National Coverage Decision (NCD) implemented by CMS as an opportunity to develop needed evidence on effectiveness. By conditioning coverage on additional evidence development, CED helps clarify policies and can therefore be seen as a regulatory approach to building a learning healthcare system. Two case studies, one on lung volume reduction surgery (LVRS) for emphysema and another on PET (positron emission tomography) scans for staging cancers, illustrate this approach. To clarify issues of risk and benefit associated with LVRS and to define characteristics of patients most likely to benefit, the National Emphysema Treatment Trial (NETT), was funded by CMS, and implemented as a collaborative effort of CMS, the National Institutes of Health (NIH), and the Agency for Healthcare Research and Quality (AHRQ). Trial results enabled CMS to cover the procedure for groups with demonstrated benefit and clarified risks in a manner helpful to patient decisions, and from January 2004 to September 2005, only 458 Medicare patients filed a total of $10.5 million in LVRS claims, far lower than estimated. In the case of

PET scanning to help diagnose cancer and determine its stage, a registry has been established for recording experience on certain key dimensions, ultimately allowing payers, physicians, researchers, and other stakeholders to construct a follow-on system to evaluate long-term safety and other aspects of real-world effectiveness. This work is in progress.

Use of Large System Databases

With the adoption and use of the full capabilities of EHRs, hypothesis-driven research utilizing existing clinical and administrative databases in large healthcare systems can answer a variety of questions not answered when drugs, devices, and techniques come to market (Trontell 2004). Jed Weissberg of the Permanente Federation described a nested, case-control study on the cardiovascular effects of the COX-2 inhibitor rofecoxib (Vioxx) within Kaiser Permanente's patient population, identifying increased risk of acute myocardial infarction and sudden cardiac death (Graham 2005). Kaiser's prescription and dispensing data, as well as longitudinal patient data (demographics, lab, pathology, radiology, diagnosis, and procedures), were essential to conduct the study and contributed to the manufacturer's decision to withdraw the drug from the marketplace. The case illustrates the potential for well-designed EHRs to generate data as a customary by-product of documented care and to facilitate the detection of rare events as well as provide insights into factors that drive variation. Weissberg also concluded that perhaps the most important requirement for reaping the benefits is that data collection be embedded within a healthcare system that can serve as a "prepared mind"—a culture that seeks learning.

Quasi-Experimental Designs

Randomized controlled trials are often referred to as the "gold standard" in trial design, while other trial designs are noted as "alternatives" to RCTs. Stephen Soumerai of Harvard Pilgrim Health Care argued that this bifurcation is counterproductive. All trial designs have widely differing ranges of applicability and validity, depending on circumstances. Although RCTs, if carefully developed, may produce the most reliable estimates of the outcomes of health services and policies, strong quasi-experimental designs (e.g., interrupted time series) are rigorous and feasible alternative methods, especially for evaluating the effects of sudden changes in health policies occurring in large populations. Because these are natural experiments that use existing data and can be conducted in less time and for less expense than many RCTs, they have great potential for contributing to the evidence base. For example, using interrupted time series to examine the impact of a statewide Medicaid cap on nonessential drugs in New Hampshire revealed that prescriptions filled by Medicaid patients dropped sharply for both essential and nonessential drugs, while nursing home admissions among chronically ill elderly increased (Soumerai et al. 1987). Similar study designs have been used to assess the impact of limitations of drug coverage on the treatment of schizophrenia and the need for acute mental health services (Soumerai et al. 1994), as well as the relationship between cost sharing changes and serious adverse events with associated emergency visits among the adult welfare population (Tamblyn 2001). He concludes that time series data allow for strong quasi-experimental designs that can address many threats to validity, and because such analyses often produce visible effects, they convey an intuitive understanding of the effects of policy decisions (Soumerai 2006 [July 20-21]).

Practical Clinical Trials

Developing valid and useful evidence for decision making requires several steps, including identifying the right questions to ask; selecting the most important questions for study; choosing study designs that are adequate to answer the questions; creating or partnering with organizations that are equipped to implement the studies; and finding sufficient resources to pay for the studies. The successful navigation of these steps is what Sean Tunis of the Health Technology Center calls "decision-based evidence making." Tunis also discussed pragmatic or practical trials as particularly useful study designs for informing choices between feasible alternatives or two different treatment options. Key features of a practical trial include meaningful comparison groups; broad eligibility criteria with maximum opportunity for generalizability; multiple outcomes including functional status and utilization; conduct in a real-world setting; and minimal intrusion on regular care. A CMS study, PET scan for suspected dementia, was cited as an example of how an appropriately designed practical clinical trial (PCT) could help address a difficult clinical question such as the impact of diagnosis on patient management and outcomes. However the trial remains unfunded, raising issues about limitations of current organizational capacity and infrastructure to support the needed expansion of such comparative effectiveness research.

Computerized Protocols to Assist Clinical Research

The development of evidence for clinical decision making can also be strengthened by increasing the scientific rigor of evidence generation. Alan Morris noted the lack of tools to drive consistency in clinical trial methodology and discussed the importance of identifying tools to assist in the design and implementation of clinical research. "Adequately explicit methods," including computer protocols that elicit the same decision from different clinicians when they are faced with the same information, can be used to increase the ability to generate highly reproducible clinical evidence across a variety of research settings and clinical expertise. Pilot studies of computerized protocols have led to reproducible results in different hospitals in different countries. As an example, Morris noted that the use of a computerized protocol (eProtocol-insulin) to direct intravenous (IV) insulin therapy in nearly 2,000 patients led to improved control of blood glucose levels. Morris proposed that in addition to increasing the efficiency of large-scale complex clinical studies, the use of adequately explicit computerized protocols for the translation of research methods into clinical practice could introduce a new way of developing and distributing knowledge.

The Evolving Evidence Base—Methodologic and Policy Challenges

An essential component of the learning healthcare system is the capacity for constant improvement: to take advantage of new tools and methods and to improve approaches to gathering and evaluating evidence. As technology advances and the ability to accumulate large quantities of clinical data increases, new opportunities will emerge to develop evidence on the effectiveness of interventions, including on risks, on the effects of complex patterns of comorbidities, on the effect of genetic variation, and on the improved evaluation of rapidly changing interventions such as devices and procedures. A significant challenge will be piecing together evidence from the full scope of this information to determine what is best for individual patients.

Although considered the standard benchmark, RCTs are of limited use in informing some important aspects of decision making (see papers by Soumerai, Tunis, and Greenfield in Chapters 1 and 2). In part, this is because in clinical research, we tend to think of diseases and conditions in single, linear terms. However, for people with multiple chronic illnesses and those that fall outside standard RCT selection criteria, the evidence base is quite weak (Greenfield and Kravitz 2006 [July 20-21]). In addition, the time and expense of an RCT may be prohibitive for the circumstance. A new clinical research paradigm that takes better advantage of data generated in the course of healthcare delivery would speed and improve the development of evidence for real-world decision making (Califf 2006 [July 20-21]; Soumerai 2006 [July 20-21]). New methodologies such as mathematical modeling, Bayesian statistics, and decision modeling will also expand our capacity to assess interventions.

Finally, engaging the policy issues necessary to expand post-market surveillance—including the use of registries and mediating an appropriate balance between patient privacy and access to clinical data—will make new streams of critical data available for research. Linking data systems and utilizing clinical information systems for expanded post-marketing surveillance have the potential to accelerate the generation of evidence regarding risk and effectiveness of therapies. Furthermore, this could be a powerful source of innovation and refinement of drug development, thereby increasing the value of health care by tailoring therapies and treatments to individual patients and subgroups of risk and benefit (Weisman 2006 [July 20-21]).

Evolving Methods: Alternatives to Large RCTs

All interventions carry a balance of potential benefit and potential risk, and many trial methodologies can reveal important information on these dimensions when the conduct of a large RCT is not feasible. Robert Califf from the Duke Clinical Research Institute discussed some issues associated with RCTs and the trial methodologies that will increasingly be used to supplement the evidence base. Large RCTs are almost impossible to conduct, and Califf supported use of the term practical clinical trial for those in which the size must be large enough to answer the question posed in terms of health outcomes—whether patients live longer or feel better. A well-designed PCT has many characteristics that are frequently missing from current RCT design and is the first alternative to a "classical" RCT. Questions should be framed by those who use the information, and the methodology of design should include decision makers. PCTs however are also not feasible for a good portion of the decisions being made every day by administrators and clinicians. To answer some of these questions, nonrandomized analyses are needed. Califf reviewed four methodologies: (1) the cluster randomized trial, which randomizes on a practice level; (2) observational treatment comparisons, for which confounding from multiple sources is an important consideration (but should be aided by the development of National Electronic Clinical Trials and Research (NECTAR), the planned NIH network that will connect practices with interoperable data systems); (3) the interrupted time series, especially for natural experiments such as policy changes; and (4) the use of instrumental variables, or variables unrelated to biology, to produce a contrast in treatment that can be characterized. Califf indicated that such alternative methodologies have a role to play in the development of evidence, but for proper use, we also need to cultivate the expertise that can guide the use of these methods.

Evolving Methods: Evaluating Interventions in a Rapid State of Flux

As the pace of innovation accelerates, methodologic issues will increasingly hamper the straightforward use of clinical data to assess safety and effectiveness. This is particularly relevant to the iterative development process for new medical device interventions. Evaluation of interventions in a rapid state of flux requires new methods. Telba Irony of the Center for Devices and Radiologic Health (CDRH) at the Food and Drug Administration (FDA) discussed some new statistical methodologies used at FDA, including Bayesian analysis, adaptive trial design, and formal decision analysis to speed approaches. Because the Bayesian approach allows the use of prior information and the performance of interim analyses, this method is particularly useful to evaluate devices, with the possibility of smaller and shorter trials and increased information for decision making. Formal decision analysis is also a mathematical decision analysis tool that has the potential to enhance the decision-making process by better accounting for the magnitude of advantage compared to the risks of an intervention (see Irony, Chapter 2).

Evolving Methods: Mathematical Models to Help Fill the Gaps in Evidence

Ideally, every important question could be answered with a clinical trial or other equally valid source of empirical observations. Because this is not feasible, an alternative approach is to use mathematical models, which have proven themselves valuable for assessing, as examples, computed tomography (CT) scans and magnetic resonance imaging (MRI), radiation therapy, and EHRs. Working through Kaiser Permanente, David M. Eddy developed a modeling system, Archimedes, that has demonstrated the promise of such systems for developing evidence for clinical decision making. Eddy notes that models will never be able to completely replace clinical trials, which as observations of real events are a fundamental anchor to reality. One step removed, models cannot exist without empirical observations. Thus, if feasible, the preferred approach is to answer a question with a clinical trial. However, in initial work on approaches to diabetes management, the Archimedes model has been validated against trial data with a very close match to the actual results (Eddy and Schlessinger 2003). Eddy maintains that in the future, the quality of models will improve, and as they do, with better data from EHRs, mathematical models can help fill more and more of the gaps in the evidence base for clinical medicine.

Heterogeneity of Treatment Effects: Subgroup Analysis

Heterogeneity of treatment effects (HTE) describes the variation in results from the same treatment in different patients. Sheldon Greenfield notes that HTE, the emerging complexity of the medical system, and the nature of health problems have contributed to the decreasing utility of

RCTs. Greenfield presented three evolving phenomena that make RCTs increasingly inadequate for the development of guidelines, for payment, and for creating quality-of-care measures. First, with an aging population, patients now eligible for trials have a broader spectrum of illness severity than previously. Second, due to the changing nature of chronic disease along with increased patient longevity, more patients now suffer from multiple comorbidities. These patients are frequently excluded from clinical trials. Both of these phenomena make the results from RCTs useful to an increasingly small percentage of patients. Third, powerful new genetic and phenotypic markers that can predict patients' responsiveness to therapy and vulnerability to adverse effects of treatment are now being discovered. In clinical trials, these markers have the potential for identifying patients' potential for responsiveness to the treatment to be investigated. The current research paradigm underlying evidence-based medicine, guideline development, and quality assessment is therefore fundamentally limited (Greenfield and Kravitz 2006 [July 20-21]). Greenfield notes that to account for HTE, trial designs must include multivariate pretrial risk stratification based on observational studies, and for patients not eligible for trials (e.g., elderly patients with multiple comorbidities), observational studies will be needed.

Heterogeneity of Treatment Effects: Prospects for Pharmacogenetics

Recent advances in genomics have focused attention on its application to understanding common diseases and identifying new directions for drug or intervention development. David Goldstein of the Duke Institute for Genome Sciences and Policy discussed the potential role of pharmacogenetics in illuminating heterogeneity in responses to treatment and defining subgroups for appropriate care. While pharmacogenetics has previously focused on describing variations in a handful of proteins and genes, it is now possible to assess entire pathways that might be relevant to disease or to drug responses. The clinical relevance of pharmacogenetics will be in the identification of genetic predictors of a patient's response to treatment with direct diagnostic utility (Need 2005), and the resulting expansion in factors to consider based on an individual's response to treatment (see Figure S-1) could be substantial. The CATIE trial (Clinical Antipsychotic Trials of Intervention Effectiveness), comparing different antipsychotics, is illustrative.

While no drug was superior with respect to discontinuation of treatment, certain drugs were worse for certain patients in causing adverse reactions, illustrating the clear potential if genetic markers for possible adverse reactions could be used as a diagnostic tool. In addition to helping to specify disease subgroups and treatment effects, pharmacogenetics could benefit drug development. If predictors of adverse events could prevent the exposure of genetically vulnerable patients and preserve even a single drug,

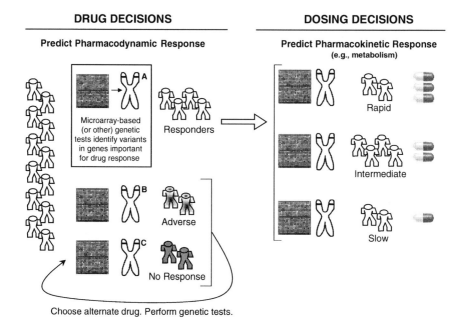

FIGURE S-1 Possible implications of pharmacogenetics on clinical decision making. The appropriate drug for an individual could be determined by microarray-based (or other) genetic tests that reveal variants in genes that affect how a drug works (pharmacodynamics) or how the body processes a drug (pharmacokinetics), such as absorption, distribution, metabolism, and excretion. Note that individual metabolic response is commonly more complicated than the simplified case presented here for conceptual clarity.

the costs of any large-scale research effort in pharmacogenetics could be fully recovered.

Broader Post-Marketing Surveillance

Although often thought of as a mechanism to detect rare adverse treatment effects, post-marketing surveillance also has enormous potential for the development of real-world data on the long-term value of new, innovative therapies. Harlan Weisman of Johnson & Johnson noted that the limited generalizability of the RCTs required for product approval means that post-marketing surveillance is the major opportunity to reveal the true value of healthcare innovations for the general population. Electronic health records, embedded as part of a learning healthcare system, would enable the development of such evidence on treatment outcomes and the effects of increasingly complex health states, comorbidities, and multiple indications. These data could also be used toward the conduct of comparative analysis. Weisman also discussed how the landscape of information needed changes rapidly and continuously, and called for the development of transparent methods and guidelines to gather, analyze, and integrate evidence—as well as consideration of how this new form of clinical data will be integrated into policies and treatment paradigms. To ensure that the goals of a learning healthcare system are achieved without jeopardizing patient benefit or medical innovation, Weisman suggested the importance of a road map establishing a common framework for post-marketing surveillance, to include initial evidence evaluation, appropriate and timely reevaluations, and application. Where possible, post-marketing data requirements of different agencies or authorities should be harmonized to reduce costs of collection and unnecessary duplication. He suggested multiple uses of common datasets as a means to accelerate the application of innovation.

Adjusting Evidence Generation to the Scale of the Effects

With new technologies introduced fast on the heels of effective older technologies, the demand for high-quality, timely comparative effectiveness studies is exploding (Lubitz 2005; Bodenheirmer 2005). Well-done comparative effectiveness studies identify which technology is more effective or safer, or for which subpopulation and/or clinical situation a therapy is superior. Steven Teutsch and Marc Berger of Merck & Co. advanced their perspective on the importance of developing strategies for generating comparative effectiveness data that improve the use of healthcare resources by considering the magnitude of potential benefits and/or risks related to the clinical intervention. Even when available, most comparative effectiveness studies do not directly provide estimates of absolute benefit or harms applicable to all relevant populations. Because of the impracticality and lack of timeliness of head-to-head trials for more than a few therapeutic alternatives, it is important that other strategies for securing this information be developed. Observational study designs and models can provide perspective on these issues, although the value of the information gleaned must be balanced against potential threats to validity and uncertainty around estimates of benefit. General consensus on the standards of evidence to apply to different clinical recommendations will be important to moving forward. Development of a taxonomy of clinical decision making would help to ensure transparency in decision making.

Linking Patient Records: Protecting Privacy, Promoting Care

Critical medical information is often nearly impossible to access both in emergencies and during routine medical encounters, leading to lost time, increased expenses, adverse outcomes, and medical errors. Having health information available electronically is now a reality and offers the potential for lifesaving measures not only through access to critical information at the point of care but also by providing a wealth of information on how to improve care. However, for many, the potential benefits of a linked health information system are matched in significance by the potential drawbacks such as threats to the privacy and security of people's most sensitive information. The HIPAA privacy rule challenged decision makers and researchers to grapple with the questions of how to foster a national system of linked health information necessary to provide the highest-quality health care. Janlori Goldman of the Privacy Project and others presented the patient perspective on these issues, supporting the concept of data linkage as a way to improve health care, provided that appropriate precautions are undertaken to ensure the security and privacy of patient data and options are offered to patients with respect to data linkage. Such guarantees are critical to developing the access to clinical information that is important for systematic generation of new insights, and practical approaches are needed to both ensure the public's confidence and address the regulatory requirement governing clinical information.

Narrowing the Research-Practice Divide—System Considerations

Capturing and utilizing data generated in the course of care offers the opportunity to bring research and practice into closer alignment and propagate a cycle of learning that can enhance both the rigor and the relevance of evidence. Presentations in this session suggest that if healthcare delivery is to play a more fundamental role in the generation and application of evidence on clinical effectiveness, process and analytic changes are needed in the delivery environment. Some considerations included strengthening feedback loops between research and practice to refine research questions and improve study timeliness and relevance, improving the structure and management of clinical data systems both to support better decisions and to provide quality data at the level of the practitioner, facilitating "built-in" study design, defining appropriate levels of evidence needed for clinical decision making and how they might vary by the nature of the intervention and condition, and changes in clinical research that might help accelerate innovation.

Feedback Loops to Expedite Study Timeliness and Relevance

An emerging model of care delivery is one focused around management of care, instead of expertise. Brent James of Intermountain Healthcare discussed the three elements of quality enhancement: quality design, quality improvement, and quality control. Of these, quality control is the key, but underappreciated, factor in developing stringent care delivery models. In this respect, process analysis is important to a care delivery model. Use of process analysis at Intermountain Healthcare revealed that a small percentage of clinical issues accounted for most care delivery shortfalls, and these became the first foci for initiation of a care management system. Although the original intent of this system was to achieve excellence in caregiving, a notable side benefit has been its use as a research tool (see James, Chapter 3). It has allowed for feedback systems, in which clinical questions can be addressed through interdisciplinary evaluation, examination of databases, prospective pilot projects, and finally, broad implementation when shown to be beneficial. Because the data management system is designed for a high degree of flexibility, data content can rapidly be changed around individual clinical scenarios. When a high-priority care process is identified, a flow chart is designed for that process, with tracking of a key targeted outcome for feedback and care management adjustment. The approach actively involves the patient and successively escalates care as needed, in a sort of "care cascade." Each protocol is developed by a team of knowledge experts that oversee implementation and teaching. Once these systems are established for individual parameters of care, they are utilized in several different ways to generate evidence, such as quasi-experimental designs to evaluate policy decisions using pilot programs. Because RCTs are not practical, ethical, feasible, or appropriate to all circumstances, these large data systems with built-in study design and feedback loops allow for investigations that have real rigor, utility, and reliability in large populations.

Use of Electronic Health Records to Bridge the Inference Gap

Clinical decisions are made every day in the context of a certain inference gap—the gap between what is known at the point of care and what evidence is required to make a clinical decision. Physicians and other healthcare providers implicitly or explicitly are required to fill in where knowledge falls short. Walter Stewart of the Geisinger Health System discussed how the electronic health record can help to narrow this gap, increasing real-time access to knowledge in the practice setting and creating evidence relevant to everyday practice needs (see Stewart, Chapter 3). As such, it will bring research and practice into much closer alignment. EHRs can change both evidence and practice through the development of new methods to extract valid evidence from analysis of retrospective longitudinal patient data; the translation of these methods into protocols that can rapidly and automatically evaluate patient data in real time as a component of decision support; and the development of protocols designed to conduct clinical trials as a routine part of care delivery. By linking research seamlessly to practice, EHRs can help address the expanding universe of practice-based questions, with a growing need for solutions that are inexpensive and timely, can meet the daily needs of practice settings, and can help drive incentives to create value in health care.

Standards of Evidence

The anchor element in evidence-based medicine is the clinical information on which determinations are based. However the choice of evidence standards used for decision making has fundamental implications for decisions about the use of new interventions, the selection of study designs, safety standards, the treatment of individual patients, and population-level decisions regarding insurance coverage. Steven Pearson of America's Health Insurance Plans discussed the development of standards of evidence, how they must vary by circumstance, and how they must be adjusted when more evidence is drawn from the care process. At the most basic level, confidence in evidence is shaped by both its quality and its strength, and its application is shaped by whether it is being used for a decision about an individual patient or about a population group through policy initiatives and coverage determinations. In part, the current challenge to evidence-based coverage decisions is that good evidence is frequently lacking, and traditional evidence hierarchies also fit poorly for diagnostics and for assessing value in real-world patient populations (see Pearson, Chapter 3). However advances are also needed in understanding how information is or should be used by decision-making bodies. Using CED as an example, Pearson discussed how similar practice-based research opportunities inherent to a learning healthcare system could affect the nature of evidence standards and bring into focus certain policy questions.

Implications for Innovation Acceleration

Evidence-based medicine has sometimes been characterized as a possible barrier to innovation, despite its potential as means of accelerating innovations that add value to health care. Robert Galvin from General Electric discussed this issue, pointing out that employers seek value—the best quality at the most controlled cost—and their goal is to spend healthcare dollars most intelligently. This has sometimes led employers to ignore innovation in their efforts to control the drivers of cost. There are numerous examples of beneficial innovations whose coverage was long delayed due to lack of evidence, as well as of innovations that, although beneficial to a subset of patients, were overused. A problem in introducing a more rational approach to these decisions is what Galvin terms the "cycle of unaccountability." Each group in the chain—manufacturers, clinicians, healthcare delivery systems, patients, government regulators, and payers—desires system change but has not, to date, taken on specific responsibilities or been held accountable for roles in instituting change. General Electric has initiated a program Access to Innovation as a way to adopt the principles of coverage with evidence development in the private sector. Using a specific investigational intervention, reimbursement for certain procedures is provided in a limited pilot population to allow for the development of evidence in real time and inform a definitive policy on coverage of the intervention. Challenges encountered include content knowledge gaps; the difficulty of engaging purchasers to increase their expenditures, despite discussions of value; finding willing participants; and the growing culture of distrust between manufacturers, payers, purchasers, and patients (see Galvin, Chapter 3). Some commonality is needed on what is meant by evidence and accountability for change within each sector.

Learning Systems in Progress

Incorporation of data generation, analysis, and application into healthcare delivery can be a major force in accelerating understanding of what constitutes "best care." Many existing efforts to use technology and create research networks to implement evidence-based medicine have produced scattered examples of successful learning systems. This session focused on the experiences of healthcare systems that highlight the opportunities and challenges of integrating the generation and application of evidence for improved care. Premier visions of how systems might effectively be used to realize the benefit of integrated systems of research and practice include the care philosophy and initiative at the Department of Veterans Affairs (VA), the front-line experience of the Practice-Based Research Networks in aligning the resources and organizations to develop learning communities, and initiatives at the AQA (formerly the Ambulatory Care Quality Alliance) to develop consensus on strategies and approaches that promote systems cooperation, data aggregation, accountability, and the use of data to bring research and practice closer together. These examples suggest a vision for a learning healthcare system that builds upon current capacity and initiatives and identifies important elements and steps that can take progress to the next level.

Implementing Evidence-Based Practice at the VA

The Department of Veterans Affairs has made important progress in implementing evidence-based practice, particularly via use of the electronic health record. Elements fostering the development of this learning system, cited by Joel Kupersmith, the chief research and development officer at the Veterans Health Administration, include an environment that values evidence, quality, and accountability through performance measures, the leadership to create and sustain this environment, and the VA's research culture and infrastructure (see Kupersmith, Chapter 4). Without this appropriate culture and setting, EHRs may simply be a graft onto computerized record systems and will not help to foster evidence-based practice. Kupersmith presented the VA's work with diabetes as an example demonstrating the range of possibilities in using the EHR for developing and implementing evidence at the point of care. This includes assistance in education and management of patients through automated decision support and evidence-based clinical reminders, as well as advancing research through the Diabetes Epidemiology Cohort (DEpiC). The cohort database consists of longitudinal record data on 600,000 diabetic patients receiving VA care, which is a key resource for a wide range of research projects. In addition, the recent launch of My HealtheVet, a web portal through which veterans will be able to view personal health records and access health information, allows patient-centered care and self-management and the ability to evaluate the effectiveness of these approaches. The result to date has been better control and fewer amputations. There are plans to link genomic information with this database to further expand research capabilities and offer increased insights toward individualized medicine.

Learning Communities and Practice-Based Research Networks

A culture change is necessary in the structure of clinical care, if the learning healthcare system is to take hold. Robert Phillips of the American Academy of Family Physicians described the formation of Practice-Based Research Networks (PBRNs) as a response to the disconnect between national biomedical research priorities and questions at the front line of clinical care. Many of the networks formed around collections of clinicians who found that studies of efficacy did not necessarily translate into effectiveness in their practices or that questions arising in their practices were not addressed in the literature. PBRNs began to appear formally more than two decades ago to support better science and fill these gaps, offering many lessons and models to inform the development of learning systems (see Phillips, Chapter 4). Positioned at the point of care, PBRNs integrate research and practice to improve the quality of care. By linking practicing clinicians with investigators experienced in clinical and health services research, PBRNs move quality improvement out of the single practice and into networks, pooling intellectual capital, resources, and motivation and allowing measures to be compared and studied across clinics. The successful learning communities of PBRNs have definite characteristics, including a shared mission and values, a commitment to collective inquiry, collaborative teams, an action orientation that includes experimentation, continuous improvement, and a results orientation.

National Quality Improvement Process and Architecture

While there are many examples of integrated health systems, such as HealthPartners, the VA, Mayo, Kaiser Permanente, and others, a learning healthcare system for the nation requires thinking and working beyond individual organizations toward the larger system of care. George Isham of HealthPartners outlined the national quality improvement process and architecture needed for system-wide, coordinated, and continual gains in healthcare quality. Also discussed was the ongoing work at AQA that has assembled key stakeholders to agree on a strategy for measuring performance at the physician or group level, collecting and aggregating data in the least burdensome way, and reporting meaningful information to consumers, physicians, and stakeholders to inform choices and improve outcomes. The aim is for regional collaboration that can facilitate improved performance at lower cost; improved transparency for consumers and purchasers, involving providers in a culture of quality; buy-in for national standards; reliable and useful information for consumers and providers; quality improvement skills and expertise for local provider practices; and stronger physician-patient partnerships. Initial steps include the development of criteria and performance measures, such as those endorsed by the National Quality Forum, and the design of an approach to aggregate information across the nation through a data-sharing mechanism, directed by an entity such as a national health data stewardship entity that sets standards, rules, and policies for data sharing and aggregation.

Envisioning a Rapid Learning Healthcare System

The pace of evidence development is simply inadequate to begin to meet the need. Lynn Etheredge of George Washington University discussed the need for a national rapid learning system—a new model for developing evidence on clinical effectiveness. Already the world's highest health expenditure, healthcare costs in the United States continue to grow, largely driven by technology. Short of rationing, any prospect of progress hinges on the development of an evidence base that will help identify the diagnosis and treatment approaches of greatest value for patients (see Etheredge, Chapter 4). Building on current infrastructure and resources, it should be possible to develop a rapid learning health system to close the evidence gaps. Computerized EHR databases enable real-time learning from tens of millions of patients that offers a vital opportunity to rapidly generate and test hypotheses. Currently the greatest capacities lie in the VA and the Kaiser Permanente integrated delivery systems, with more than 8 million EHRs apiece, national research databases, and search software under development. Research networks such as the Health Maintenance Organization (HMO) Research Network (HMORN), the Cancer Research Network at the National Cancer Institute (NCI), and the vaccine safety data link at the Centers for Disease Control and Prevention (CDC) also add substantially to the capacity. Medicaid currently represents the biggest gap, with no state yet using EHRs. An expansion of the infrastructure could be led by the Department of Health and Human Services and the VA, beginning with the use of their standards, regulatory responsibilities, and purchasing power to foster the development of an interconnected national EHR database with accommodating privacy standards. In this way, all EHR research databases could become compatible and multiuse and lead to substantial expansion of the clinical research activities of NIH, AHRQ, CDC, and FDA. In addition, NIH and FDA clinical studies could be integrated into national computer-searchable databases, and Medicare's evidence development requirements for coverage could be expanded into a national EHR-based model system for evaluating new technologies. Leadership and stable funding are needed as well as a new way of thinking about sharing data.

Developing the Test Bed: Linking Integrated Service Delivery Systems

Many extensive research networks have been established to conduct clinical, basic, and health services research and to facilitate communication between the different efforts. The scale of these networks ranges from local, uptake-driven efforts to wide-ranging efforts to connect vast quantities of clinical and research information. This section explores how various integrated service delivery systems might be better linked to expand our nation's capacity for structured, real-time learning—in effect, developing a test bed to improve development and application of evidence in healthcare decision making. The initiatives of two public and two private organizations serve as examples of the progress in linking research, translational, and clinical systems. A new series of grants and initiatives from NIH and AHRQ (NECTAR and Accelerating Change and Transformation in Organizations and Networks [ACTION], respectively—see below) highlight the growing emphasis on the need to integrate and communicate the results of research endeavors. The ongoing activities of the HMO Research Network and the Permanente Foundation-Council of Accountable Physician Practices demonstrate that there is considerable interest at the interface of public and private organizations to further these goals. For each, there are organizational, logistical, data system, reimbursement, and regulatory considerations.

NIH and Reengineering Clinical Research

The NIH (http://nihroadmap.nih.gov/) Roadmap for Medical Research was developed to identify major opportunities and gaps in biomedical research, to identify needs and roadblocks to the research enterprise, and to increase synergy across NIH in utilizing this information to accelerate the pace of discoveries and their translation. Stephen Katz of the National Institutes of Health explained that a significant aim of this endeavor is to address questions that none of the 27 different institutes or centers that make up the NIH could examine on its own, but that could be addressed collectively. Within this context, there are several initiatives grouped as the Reengineering the Clinical Research Enterprise components of the Road-map Initiative. They are oriented around translational science, clinical informatics, and clinical research network infrastructure and utilization. A major activity is the Clinical and Translational Science Awards (CTSAs), which represent the largest component of NIH Roadmap funding for medical research. The CTSAs are aimed at creating homes that lower barriers between disciplines, clinicians, and researchers and encourage creative, innovative approaches to solve complex medical problems at the front lines of patient care. A second component is the development of integrated clinical research networks through formation of the National Electronic Clinical Trials and Research (NECTAR) network. This initiative includes an inventory of 250 clinical research networks, as well as pilot projects to bring the NECTAR framework into action for a wide range of disease entities, populations, settings, and information systems.

AHRQ and the Use of Integrated Service Delivery Systems

Large integrated delivery systems are important as test beds not only for generating evidence, but for applying it as well. Cynthia Palmer of the Agency for Healthcare Quality and Research described its program ACTION, designed to foster the dissemination and adoption of best practices through the use of demand-driven, rapid-cycle grants that focus on practical and applied work across a broad range of topics. ACTION is the successor to the Integrated Delivery System Research Network (IDSRN), a five-year implementation initiative that was completed in 2005 and is based on the finding that the organizations that conduct health services research are also the most effective in accelerating its implementation. One report suggested that it may take as long as 17 years to turn some positive research results to the benefit of patient care (Balas and Boren 2000), so working to reduce the lag time between innovation and its implementation is another primary goal of ACTION (see Palmer, Chapter 5). Features among participating organizations include size (the volume it takes to initiate change and assess its implementation), diversity (with regard to payer type, geographic location, and demographic characteristics), database capacity (large, robust databases with nationally recognized academic and field-based researchers), and speed (the ability to go from request for proposal to an award in 9 weeks and average project completion in 15 months).

The Health Maintenance Organization Research Network

Health maintenance organizations represent an important resource for innovative work in testing the effectiveness of new interventions. Eric Larson of Group Health Cooperative discussed HMORN, a consortium of 15 integrated delivery systems assembled to bring together their combined resources for clinical and health services research. Together these systems contain more than 15 million people, and as contained systems, natural experiments are going on every day. The formal research programs of HMORN include research centers at each of the participating sites, with a total of approximately 200 researchers and more than 1,500 ongoing research projects. All sites have standardized and validated datasets, and some have become standardized to each other. HMORN's advantages include the close ties between care delivery, financing, administration, and patients, which aligns incentives for ongoing improvement of care as well as shared administrative claims and clinical data, including some degree of electronic health record (Larson 2006 [July 20-21]). The ongoing research initiatives are all public interest, nonproprietary, open-system research projects that include the ability to structure clinical trials with individual or cluster randomization around real-world care as opposed to the idealized world of the RCT. These studies can be formed prospectively, with the potential for longitudinal evaluation. Examples of HMORN's work toward real-time learning include post-marketing surveillance and drug safety studies, population-based chronic care improvement studies, surveillance of acute diseases including rapid detection of immediate environmental threats, and health services research demonstration projects.

Council of Accountable Physician Practices

Physicians remain the central decision makers in the nation's medical care enterprise. Michael Mustille of the Permanente Federation described the work of the Council of Accountable Physician Practices (CAPP), organized in 2002 to enhance physician leadership in improving the healthcare delivery system. The organization is made up of 35 multispecialty group practices from all over the United States that share a common vision as learning organizations dedicated to the improvement of clinical care. Their features include physician leadership and governance, dedication to evidence-based care management processes, well-developed quality improvement systems, team-based care, the use of advanced clinical information technology, and the collection, analysis, and distribution of clinical performance information (see Mustille, Chapter 5). The formation of CAPP was initiated because multispecialty medical groups are well-designed learning systems at the forefront of using health information technology and electronic health records to provide advanced systems of care. One of the central organizing principles of CAPP is that physicians are responsible not only to the patient they are currently treating, but also to a group of patients, and to their colleagues, to provide the best care and contribute to the quality of care overall. Mustille described many of the ongoing activities of CAPP, including lending medical group expertise and leadership in the public policy arena, enabling physicians to lead change, facilitating research, and translating research and epidemiology into actual practice at the group setting level.

The Patient as a Catalyst for Change

There is a growing appreciation of the centrality of patient involvement as a contributor to positive healthcare outcomes and as a catalyst for change in healthcare delivery. This session focused on the changing role of the patient in the era of the Internet and the personal health record. It explored the potential for increased patient knowledge and participation in decision making and for expediting improvements in healthcare quality. It examined how patient accessibility to information could be engaged to improve outcomes; the roles and responsibilities that come with increased patient access and use of information in the electronic health record; privacy assurance and patient comfort as the EHR is used for evidence generation; and the accommodation of patient preferences. The types of evidence and decision aids needed for improved shared decision making, and how the communication of evidence might be improved, were also discussed. All of these are key issues in the emergence of a learning healthcare system focused on patient needs and built around the best care.

The Internet, eHealth, and Patient Empowerment

Information technology (IT) has the potential to support a safer, higher-quality, more effective healthcare system. By offering patients and healthcare consumers unprecedented access to information and personal health records, IT will also impact patient knowledge and decision making. Janet Marchibroda, from the eHealth Initiative, offered an overview of federal, state, and business initiatives contributing to the development of a national health information network that aims to empower the patient to be a catalyst for change and drive incentives centered around value and performance. For example, the National Coordinator for Health Information Technology was established to foster development of a nationwide interoperable health information technology (HIT) infrastructure, and about half of the states have either an executive order or a legislative mandate in place that is designed to stimulate the use of HIT. Employers, health plans, and patient groups are also engaged in various cooperative initiatives to develop a standardized minimum data content description for electronic health records, as well as the processing rules and standards required to ensure data consistency, data portability, and EHR interoperability. Most consumers—60 percent according to an eHealth Initiative survey (see Marchibroda, Chapter 6)—are interested in the benefits that personal and electronic health records have to offer and would utilize tools to mange many aspects of their health care. While Marchibroda felt that the United States is not yet at the point of a consumer revolution in shaping health care, it is clear that the patient is an integral part of expediting healthcare improvements and that the Internet and EHR-related tools will facilitate this progress.

Joint Patient-Provider Management of the Electronic Health Record

As patients, family members, other caregivers, and clinicians all begin viewing, using, contributing to, and interacting with information in the personal and electronic health record, new roles and responsibilities emerge. Andrew Barbash of Apractis Solutions noted that moving toward true patient-provider collaboration in health care may be less a data and infrastructure issue than a communication issue. What is needed is not the organization's view of how to communicate with patients, but the patients' view of how to communicate with the organization. Personal health records are only a small piece of the consumer's world; and the technologies, demographics, and knowledge base are constantly changing, creating a very complex dynamic to navigate when making shared and often complex decisions about health care. A first obligation is defining what different users need to know, how best to convey this information to them, and what information models will be most useful. Existing collaboration tools are "web-centric," but the next step is to leverage the web as a vehicle for becoming "communication-centric." There is significant potential for the Internet and EHRs to bring about changes in patient-provider communication and collaboration that will require forethought regarding the processes for governing, shared privacy management, liability, and self-education.

Evidence and Shared Decision Making

When medical evidence is imperfect, and its application must account for preferences, a collaborative approach by providers and patients is essential. James Weinstein of Dartmouth described what has been learned about discerning patient preferences as a part of shared decision making. Variation in care is a common feature of the healthcare system (Figure S-2). In emergency situations, such as hip fracture, patients both understand and desire the need for specific, directed intervention, and the choice to have a specific treatment is all but decided. However for other conditions such as chronic back pain, early-stage breast or prostate cancer, benign prostatic enlargement, or abnormal uterine bleeding, the decision to have a medical or surgical intervention is less clear and the path of watchful waiting is often an option. When patients delegate their decision making to their physicians, which is generally the case, the decisions often reflect providers' options

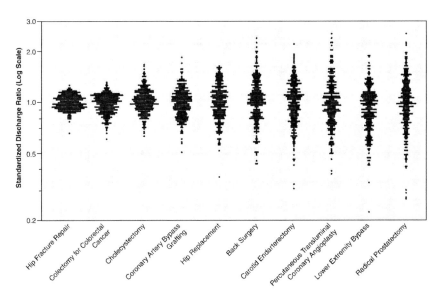

FIGURE S-2 Profiles of variation for 10 common (surgical) procedures.
SOURCE: Dartmouth Atlas Healthcare.

rather than patients'. One result is that the likelihood of having a prosta-tectomy or hysterectomy varies two- to fivefold from one region to another; that is, "geography is destiny" (Wennberg and Cooper 1998; Wennberg et al. 2002). Many of these are "preference-sensitive" decisions, with the best choice depending on a patient's values or preferences, given the benefits and harms and the scientific uncertainty associated with the treatment options. The Shared Decision Making Center at the Dartmouth-Hitchcock Medical Center seeks to engage the patient in these decisions by better informing patient choice through the use of interactive decision aids. One example given by Weinstein is SPORT (Spine Patient Outcomes Research Trial), a novel practical clinical trial that utilizes shared decision making as part of a generalizable, evidence-based enrollment strategy. Patients are offered interactive information about treatments and then offered enrollment in a clinical trial; those with strong treatment preferences who do not want to enter the RCT are asked to enroll in a cohort study. Shared decision making of this sort can lead to improved patient satisfaction, improved outcomes, and better evidence.

Training the Learning Health Professional

In a system that learns from data collected at the point of care and ap-plies the lessons to patient care improvement, healthcare professionals will continue to be the key components at the front lines, assessing the needs, directing the approaches, ensuring the integrity of the tracking and quality of the outcomes, and leading innovation. However, what these practitioners will need to know and how they learn will change dramatically. Orienting practice around a continually evolving evidence base requires new ways of thinking about how to create and sustain a healthcare workforce that recognizes the role of evidence in decision making and is attuned to life-long learning. Our current system of health professions education offers minimal integration of the concepts of evidence-based practice into core curricula and relegates continuing medical education to locations and top-ics distant from the issues encountered at the point of care. Advancements must confront the barriers presented by the current culture of practice and the potential burden to practitioners presented by the continual acquisition and transfer of new knowledge. Opportunities identified by presentations in this session include developing tools and systems that embed evidence into practice workflow, reshaping formal educational curricula for all healthcare practitioners, and shifting to continuing educational approaches that are integrated with care delivery and occur each day as a part of practice.

The Electronic Health Record and Clinical Informatics as Learning Tools

As approaches shift to individualized care, changes will be needed in the roles and nature of the learning process of health professionals. William Stead from Vanderbilt University discussed the use of informatics and the EHR to bring the processes of learning, evidence development, and application into closer alignment by changing the practice ecosystem. Currently, the physician serves as an integrator, aggregating information, recognizing patterns, making decisions, and trying to translate those decisions into action. However, the human mind can handle only about seven facts at a time, and by the end of this decade, there will be an increase of one or two orders of magnitude in the number of facts needed to coordinate any given medical encounter (Stead 2006 [July 20-21]). Future clinical decision making will need not just a personal health record but a personal health knowledge base that is an intelligent integration of information about the individual with evidence related to that individual, presented in a way that lets the provider and the patient make the right decisions. Also necessary is a shift from an educational model in which learning is a just-in-case proposition to one in which it is just-in-time—that is, current, competent, and appropriate to the circumstance. A model for a learning process, continuous learning during performance, details how learning can use targeted curricula to drive competency and outcomes. The potential uses of the EHR to manage information and support learning strategies include data-driven practice improvement, alerts and reminders in clinical workflow, identification of variability in care, patient-specific alerts to change in practice, links to evidence within clinical workflow, detection of unexpected events and identifying safety concerns, and large-scale phenotype-genotype hypothesis generation. These systems will also provide a way to close the loop by identifying relevant order sets, tracking order set utilization, and routinely feeding this performance data back into order set development. Achieving this potential will require a completely new approach, with changes in how we define the roles of health professionals and how the system facilitates their lifelong learning (see Stead, Chapter 7).

Embedding an Evidence Perspective in Health Professions Education

Evidence-based practice allows health professionals to deliver care of high value even within a landscape of finite resources (Mundinger 2006 [July 20-21]). With rapid advances in medical knowledge, teaching health professionals to evaluate and use evidence in clinical decision making becomes one of the most crucial aspects of ensuring efficacy of care and patient safety. To adequately prepare the healthcare workforce, their training must familiarize them with the dynamic nature of evolving evidence and position them to contribute actively to both the generation and the application of evidence through healthcare delivery. Mary Mundinger from the Columbia University School of Nursing presented several examples of curricula currently used at Columbia University by the medical, nursing, and dentistry schools to educate their students about evidence. One successful approach taken by the Columbia Nursing School was to adopt translational research as a guiding principle leading to a continuous cycle in which students and faculty engage in research, implementation, dissemination, and inquiry. This principle extends beyond the traditional linear progression of research from the bench to the bedside and also informs policy and curriculum considerations. Topics emphasized in these curricula included developing the skills needed to become sophisticated readers of the literature; understanding the different levels of evidence; understanding the relationship between design methods and conclusions and recommendations; understanding the science; knowing how care protocols evolve; and knowing when to deviate from protocols because of patient responses. To take advantage of a workforce trained in evidence-based practice, changes are needed in the culture of health care to emphasize the importance of evidence management skills (see Mundinger, Chapter 7).

Knowledge Translation: Redefining Continuing Education

Evidence-based practice will require a shift in medical thinking that deemphasizes personal expertise and intuition in favor of the ability to draw upon the best available evidence for the situation, in an environment in which knowledge is very dynamic. Mark Williams from Emory University described the potential role of continuing education in such a transformation. Continuing medical education (CME) seeks to promote lifelong learning in the physician community by providing opportunities to learn current best evidence. However, technology development and the creation of new knowledge have increased dramatically in both volume and pace (Figure S-3), nearly overwhelming practicing clinicians (Williams 2006 [July 20-21]). While CME aims to alleviate this burden, the current format is based on a static model of evidence development that will become increasingly inadequate to support the delivery of timely, up-to-date care. New approaches to CME are being developed to engage these critical dimensions of a learning system. One variation is the knowledge translation approach in which CME is moved to where care is delivered and is targeted at all participants—patients, nurses, pharmacists, and doctors—and the content consists of initiatives to improve health care (Davis et al. 2003). By emphasizing teamwork and pulling physicians out of the autonomous role and into collaborations that are cross-departmental and cross-institutional,

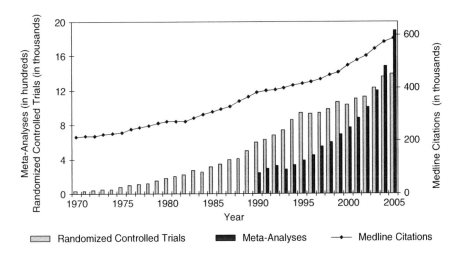

FIGURE S-3 Trends in Medline citations and Medline citations for randomized controlled trials and meta-analyses per year.
SOURCE: National Library of Medicine public data, http://www.nlm.nih.gov/bsd/pmresources.html.

new approaches to CME support the necessary culture change and help shift toward practice-based learning that is integrated with care delivery and is ongoing.

Structuring the Incentives for Change

A fundamental reality in the prospects for a learning healthcare system lies in the nature of the incentives for inducing the necessary changes. Incentives are needed to drive the system and culture changes, as well as to establish the collaborations and technological developments necessary to build learning into every healthcare encounter. Public and private insurers, standards organizations such as the National Committee for Quality Assurance (NCQA) and the Joint Commission (formerly JCAHO), and manufacturers have the opportunity to shape policy and practice incentives to accelerate needed changes. Incentives that support and encourage evidence development and application as well as innovation are features of a learning healthcare system. Change can be encouraged through incentives at all layers—giving providers incentive to use established guidelines and drive better outcomes; giving healthcare delivery systems incentives for increased efficiency; giving manufacturers and developers incentives for bringing the safest, most effective and efficient products to market; and giving patients incentives for increased engagement as decision-making participants.

Opportunities for Private Insurers

Ultimately, the strongest incentives are economic, and a variety of opportunities exist for insurers to structure payment approaches that encourage both the development of evidence and the application of the best available evidence. Alan Rosenberg of Wellpoint discussed several inducements through the services and methodologies included in physician and hospital reimbursement: the structure of benefit plans; the encouragement of technology use, including the EHR; rewarding the capacity to generate evidence as a by-product of care; and adoption of a consumer-focused healthcare policy. With respect to physician and hospital reimbursement, there is an increasing trend for payment for care associated with clinical trials, with participation in national registries, or in conjunction with centers of excellence, including aligning policies with the investigational processes (Rosenberg 2006 [July 20-21]). These shifts provide an opportunity for private insurers to participate in evidence development, both in coverage decision making and in willingness to provide data for these efforts. Rosenberg also supported the use of claims data analysis by private insurers to support evidence development. For example, the use of pharmacy claims data allows for one form of post-marketing surveillance that can provide valuable insights into both the safety and the effectiveness of drugs when used on a large scale. Claims data analysis can also drive quality improvement initiatives. Hurdles to progress noted include large dollar court settlements that do not align with evidence; desire to avoid these public court proceedings; and lack of trust between the consumer, medical community, and insurers.

Opportunities for CMS

As the world's largest health insurer, the Centers for Medicare and Medicaid Services has the greatest potential to enhance the role of evidence development and application in medical care. Steve Phurrough from CMS pointed out that the agency has fundamentally two mechanisms to influence healthcare behavior: using the system of payment to direct what people do in practice, and using regulatory responsibilities and authorities to require system changes. In the latter respect, better use of claims data can bring about significant changes in how healthcare services are evaluated. The movement of claims data from ICD-9 (International Classification of Diseases, Ninth Revision) to ICD-10 will help bring a greater level of detail to diagnoses and procedures than is currently available and help provide greater resolution of the information gleaned from these data. In addition to pay-for-performance, there is also the concept of pay-for-reporting, currently under way in several examples under the Coverage with Evidence Development initiative at CMS. These efforts have allowed the evaluation of data demonstrating effects and outcomes that would not have been foreseen by RCTs. There is a leadership role for government as individual policies are implemented, with the expectation that some key decisions made in the setting of CMS will be adopted in other settings. To make every healthcare experience a learning experience, technologies will have to be adopted, some of which can be encouraged by CMS. There will also have to be an understanding and acceptance of methodologies for collecting data in a form that is not the randomized controlled trial.

Opportunities for Pharmaceutical Companies

Healthcare product manufacturers are major sponsors of the collection of evidence important to better understanding the effectiveness of diagnostic and treatment interventions. The pre-market requirements for testing of efficacy and safety represent the most obvious contribution, but it is also possible for manufacturers to structure their studies in a fashion that might better anticipate some of the issues about effectiveness and efficiency that are important for coverage decisions and a smooth transition to the post-market surveillance phase. Wayne A. Rosenkrans of AstraZeneca pointed out that when assessing the comparative effectiveness of various therapeutic options, all of the evidence needed to fully assess the options is rarely available to decision makers. In the face of insufficient information, the decisions often seem arbitrary and the rules seem unclear from the manufacturers' perspective. Rosenkrans felt that greater clarity is needed on the standards of evidence to be met for different purposes, as well as greater transparency in the process of how evidence is used to make reimbursement and treatment guidelines decisions. With respect to investment in comparative outcomes research, one of the barriers is the presumption that manufacturers, to ensure credibility, must employ a traditional clinical trial approach, yet that approach may be both impractical and prohibitively expensive. There is a need to develop either a credible third party to help make those determinations or some other creative approach to this problem. One possibility might be an industry-wide approach to evidence-based drug development, in which the creation of effectiveness data, in addition to efficacy and safety data, is a central component of the process of drug development—rather than an afterthought or part of post-marketing surveillance. Especially with the pending developments in information technology, electronic health records, biomarkers, surrogate markers, and simulations, this may be the time to explore new approaches.

Opportunities for Standards Organizations

When it comes to improving medical care, the notion that what gets measured gets done raises the issue of what to measure and how to judge the result. Margaret O'Kane of the National Committee for Quality Assurance discussed the relationships between new approaches to evidence development and accountability for quality. In order to achieve the goal of improvement through standards and measurement, several parameters are combined for accreditation, including standards for structural and procedure activities, means to ensure consumer protection, measures of care received (the Health Plan Employer Data and Information Set [HEDIS]), and the evaluation of consumer satisfaction and experience (Consumer Assessment of Health Providers and Systems [CAHPS]). New efforts include metrics for physician practices, to accomplish for physician practice what has been done for health plans through pilot programs across the country. Despite this progress, O'Kane noted that there are significant gaps in measurement initiatives as a result of lack of funding, lack of evidence, failure to develop consensus, unusable guidelines, and lack of interest on the part of some payers. Standards organizations then have a strong stake in efforts to generate better evidence, and they can both provide incentives for its application and, through the monitoring process, add to the body of evidence.

REFERENCES

AcademyHealth. 2005 (September). *Placement, Coordination, and Funding of Health Services Research Within the Federal Government*. Committee on Placement, Funding, and Coordination of Health Services Research within the Federal Government.

Balas, E, and S Boren. 2000. Managing clinical knowledge for healthcare improvements. In *Yearbook of Medical Informatics*, edited by V Schatauer. Stuttgart, Germany: Schattauer Publishing.

Bodenheirmer, T. 2005. High and rising health care costs. Part 2: Technologic innovation. *Annals of Internal Medicine* 142:932-937.

Califf, R. 2006 (July 20-21). *Session 2: The Evolving Evidence-Base—Methodologic and Policy Challenges, Alternatives to Large RCTs*. Presentation at the Roundtable on Evidence-Based Medicine Workshop, The Learning Health Care System. Washington, DC: Institute of Medicine, Roundtable on Evidence-Based Medicine.

Clancy, C. 2006 (July 20-21). *Session 1: Hints of a Different Way—Case Studies in Practice-Based Evidence, Opening Remarks*. Presentation at the Roundtable on Evidence-Based Medicine Workshop, The Learning Health Care System. Washington, DC: Institute of Medicine, Roundtable on Evidence-Based Medicine.

Davis, D, M Evans, A Jadad, L Perrier, D Rath, D Ryan, G Sibbald, S Straus, S Rappolt, M Wowk, and M Zwarenstein. 2003. The case for knowledge translation: shortening the journey from evidence to effect. *British Medical Journal* 327(7405):33-35.

Devereaux, P, M Bhandari, M Clarke, V Montori, D Cook, S Yusuf, D Sackett, C Cina, S Walter, B Haynes, H Schunemann, G Norman, and G Guyatt. 2005. Need for expertise based randomised controlled trials. *British Medical Journal* 330(7482):88.

Eddy, D, and L Schlessinger. 2003. Validation of the Archimedes diabetes model. *Diabetes Care* 26(11):3102-3110.

Fisher, E, D Wennberg, T Stukel, D Gottleib, F Lucas, and E Pinder. 2003. The implications of regional variations in Medicare spending. Part 2: health outcomes and satisfaction with care. *Annals of Internal Medicine* 138(4):288-299.

Graham, D, D Campen, R Hui, M Spence, C Cheetham, G Levy, S Shoor, and W Ray. 2005. Risk of acute myocardial infarction and sudden cardiac death in patients treated with cyclo-oxygenase 2 selective and non-selective non-steroidal anti-inflammatory drugs: nested case-control study. *Lancet* 365:475-481.

Green, L. 2006. Public health asks of systems science: to advance our evidence-based practice, can you help us get more practice-based evidence? *American Journal of Public Health* 96(3):406-409.

Greenfield, S, and R Kravitz. 2006 (July 20-21). *Session 2: The Evolving Evidence-Base—Methodologic and Policy Challenges, The Increasing Inadequacy of Randomized Trials for Guide-lines, Payment and Quality.* Presentation at the Roundtable on Evidence-Based Medicine Workshop, The Learning Health Care System. Washington, DC: Institute of Medicine, Roundtable on Evidence-Based Medicine.

IOM (Institute of Medicine). 2000. *To Err Is Human: Building a Safer Health System.* Washington, DC: National Academy Press.

———. 2001. *Crossing the Quality Chasm: A New Health System for the 21st Century.* Washington, DC: National Academy Press.

Kupersmith, J, N Sung, M Genel, H Slavkin, R Califf, R Bonow, L Sherwood, N Reame, V Catanese, C Baase, J Feussner, A Dobs, H Tilson, and E Reece. 2005. Creating a new structure for research on health care effectiveness. *Journal of Investigative Medicine* 53(2):67-72.

Larson, E. 2006 (July 20-21). *Session 6: Developing the Test-Bed: Linking Integrated Delivery Systems, HMO Research Network.* Presentation at the Roundtable on Evidence-Based Medicine Workshop, The Learning Health Care System. Washington, DC: Institute of Medicine, Roundtable on Evidence-Based Medicine.

Lubitz, J. 2005. Health, technology, and medical care spending. *Health Affairs* Web exclusive (W5-R81).

McCulloch, P, I Taylor, M Sasako, B Lovett, and D Griffin. 2002. Randomised trials in surgery: problems and possible solutions. *British Medical Journal* 324(7351):1448-1451.

McGlynn, E, S Asch, J Adams, J Keesey, J Hicks, A DeCristofaro, and E Kerr. 2003. The quality of health care delivered to adults in the United States. *New England Journal of Medicine* 348(26):2635-2645.

Moses, H, 3rd, E Dorsey, D Matheson, and S Thier. 2005. Financial anatomy of biomedical research. *Journal of the American Medical Association* 294(11):1333-1342.

Mundinger, M. 2006 (July 20-21). *Session 8: Training the Learning Healthcare Professional, Health Professions Education and Teaching About Evidence.* Presentation at the Roundtable on Evidence-Based Medicine Workshop, The Learning Health Care System Washington, DC: Institute of Medicine, Roundtable on Evidence-Based Medicine.

Need, A, A Motulsky, and D Goldstein. 2005. Priorities and standards in pharmacogenetic research. *Nature Genetics* 37(7):671-681.

Rosenberg, A. 2006 (July 20-21). *Session 9: Structure Incentives for Change, Opportunities for Private Insurers.* Presentation at the Roundtable on Evidence-Based Medicine Workshop, The Learning Health Care System. Washington, DC: Institute of Medicine, Roundtable on Evidence-Based Medicine.

Rosser, W. 1999. Application of evidence from randomised controlled trials to general practice. *Lancet* 353(9153):661-664.

Sackett, D, W Rosenberg, J Gray, R Haynes, and W Richardson. 1996. Evidence-Based medicine: what it is and what it isn't. *British Medical Journal* 312(7023):71-72.

Soumerai, S. 1987. Payment restrictions for prescription drugs under Medicaid. Effects on therapy, cost, and equity. *New England Journal of Medicine* 317(9):550-556.

———. 1994. Effects of limiting Medicaid drug-reimbursement benefits on the use of psychotropic agents and acute mental health services by patients with schizophrenia. *New England Journal of Medicine* 331(10):650-655.

———. 2006 (July 20-21). Session 1: Hints of a Different Way—Case Studies in Practice-Based Evidence, Potential of Quasi-Experimental Trial Designs for Evaluating Health Policy. Presentation at the Roundtable on Evidence-Based Medicine Workshop, The Learning Health Care System. Washington, DC: Institute of Medicine, Roundtable on Evidence-Based Medicine.

Stead, W. 2006 (July 20-21). Session 8: Training the Learning Healthcare Professional, Providers and the EHR as a Learning Tool. Presentation at the Roundtable on Evidence-Based Medicine Workshop, The Learning Health Care System. Washington, DC: Institute of Medicine, Roundtable on Evidence-Based Medicine.

Tamblyn, R. 2001. Adverse events associated with prescription drug cost-sharing among poor and elderly persons. *Journal of the American Medical Association* 285(4):421-429.

Trontell, A. 2004. Expecting the unexpected—drug safety, pharmacovigilance, and the prepared mind. *New England Journal of Medicine* 351(14):1385-1387.

Tunis, S. 2005. A clinical research strategy to support shared decision making. Health Affairs 24(1):180-184.

Weisman, H. 2006 (July 20-21). Session 2: The Evolving Evidence-Base—Methodologic and Policy Challenges, Broader Post-Marketing Surveillance for Insights on Risk and Effectiveness. Presentation at the Roundtable on Evidence-Based Medicine Workshop, The Learning Health Care System. Washington, DC: Institute of Medicine, Roundtable on Evidence-Based Medicine.

Wennberg, J, and M Cooper. 1998. Chapter 5: The surgical treatment of common disease. *The Dartmouth Atlas of Healthcare*. Chicago: American Hospital Publishing. Available from http://www.dartmouthatlas.org/atlases/98Atlas.pdf. (accessed April 4, 2007).

Wennberg, J, E Fisher, and J Skinner. 2002. Geography and the debate over Medicare reform. *Health Affairs* Supplemental Web Exclusives:W96-W114.

Williams, M. 2006 (July 20-21). *Session 8: Training the Learning Healthcare Professional, Redefining Continuing Medical Education Around Evolving Evidence.* Presentation at the Roundtable on Evidence-Based Medicine Workshop, The Learning Health Care System. Washington, DC: Institute of Medicine, Roundtable on Evidence-Based Medicine.

Wilson, S, B Delaney, A Roalfe, L Roberts, V Redman, A Wearn, and F Hobbs. 2000. Randomised controlled trials in primary care: case study. *British Medical Journal* 321(7252):24-27.

1

Hints of a Different Way—
Case Studies in Practice-Based Evidence

OVERVIEW

The Institute of Medicine Roundtable on Evidence-Based Medicine seeks "the development of a learning healthcare system that is designed to generate and apply the best evidence for the collaborative healthcare choices of each patient and provider; to drive the process of discovery as a natural outgrowth of patient care; and to ensure innovation, quality, safety, and value in health care" (Roundtable on Evidence-Based Medicine 2006). Generating evidence by driving the process of discovery as a natural outgrowth and product of care is the foundational principle for the learning healthcare system. This has been termed by some "practice-based evidence" (Greene and Geiger 2006). Practice-based evidence focuses on the needs of the decision makers, and narrowing the research-practice divide by identifying questions most relevant to clinical practice and conducting effectiveness research in typical clinical practice environments and unselected populations (Clancy 2006 [July 20-21]).

This chapter highlights several examples of the use of healthcare experience as a practical means of both generating and successfully applying evidence for health care. In the first paper, Peter B. Bach discusses how the Coverage with Evidence Development policy at Centers for Medicare and Medicaid Services (CMS) has aided the development of important evidence on effectiveness for a range of interventions, including lung volume reduction surgery (LVRS), PET (positron emission tomography) scanning for oncology, and implantable cardioverter defibrillators. By identifying information needed for improved understanding of intervention risks and benefits and designing appropriate trials or mechanisms to accumulate such evidence, CMS has accelerated access to health innovations. Moreover, generation of needed evidence from clinical practice is a means to better inform some of the many difficult clinical decisions inherent to medical practice. In the specific case of LVRS, the work of CMS identified an unproven approach that could have had an adverse impact on many patients before enough evidence was collected. By taking the lead, CMS helped develop timely information useful to other payers, clinicians, and patients.

Many risks or benefits of health technologies are not evident when initially introduced into the marketplace, and Jed Weissberg demonstrates the value of collecting, linking, and utilizing data for pharmacovigilance purposes in his paper on Kaiser Permanente's use of accumulated data for a post-market evaluation of cyclooxygenase-2 (COX-2) inhibitors. In this case, analysis was hypothesis driven and Weissberg notes that substantial work is needed to achieve a system in which such insights are generated customarily as a by-product of care. For such a transformation, we must improve our ability to collect and link data but also make the organizational and priority changes necessary to create an environment that values "learning"—a system that understands and values data and has the resources to act upon such data for the betterment of care.

Stephen Soumerai discusses the potential for quasi-experimental study designs to inform the entire process of care. His examples highlight well-designed studies that have been used to analyze health outcomes and demonstrate unintended consequences of policy decisions. He notes that widespread misperception of observational trials belies their strength in generating important information for decision making. Sean Tunis expands this argument by illustrating how practical clinical trials (PCTs) could serve as an effective means to evaluate issues not amenable to analyses by randomized controlled trials (RCTs), using the example of a PCT designed to evaluate the use of PET for diagnosing Alzheimer's disease. Alan H. Morris' work with computerized protocols—termed adequately explicit methods—demonstrates the considerable potential for such protocols to enhance a learning healthcare system. In his example, protocols for controlling blood glucose with IV insulin (eProtocol-insulin) provide a replicable and exportable experimental method that enables large-scale complex clinical studies at the holistic clinical investigation scale while reducing bias and contributing to generalizability of trial results. These protocols were also integrated into clinical care electronic health records (EHRs) demonstrating their utility to also improve the translation of research methods into clinical practice. Additionally, they could represent a new way of developing and distributing knowledge both by formalizing experiential learning and by enhancing education for clinicians and clinical researchers.

COVERAGE WITH EVIDENCE DEVELOPMENT

Peter B. Bach, M.D., M.A.P.P.[1]
Centers for Medicare and Medicaid Services

Coverage with Evidence Development (CED) is a form of National Coverage Decision (NCD) implemented by CMS that provides an opportunity to develop evidence on the effectiveness of items or services that have great promise but where there are potentially important gaps between efficacy and effectiveness, the potential for harm without benefit in subpopulations, or an opportunity to greatly enrich knowledge relevant to everyday clinical decision making. Most Medicare coverage determinations are made at a local level through carriers and fiscal intermediaries under contract with CMS. However, a few times each year, an NCD is made at the central level that dictates coverage policy for the entire country.

Whether the coverage determination is made locally or through an NCD, these determinations are based on historical data regarding the risks and benefits of items or services. Once coverage decisions are made, Medicare very rarely evaluates utilization, whether or not beneficiaries receiving the services are similar to those studied, or assesses whether outcomes of the covered services match those in the reports used to make the determination. At the extreme, there are many instances in Medicare coverage where determinations are made regarding coverage based on a brief trial of a handful of volunteer research subjects and then the service is provided to hundreds of thousands of patients for a far greater duration, where the patients are also more elderly and have a greater degree of comorbid illness than any of the patients included in the original study. This lack of information collection about real-world utilization and outcomes, the potential for differences between effectiveness and efficacy, and different trade-offs between benefits and risks is viewed by many as an important "forgone opportunity" in health care.

CED aims to integrate further evidence development into service delivery. Technically, CED is one form of "coverage with restrictions," where the restrictions include limiting coverage to specific providers or facilities (e.g., the limitation on which facilities can perform organ transplants), limiting coverage to particular patients, or in the case of CED, limiting coverage to contexts in which additional data are collected. From an implementation standpoint, CED requires that, when care is delivered, data collection occurs. Not a requirement of CED per se, but an expectation of it, is that

---

[1]Dr. Bach is an attending physician at Memorial Sloan-Kettering Cancer Center in New York City. He served as senior adviser to the administrator of the Centers for Medicare and Medicaid Services from February 2005 to November 2006.

the additional data generated will lead to new knowledge that will be integrated both into the CMS decision-making process to inform coverage reconsideration and into the knowledge base available for clinical decision making. Two case studies illustrate how CED can be used to directly or indirectly develop evidence that augments healthcare decision-making and CMS coverage policy.

Specific Examples of CED

The National Emphysema Treatment Trial (NETT), funded by CMS, was a multicenter clinical trial designed to determine the role, safety, and effectiveness of bilateral lung volume reduction surgery (LVRS) in the treatment of emphysema. The study had, as a secondary objective, to develop criteria for identifying patients who are likely to benefit from the procedure. While conducted prior to the coinage of the term "coverage with evidence development," the trial was implemented through a CMS NCD that eliminated coverage of LVRS outside of the trial but supported coverage for the surgery and routine clinical costs for Medicare beneficiaries enrolled in the trial. NETT demonstrates how coverage decisions can be leveraged to directly drive the development of evidence necessary for informed decision making by payers, physicians, and patients. The trial clarified issues of risk and benefit associated with the procedure and defined characteristics to help identify patients who were likely to benefit—information that was incorporated into the revised CMS NCD on lung volume reduction surgery and had significant impact on guidance offered for treatment of emphysema.

Emphysema is a major cause of death and disability in the United States. This chronic lung condition leads to the progressive destruction of the fine architecture of the lung that reduces its capacity to expand and collapse normally—leaving patients increasingly unable to breathe. The presence of poorly functioning portions of the lung is also thought to impair the capacity of healthy lung tissue to function. For patients with advanced emphysema, LVRS was hypothesized to confer benefit by removing these poorly functioning lung portions—up to 25-30 percent of the lung—and reducing lung size, thus pulling airways open and allowing breathing muscles to return to normal positioning, increasing the room available for healthy lung function, and improving the ability of patients to breathe. Prior to the trial, evidence for LVRS consisted of several case series that noted high upfront mortality and morbidity associated with the surgery and anecdotes of sizable benefit to some patients. At the time of the NCD, the procedure was a high-cost item with the operation and months of rehabilitation costing more than $50,000 on average. Many health economists predicted that utilization would rise rapidly with tens of thousands of patients eligible for the procedure and an estimated cost to Medicare predicted to be as much as $15 billion per year (Kolata 2006).

Because of the surgery's risks and the absence of clear evidence on its efficacy, patient selection criteria, and level of benefit, CMS initiated an interagency project with the National Heart, Lung, and Blood Institute (NHLBI) and the Agency for Healthcare Research and Quality (AHRQ). AHRQ's Center for Health Care Technology and NHLBI carried out independent assessments of LVRS; they concluded that the current data on the risks and benefits were inconclusive to justify unrestricted Medicare reimbursement for the surgery and suggested a trial to assess the effectiveness of the surgery. NHLBI conducted a scientific study of LVRS to evaluate the safety and efficacy of the current best available medical treatment alone and in conjunction with LVRS by excision. CMS funded the routine and interventional costs. The trial was conducted with the expectation that it would provide answers to important clinical questions about the benefits and risks of the surgery compared with good medical therapy, including the duration of any benefits, and clarification of which subgroups experienced benefit. Some initial barriers included resistance by the public, which considered it unethical to pay for some patients but not others to receive treatment.

The trial evaluated four subgroups prespecified by the case series studies and physiological hypotheses. One group was dropped early (homogeneous lung, severe obstruction, very low diffusing capacity) due to severe adverse outcomes including a high up-front mortality. The other three subgroups experienced some level of benefit and patients were followed for two years. On average, patients with severe emphysema who underwent LVRS with medical therapy were more likely to function better and did not face an increased risk of death compared to those who received only medical therapy. However results for individual patients varied widely. The study concluded that overall, LVRS increased the chance of improved exercise capacity but did not confer a survival advantage over medical therapy. The overall mortality was the same for both groups, but the risk of up-front mortality within the first three months was significantly increased for those receiving therapy (Ries et al. 2005). In addition to identifying patients that were poor candidates for the procedure, the trial identified two characteristics that could be used to predict whether an individual participant would benefit from LVRS, allowing clinicians to better evaluate risks and benefits for individual patients. CMS responded by covering the procedure for all three subgroups with any demonstrated benefit.

In this case, a well-designed and implemented CED NCD led to the creation of data that clarified the CMS coverage decision, refined questions in need of future research, and provided the types of evidence important to guide treatment evaluation by clinicians (subgroups of patients who might benefit or be at increased risk from LVRS) and patients (symptoms and quality-of-life data not previously available). Such evidence development led to informal and formative impressions among patients and providers that caused them to reconsider the intervention's value. As a result, from January 2004 to September 2005, only 458 Medicare beneficiaries received LVRS at a total cost to the government of less than $10.5 million (Kolata 2006).

Alternatively, CED can indirectly provide a basis for evidence development. PET is a diagnostic imaging procedure that has the ability to differentiate cancer from normal tissue in some patients, and thus can help in diagnosing and staging cancer and monitoring a patient's response to treatment. While the available evidence indicated that PET can provide more reliable guidance than existing imaging methods on whether the patient's cancer has spread, more data were required to help physicians and patients make better-informed decisions about the effective use of PET scanning.

CMS implemented an NCD to cover the costs of PET scanning for diagnosis, staging, re-staging, and monitoring of cancer patients, with the requirement that additional clinical data be collected into a registry. This type of CED allowed CMS to ensure patients would receive treatment benefit and build upon emerging evidence that PET was safe and effective by creating a platform from which other questions of clinical interest could be addressed. The NCD articulated questions that could lead to a reevaluation of the NCD, such as whether and in what specific instances PET scanning altered treatment decisions or other aspects of management of cancer patients. CMS required that information about PET scan be submitted to a registry. The registry then conducted research by following up with physicians to ask why a PET scan was ordered and whether the results of the PET scan altered disease outcomes. Participating patients and physicians were given the opportunity to give consent for their data to be used for research purposes, and other HIPAA (Health Insurance Portability and Accountability Act) issues were avoided by restricting research to the registry. While such research questions are simple and not likely to be independently pursued by agencies engaged in broader investigations such as the National Institutes of Health (NIH), they are typical of the kinds of evidence often needed to ensure the delivery of appropriate and effective health care.

Overarching Issues Affecting CED

Several overarching issues will affect the long-term viability of CED as a robust policy that spurs the development of a learning healthcare system. Of particular interest are the statutory authorities on which CED is based, the implications for patients who are eligible for services covered under CED, the role that the private-public interface must play for the learning to take place, and the issue of capacity in the healthcare system more broadly for such data collection, analysis, interpretation, and dissemination. Each of these issues has been extensively considered in the development of existing CED determinations, so moving forward the implementation of further CED determinations should be somewhat more straightforward.

Statutory Authority

In describing CED, CMS released a draft guidance followed by a final guidance that articulated the principles underpinning CED and the statutory authorities on which it is based. Both are available on the CMS coverage web site (www.cms.hhs.gov/coverage). In truth, there are two separate authorities, depending on the type of CED determination. When participation in a clinical trial is required as part of coverage, as in the NETT, the authority being used by CMS is based on section 1862(a)(1)(E) of the Social Security Act. CMS terms this "Coverage with Clinical Study Participation (CSP)." This section of the act allows CMS to provide coverage for items or services in the setting of a clinical research trial, and the use of this authority clarifies further that the item or service is not "reasonable and necessary" under section 1862(a)(1)(A) of the Social Security Act—the authority under which virtually all routine services are covered. The CED guidance further articulates that decisions such as NETT, in which coverage is provided only within the context of a clinical study, is meant as a bridge toward a final coverage determination regarding the service being "reasonable and necessary" under section 1862(a)(1)(A). Coverage, such as that provided for the PET registry, is based on the 1862(a)(1)(A) section of the Social Security Act because CMS has made the determination that the service is reasonable and necessary for the group of patients and indications that are covered, but that additional data are required to ensure that the correct service is being provided to the correct patient with the correct indications. As such, the registry is being used to collect additional data elements needed to better clarify the details of the service, patient, and indication. CMS terms this type of CED "Coverage with Appropriateness Determination" (CAD).

Implications for Patients

Unlike an NCD that provides coverage without restrictions, all NCDs that include restrictions affect how or where or which beneficiaries can receive services. As in coverage for organ transplants being provided only in certain hospitals, CED requires that patients receive services in locales where evidence can be collected. This limitation may be quite significant in terms of its effect on access or not significant at all. For instance, the NETT was conducted at only a handful of centers throughout the United States, so Medicare beneficiaries who wanted to receive the service had to travel to one of these centers and be evaluated. The coverage of fluorodeoxyglucose (FDG) PET for cancer is also limited to those PET facilities that have put in place a registry; but in this case, virtually all facilities in the country have been able to do so relatively easily. Not only can CED in some cases limit geographic access, but when CED requires clinical research participation, patients may have to undergo randomization in order to have a chance to receive the service. In the case of the NETT trial, some patients were randomized to best medical care instead of the surgery. In general, it is not unethical to offer services that are unproven only in the context of a clinical trial, when the scientific community is in equipoise regarding the risks and benefits of the service versus usual care and the data are insufficient to support a determination that the service is reasonable and necessary. Sometimes, patients may also be asked to provide "informed consent" to participate in research as part of CED, as in the NETT. However, patients have not been required to allow their data to be used for research when receiving a service such as the FDG-PET scan under CED. Rather, patients have been able to elect to have their data used for research, or not, but their consent has not been required for the service to be covered. (Early reports suggest that about 95 percent of Medicare beneficiaries are consenting to have their data used for research.) Theoretically, under some scenarios in which registries are being used to simply gather supplementary medical information, a requirement for informed consent could be waived due to the minimal risk posed and the impracticability of obtaining it.

The Private-Public Interaction Necessitated by CED

Because CED leads only to the requirement for data collection, but not to the requirement for other steps needed for evidence development, such as data analysis, scientific hypothesis testing, or publication and dissemination, CED requires a follow-on process to achieve its broader policy goals. To date, these goals have been achieved through partnerships with other federal agencies, providers, professional societies, academic researchers, and manufacturers. For instance, in the NETT, as noted above, the scientific design of data collection and the analysis and publication of study results were orchestrated through NHLBI, which engaged and funded investigators at multiple participating institutions. The involvement of the NHLBI and investigators from around the country ensured that CED would lead to a better understanding of the clinical role of LVRS in the Medicare population. In the case of the FDG-PET registry, the registry was required by CED, but was set up through a collaboration involving researchers at several academic institutions, and professional societies, to form the National Oncologic PET Registry (NOPR). These researchers constructed a research study design around the CED requirement, such that there is a high probability that both clinicians and CMS will have a far better understanding of the role of FDG-PET scans in the management of Medicare patients with cancer.

Recently, CMS issued another CED decision covering implantable cardiac defibrillators (ICDs), in which all patients in Medicare receiving ICDs for primary prevention are required to submit clinical data to an ICD registry. The baseline registry, which captures patient and disease characteristics for the purpose of gauging appropriateness (i.e., CAD) forms the platform for a 100 percent sample of patients receiving this device for this indication in Medicare. The entity running the registry has since engaged other private payers, cardiologists, researchers, and device manufacturers in order that a follow-on data collection can be put in place to capture the frequency of appropriate ICD "firings" (where the device restores the patient's heart to an appropriate rhythm). In other words, because CMS requires only the core data elements to be submitted, evidence development is driven only indirectly by CED. However, the establishment of the registry mechanism and baseline data creates the framework for a powerful and important tool that, if utilized, provides the opportunity to conduct and support the kind of research necessary for a learning approach to health care.

Capacity

The NETT has been completed, and as previously noted, the results of the trial substantially altered clinical practice. The FDG-PET registry and the ICD registry, as well, are still ongoing. These are only two more examples of how needed clinical evidence could be gathered through the CED to ensure that the best available information about utilization, effectiveness, and adverse events is made available to clinicians and policy makers. It is easy to imagine that for these two decisions, it will not be difficult to find qualified researchers to analyze the data or journals interested in publishing the findings. However, these few CED decisions are just a model for what could theoretically become a far more common process in coverage, not only at CMS but more broadly. As the healthcare system moves toward increasing standardization of medical information and toward adoption of EHRs more extensively, better clinical detail should be readily available to satisfy CAD requirements, and longitudinal data should be readily accessible to address study questions. At that point, the current scientific infrastructure, the number of qualified researchers, and the appetite of peer-reviewed journals for such data analyses may constitute obstacles to a learning healthcare system. Aware of these potential system-level limitations, were CED to be implemented more broadly, CMS has cautiously applied the policy in settings where the infrastructure and science were in place or could quickly be put into place. Going forward, CMS will likely make relatively few CED determinations, judiciously choosing those areas of medical care in which routine data collection could enhance the data on which coverage determinations are made and improve the quality of clinical care.

USE OF LARGE SYSTEM DATABASES

Jed Weissberg, M.D.
Kaiser Permanente Medical Care Program

Integrated delivery systems and health maintenance organizations (HMOs) have a long history of epidemiologic and health services research utilizing linked, longitudinal databases (Graham et al. 2005; East et al. 1999; Friedman et al. 1971; Selby 1997; Platt et al. 2001; Vogt et al. 2004). Research networks currently supported by the government are examining healthcare interventions in diverse populations, representative of the U.S. citizenry. Hypothesis-driven research utilizing existing clinical and administrative databases in large healthcare systems is capable of answering a variety of questions not answered when drugs, devices, and techniques come to market. The following case study illustrates the value of collecting, linking, and utilizing data for pharmacovigilance purposes, outlines key elements necessary to encourage similar efforts, and hints at changes that might develop the potential to discover such insights as a natural outcome of care within a learning healthcare system.

A project using a nested, case-control design to look at the cardiovascular effects of the COX-2 inhibitor, rofecoxib, in a large HMO population within Kaiser Permanente (KP) (Graham et al. 2005) demonstrates the potential value of pharmacoepidemiological research and the opportunities offered with the advent of much greater penetration of full EHRs to rapidly increase knowledge about interventions and delivery system design. Much can be learned from this case study on what it will take to move to a learning system capable of utilizing data, so that valid conclusions, strong enough on which to base action, can be identified routinely. While the potential for such a system exists, many barriers including technical data issues, privacy concerns, analytic techniques, cost, and attention of managers and leaders will need to be overcome.

Nonsteroidal anti-inflammatory drugs (NSAIDs) are widely used to treat chronic pain, but this treatment is often accompanied by upper gastrointestinal toxicity leading to admission to the hospital for ulcer complications in around 1 percent of users annually (Graham et al. 2005). This is due to NSAID inhibition of both isoforms of COX: COX-1, which is associated with gastro protection as well as the COX-2 isoform, which is induced at sites of inflammation. The first COX-2 selective inhibitors, rofecoxib and celecoxib, were thus developed with the hope of improving gastric safety. In the five years from the approval and launch of rofecoxib to its withdrawal from the market, there were signs of possible cardiovascular risk associated with rofecoxib use.

Using Kaiser Permanente data, Graham et al. examined the potential adverse cardiovascular effects of "coxibs." The nested, case-control study design was enabled by the availability of a broad set of data on Kaiser Permanente members, as well as the ability to match data from impacted and non-impacted members. As a national integrated managed care organization providing comprehensive health care to more than 6.4 million residents in the State of California, Kaiser Permanente maintains computer files of eligibility for care, outpatient visits, admissions, medical procedures, emergency room visits, laboratory testing, outpatient drug prescriptions, and mortality status for all its members. While the availability of prescription and dispensing data as well as longitudinal patient data (demographics, lab, pathology, radiology, diagnosis, and procedures) was essential to conduct such a study, several other elements related to organizational culture precipitated and enabled action.

The organization and culture of KP created an environment that can be described as the "prepared mind" (Bull et al. 2002). The interest of clinicians and pharmacy managers in the efficacy, safety, and affordability of the entire class of COX-2 drugs had resulted in the relatively low market share of COX-2 drugs within KP NSAID use (4 percent vs. 35 percent in the community, Figure 1-1). This 4 percent of patients was selected based on a risk score developed in collaboration with researchers to identify appropriate patients for COX-2 therapy (Trontell 2004). Of additional importance to the investigation was the presence of a small, internally funded group within KP—the Pharmacy Outcomes Research Group (PORG)—with access to KP prescription information and training in epidemiology. These elements were brought together when a clinician expressed concern about the cardiovascular risk associated with COX-2 drugs and suggested that KP could learn more based on its own experiences. A small grant from the Food and Drug Administration (FDA), combined with the operating budget of the PORG, enabled the authors to design and execute a case-control study. The study concluded that rofecoxib usage at a dose greater than 25 mg per day increased the risk of acute myocardial infarction (AMI) and sudden cardiac death (SCD). Additional insights of the study pointed to the differences between other NSAIDs and the inability to assume cardiovascular safety for other COX-2 drugs. The conduct of this study contributed to the FDA's scrutiny of rofecoxib, which resulted in the manufacturer's decision to withdraw the drug from the marketplace. In addition, the initial release of the study abstract stimulated similar analyses that clarified the clinical risks associated with this drug class and illustrated the gap between

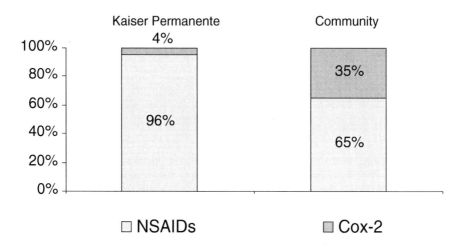

FIGURE 1-1 COX-2 market share within overall NSAID use: Kaiser Permanente and Community.

marketing promises and real-world outcomes. Similar observational studies conducted elsewhere, some including propensity scoring, have confirmed these results. In addition, a meta-analysis of related observational studies was also conducted and offers a promising method for strengthening the credibility of observational studies.

As we implement EHRs widely throughout the healthcare system, we will have unprecedented opportunities for data capture. Well-designed functionalities will allow generation of data, whether coded or though analysis of free text, as a by-product of the usual documentation of care. The benefits are obvious: detection of rare events or other insights that do not readily emerge from pre-marketing studies with small sample sizes, comparisons of practice to gain insights into what factors drive variation in outcomes, the creation of tools to track the dissemination of new technologies and health impacts, real-time feedback systems to improve healthcare system design, safety, and management, and the collection of data demonstrating compliance in process—which will provide the opportunity to demonstrate proof of the value of adherence to evidence-based guidelines. All these are critical elements as we move to a system of evidence-based medicine and management.

The accumulation and availability of data, however, is simply a start, and much work will need to be done to resolve methodological issues to ensure that the data are comprehensive and of high quality. For example, current managed care databases do not include over-the-counter medications and have incomplete information on potential confounders. The experience of Kaiser Permanente in establishing such databases indicates that the technical challenges are manifold. Within KP, epidemiologists and clinical researchers have indicated that missing data, particularly in registries, complicate analysis, and relevant data often are not collected. In KP's migration to a common EHR platform (Garrido et al. 2005) we discovered more than 12 different ways to code for gender, so standards will have to be set on even the most basic level to encourage the use of consistent data definitions. Clinicians will need to adhere to certain charting conventions in order to find relevant data, because many EHRs allow storage of the same coded or free text data elements in multiple locations. Various studies have documented that while EHR data can be richer than routine claims data, even EHR data can misclassify patients based on the gold standard of combining such data with careful, expert review of free text medical documentation (Persell et al. 2006).

Other ongoing challenges will be how to define cases and "normal ranges" for things such as viral load or different laboratory assay systems. Standardized nomenclature and messaging (e.g. SNOMED, LOINC, HL7) are vital. Additionally, unlike in clinical trials, the timing of data collection for registries and in clinical practice varies. Therefore, as we shift to collection of data as part of patient care, nonstandard time points will be a variation that will increasingly compound the issue of missing data. Quality-of-life and functional surveys are essential to evaluating outcomes of care. Routine administration via multiple modalities, storage, and association with clinical events will require standardized input from patients that still poses a challenge for current EHRs.

Finally, it will be necessary to ensure that the data are captured and routinely available in a timely fashion. In this respect, HIPAA is an issue as well as proprietary data relating to maintaining business advantage. For example, at KP, our use of various pharmaceuticals and our ability to move market share are critical in maintaining affordability for our membership. These are not data that we share lightly. We also use registry data from our total joint implant experience to drive purchasing decisions from implant vendors. Timeliness is another concern. Even something as basic as identifying when a patient dies is not straightforward. Via Social Security and Medicare death tapes, with reasonable accuracy we can determine deaths within four months of occurrence for our Medicare beneficiaries. However, death of commercial members may not appear in state death files reliably for several years.

While standardization will make data amenable to comprehensive data analysis, an even greater challenge will be to create a learning system in which meaningful insights emerge organically. Currently, data mining is the source of hundreds of associations, but analysis is most efficiently done when a particular hypothesis is pursued. Non-hypothesis-driven analysis will likely yield far more false positive associations than true positives, and each association might require further study. While improved methods or search capacity may partially alleviate this problem, there will need to be thought regarding how to prioritize which findings merit further study. Moreover, these analyses will take time, interest, and money; so as we think about expanding our capacity to conduct such research, we also need to ensure that we develop the funding resources and expertise necessary to pursue these associations. While federal, pharmaceutical, and health provider funding exists for such studies, it is often driven by regulatory requirements, business needs, or the specific interests of researchers and will not be adequate for exploratory approaches to data mining.

Reaping the benefits of large, linked systems of EHRs will require more work on interoperability, data definitions, and statistical techniques. Making health information technology (HIT) truly interoperable will require testing, utilization of standardized nomenclatures, and vendor cooperation. Users of EHRs will have to learn to document consistently in order to best aggregate data among sites of care. Also, we probably will have to develop more robust natural language processing algorithms in order to glean important medical information from noncoded sections of the EHR. However, as this case study reveals, data are only the means to an end. Data collection must be embedded within a healthcare system, like Kaiser's, that can serve as a prepared mind—an environment in which managers and clinicians are trained to discern patterns of interest and work within a system with the inclination, resources, and capacity to act upon such findings (Garrido et al. 2005). We already have the opportunity to build upon the many analyses being done for the varied purposes of quality improvement (QI), quality assurance (QA), utilization studies, patient safety, and formal research; however, only prepared minds can see patterns and data of interest beyond their own inquiries, and only a system that understands and values data will act on it for the betterment of patient care.

QUASI-EXPERIMENTAL DESIGNS FOR POLICY ASSESSMENT

Stephen Soumerai, Sc.D.
Harvard Medical School and Harvard Pilgrim Health Care

Although randomized controlled trials produce the most valid estimates of the outcomes of health services, strong quasi-experimental designs (e.g., interrupted time series) are rigorous and feasible alternative methods, especially for evaluating sudden changes in health policies occurring in large populations (Cook and Campbell 1979). These methods are currently underutilized but have the potential to inform and impact policy decision making (Wagner et al. 2002). These case examples illustrate the application of such designs to the quality and outcomes of care and demonstrate how these studies influence state and national health policies, including the Medicare drug benefit. These case studies will focus on evaluation of the unintended impacts of statewide pharmaceutical cost containment policies, and how quasi-experimental design can contribute to the understanding and modification of health policy. Since randomization of health policies is almost never feasible (Newhouse et al. 1981), quasi-experimental designs represent the strongest methods for evaluating policy effects.

We often speak of randomized controlled trials as the gold standard in research design to generate evidence and of other trial designs as alternatives to RCTs. These many alternative designs, however, should not be grouped together as "observational studies" because they provide vastly different ranges of validity of study conclusions. For example, we have previously reported that the weakest nonexperimental designs, such as uncontrolled pre-post designs or post-only cross-sectional designs frequently produce biased estimates of policy impacts (Soumerai et al. 1993; Soumerai 2004). However, there are several strong quasi-experimental designs that have been effectively used to evaluate health policies and thereby affect policy decision making. These methods have been used to analyze health services, but here, we will focus on the evaluation of health policy (Park 2005). Two strong quasi-experimental designs are the *pre-post with non-equivalent control group design* that observes outcomes before and after an intervention in a study and comparison group and the *interrupted time series design* with and without comparison series. Such designs, when carefully implemented, have the potential to control for many threats to validity, such as secular trends. Although these designs have been used for many decades, they are not often applied, in part because they are not emphasized in medical and social science training. Because these are natural experiments that use existing data and can be conducted in less time and expense than many RCTs, they have great potential for contributing to the evidence base. The following case studies will focus on the use of one of the strongest quasi-experimental designs, the interrupted time series design.

Health policy interventions can be analyzed using interrupted time series using segmented, linear regression. The interrupted time series (ITS) method assumes that the counterfactual experience of patients—or the trend had the policy not been implemented—is reflected by the extrapolation of the pre-policy trend. Changes in level of slope after the intervention as well as the immediate magnitude of change following implementation can give information on the effect of the intervention measured as a discontinuity in the time-series as compared with the counterfactual or extrapolation of the baseline trend (Figure 1-2). Because of the use of a baseline trend, one can actually control for a number of threats to validity such as

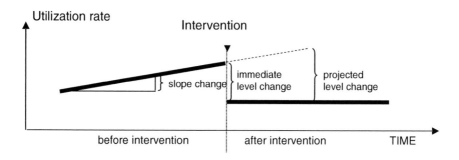

FIGURE 1-2 Hypothetical changes in level and slope of a time–series. Assumption: the (counterfactual) experience of patients, had the policy not been implemented, is correctly reflected by the extrapolation of the pre-policy trend.

history (e.g., ongoing changes in medical knowledge and practice), maturation (e.g., aging of the study population), and changing composition of the study population.

A good illustration of this, using real-world data, was a study that looked at the effects of a Medicaid drug coverage limit (cap) in New Hampshire on use of essential and nonessential drugs (Soumerai et al. 1987) (see Figure 1-3). After implementation of the cap, prescriptions filled by chronically ill Medicaid patients in New Hampshire dropped sharply and affected both essential (e.g., cardiac and antidiabetic) and nonessential drugs. The time series clearly shows a 46 percent sudden reduction in the level of medication use from the pre-intervention trend, and an immediate increase in both level and trend when the policy was suspended, adding to the internal validity of the findings (off-on-off design). A similar approach was used to look at the effects of this drug cap on nursing home admissions. Segmented survival analysis shows that this policy increased nursing home admissions among chronically ill elderly (Soumerai et al. 1991). Taken together, these data indicate the intended and unintended consequences of this policy. Similar work has been done on schizophrenia, in which the limitations on drug coverage affected the use of psychotropic agents and substantially increased utilization of acute mental health services intended to treat psychotic episodes among patients with schizophrenia (Soumerai et al. 1994). The Medicaid costs of such increased treatment exceeded the drug savings from the cap by a factor of 17 to 1. Similar time series data again show the remarkable and unintended consequences of this policy.

These types of studies can clearly provide good evidence for the effectiveness of health policies but they also have a significant effect on policy. While this is somewhat unusual for most academic research, the impact of

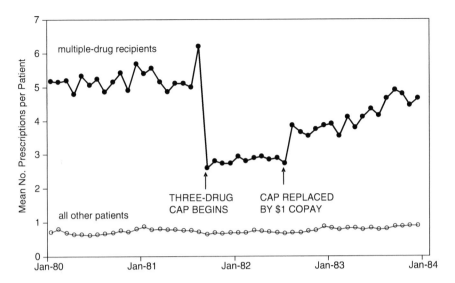

FIGURE 1-3 Time series of constant-size Rxs per continuously eligible patient per month among multiple drug recipients ($N = 860$) and other outpatients ($N = 8,002$).
SOURCE: Soumerai et al. *New England Journal of Medicine* 1987; 317:550-556.
Copyright 1987 Massachusetts Medical Society.

this study has in part supported the decision of six states and several countries in changing their health policy, was instrumental in developing reports from public advocacy groups such as the National Alliance on the Mentally Ill (NAMI) and the AARP to make the case for adequate drug benefits, and contributed to more rational state policy decisions. Recently, these data were used by CMS as evidence to support subsidies for up to 5 million poor or near-poor Medicare beneficiaries to achieve greater economic access to medications in the Medicare drug benefit (Tunis 2005). The policy impact of these studies was due, in part, to their very visible effects and because they produced usable and understandable information for policy makers. A key need however will be a system that values and actively seeks out such information. These data had significant impact but required the efforts of individuals who were trained to recognize the value of such data and able to reach out and find results that were relevant to their decision making (Soumerai et al. 1997). Based on the data reported in these two natural experiments (Soumerai et al. 1991; Soumerai et al. 1994), if the findings were applied to all 18 states with drug benefit caps today, it might be possible to reduce hundreds or thousands of nursing home admissions and psychotic episodes, while reducing net government health expenditures.

These types of quasi-experimental studies can answer a range of questions in the field of health services research and pharmacoepidemiology, and the use of interrupted time series designs is increasing (Smalley 1995; Tamblyn et al. 2001; Ray et al. 2003). One example is a study done by Tamblyn et al., in which interrupted time series analysis looked at the effect of changes in cost sharing on the elderly and welfare populations in Quebec in terms of the use of essential and nonessential drugs, rate of emergency department visits, and serious adverse events associated with reductions in drug use before and after policy implementation. The study, which has significant application to the Medicare drug benefit in the United States, showed that increased cost sharing led to a reduction in use of essential drugs, particularly among the adult welfare population. This was associated with higher rates of serious adverse events and emergency department (ED) visits. The findings of this study, combined with public advocacy pressure, caused the policy of increased cost sharing to be rescinded, with major impacts on illness and potential mortality. A similar study (Roblin et al. 2005) was used to determine the effects of increased cost sharing on oral hypoglycemic use and found that within 5 HMOs, an increase of ≥$10 in cost sharing for the intervention resulted in an immediate and persistent decline in oral hypoglycemic use, which was not observed with smaller incremental increases (see Figure 1-4).

As a final example of the potential utility of this approach, an interrupted time series (Ross-Degnan et al. 2004; Pearson 2006) examined the effect of a triplicate prescription policy on the likelihood of benzodiazepine use in Medicaid patients. To set the background, there are several clinical issues regarding the utilization of benzodiazapines, which are commonly used as hypnotics, anxiolytics, and muscle relaxants, but are also used for seizure and bipolar disorders (APA 1998; Bazil and Pedley 1998; Henriksen 1998). In elderly populations, they are considered to confer an increased risk for fall—given the side effects—and are controlled substances under schedule IV of the Drug Enforcement Administration (DEA) conferring an additional risk of dependence. Thus policies have been enacted to attempt to reduce inappropriate prescribing of this drug class. The study demonstrated that, upon initiation of a triplicate prescription policy for benzodiazapines, there was an abrupt reduction in the prescribing of the entire class of drug, with equal effects on likely appropriate (e.g., short-term, low-dose) and inappropriate use. Examination of the effect of this policy by race showed that despite the observation that black populations were about half as likely to use benzodiazapines to begin with, the triplicate prescription policy disproportionately affected blacks, with an approximately 50 percent greater likelihood of prescription stoppage due to the policy (Pearson 2006) (see Figure 1-5). Thus, while there may be a high rate of inappropriate use of this class of medication overall, the policy caused

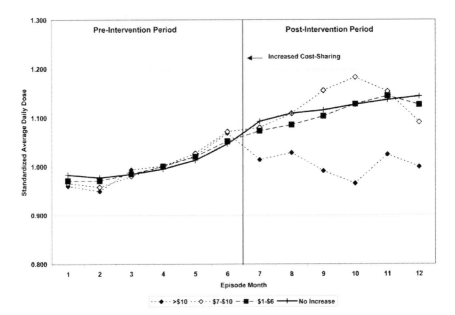

FIGURE 1-4 Trends in oral hypoglycemic use stratified by level of increased cost-sharing ($1-$6, $7-$10, and >$10). SOURCE: Roblin et al. *Medical Care* 2005; 43: 951-959 (www.lww.com).

an unintended decrease in appropriate use of benzodiazepines in a way that disproportionally affects black populations. This leads to a different sort of question: Is it ever appropriate to halt the use of an entire class of drug? Even if 50 percent of the use of that class is inappropriate, the other 50 percent may be very important for the health and well-being of those patients. To further confound the issue, our study published in the January 2007 issue of the *Annals of Internal Medicine* shows that the above reduction in benzodiazepine use among elderly Medicaid or Medicare patients did not result in any change in rates of hip fracture, which casts doubt on the conventional wisdom derived from 20 years of epidemiological research (Wagner et al. 2007 [in press]).

In summary, quasi-experimental design has many benefits and can clearly delineate effects of policy on health outcomes and healthcare utilization. Interrupted time series designs address many threats to validity. As natural experiments, these studies are cheaper and faster than RCTs, can use existing data, and are useful when RCTs are not feasible (e.g., most policies cannot be randomized). Because analysis often produces very visible

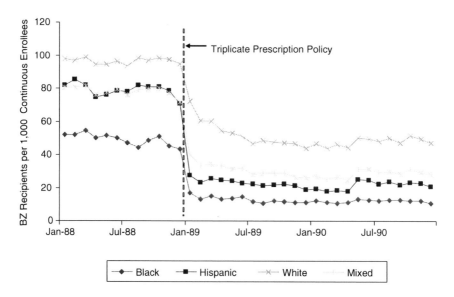

FIGURE 1-5 Reductions in benzodiazepine use after triplicate prescription policy among patients living in neighborhoods with different racial compositions.
SOURCE: Pearson et al. *Archives of Internal Medicine* 2006; 166:572-579. Copyright 2006, American Medical Association. All rights reserved.

effects (especially if interventions are applied suddenly) and these visible effects are often significant, this type of research conveys an intuitive understanding of the effects of policy decisions and has had a significant impact on changing and influencing health policy decisions. The use of comparison series increases validity and can be used to look at high-risk subgroups and unintended outcomes. In addition, these studies can also illuminate the mechanism of these effects, for example, by observing simultaneous changes in processes (e.g., adherence) and health outcomes (e.g., hospital admission). Currently much of this research is conducted at the Centers for Education and Research in Therapeutics and is funded primarily by AHRQ. More quasi-experimental studies of natural experiments are needed, especially on the effects of numerous changes in coverage, cost sharing, and utilization in the Medicare drug benefit. This will require more extensive training of clinical and social scientists, journal editors, and federal study sections to recognize the potential strengths of quasi-experimental design in health policy evaluation. In light of the substantial impact that health policies can have on the population's health, there is a need to redress the relative scarcity of scientific data on the outcomes of policy interventions.

PRACTICAL CLINICAL TRIALS

Sean Tunis, M.D., M.Sc.
Health Technology Center

Developing useful and valid evidence for decision making requires several steps, all of which must be successfully completed with full engagement of the key decision makers—patients, clinicians, and payers. These include (1) identifying the right questions to ask, (2) selecting the most important questions for study, (3) choosing study designs that are adequate to answer the questions, (4) creating or partnering with organizations that are equipped to implement the studies, and (5) finding sufficient resources to pay for the studies. This paper discusses specific case studies that highlight progress and challenges related to each of these steps from the perspective of those decision makers who are trying to decide whether particular healthcare services are worth paying for. The primary focus is on identifying relevant questions, real-world (practical, pragmatic) study designs and funding, which are listed in their logical order, as well as in the order of increasing challenge. Considerable work is needed to develop more efficient and affordable methods for generating reliable data on the comparative effectiveness of healthcare services. While observational methods may have value for selected questions, increasing attention is necessary to developing strategies to design and implement faster, larger, and more efficient prospective intervention studies. Serious attention, along with some creative thinking, will also be required to ensure that adequate and sustainable real-time funding is available to support what might be called "decision-based evidence making."

Clinical trials can be thought of as falling into two broad categories: explanatory trials and pragmatic (or practical) trials. Explanatory trials focus on the mechanism of disease and whether things can work under optimal circumstances. Pragmatic or practical clinical trials are designed to inform choices between feasible alternatives or two different treatment options by estimating real-world outcome probabilities for each (Schwartz and Lellouch 1967; Tunis et al. 2003). That is, PCTs are purposefully designed to answer the specific policy or clinical questions of those who make policy and clinical decisions. Key features of a practical trial include meaningful comparison groups (i.e., generally not placebo, but rather comparisons to other reasonable alternatives), broad patient inclusion criteria, such that the patient population offers the maximum opportunity for generalizability of study results; multiple outcome measures including functional status, resource utilization, etc., conducted in real world setting (where research is not the primary organizational purpose), and minimal interventions to ensure patient and clinician compliance with the interventions being studied.

The underlying notion of PCTs is to design studies in ways that maximize the chances that the results will be translatable and implementable. The usual concept of translation is to design studies without careful consideration of the needs of decision makers, and then use various communication techniques to encourage adoption of the results. However, the major barrier to translation may be how the research question was framed, which patients were enrolled, et cetera. PCTs make a serious effort to anticipate potential translation problems and address those through the design of the study.

One key consideration in designing a study is to determine at the onset whether a non-experimental design would be adequate to persuade decision makers to change their decision. For example, most technology assessment organizations exclude nonrandomized studies from systematic reviews because they know that payers will not consider such studies in their coverage decisions. Given that, one would need to think carefully about the value of conducting observational studies if those studies are intended to influence coverage decisions. There are certain questions of real-world significance that cannot be answered through the collection of data generated in the routine provision of care, whether administrative data or data extracted from EHRs. In those circumstances, creative methods will need to be developed for conducting prospective real-world comparative effectiveness studies.

Over the past several years, a working group of methodologists—the Pragmatic Randomized Controlled Trials in Healthcare, or PRaCTIHC, workgroup—has been working to identify a set of domains upon which trials can be rated according to the degree to which they are pragmatic or explanatory. These domains include study eligibility criteria, flexibility of the intervention, practitioner expertise, follow-up intensity, follow-up duration, participant compliance, practitioner adherence to protocol and intervention, and primary analysis scope and specification. For each domain, there are definitions that indicate whether a study is highly explanatory, highly pragmatic, or somewhere in between. For example, on the patient eligibility domain, a maximally pragmatic approach would enroll "all comers" who might benefit from the intervention regardless of prior information about their risk, responsiveness to the intervention, or past compliance. The maximally explanatory trial would enroll only individuals or clusters thought, on the basis of prior information, to be at high risk, highly responsive to the intervention, *and* who have demonstrated high compliance in a pre-trial test. Similarly, the highly pragmatic and highly explanatory descriptors for the expertise of practitioners taking care of the patients are as follows: A maximally pragmatic approach would involve care applied by *usual practitioners* (regardless of expertise), with only their *usual monitoring* for dose setting and side effects (and *no* external monitoring). The explanatory approach would involve care applied by *expert practitioners who monitor patients more closely than usual* for optimal dose setting and the early detection of side effects. These domains can be represented pictorially on numbered scales, creating a two-dimensional image that provides information about the degree to which the trial is pragmatic or explanatory, and on what specific domains. These maps then convey the nature of a trial and give a sense to clinical or health policy makers on how best to consider that trial in informing their decisions. For example, mapping a highly pragmatic trial such as the Directly Observed Therapy for TB study, gives a very different map than that of the highly explanatory North American Symptomatic Carotid Endarterectomy Trial. Such a visual representation could be very useful for decision makers in evaluating evidence by providing a common framework in which to understand strengths and weaknesses of evidence. The instrument is currently being piloted and refined by a Cochrane workgroup and various other Evidence-Based Medicine (EBM) experts, with the goal of developing a valid and reliable instrument for scoring the studies included in systematic reviews.

The Medicare program has attempted to build interest in pragmatic clinical trials by highlighting the value of such trials in making national coverage decisions. Once such example is the pragmatic trial of FDG-PET for suspected dementia—which Medicare called for in the context of an NCD in 2004. The original noncoverage decision for use of FDG-PET in the context of suspected dementia was issued in April 2003. The decision was based in part on a decision analysis conducted for and reviewed by the Medicare Coverage Advisory Committee. It was concluded that, even though FDG-PET had greater sensitivity and specificity than expert evaluation by a neurologist, the scan provided no measurable benefit because existing treatments are very safe and of limited benefit. The improved accuracy of the diagnosis therefore offered no clinical benefit to the patient undergoing the study. Because this was a controversial decision, CMS agreed to continue to review the technology with the assistance of an expert panel convened by NIH. CMS also committed to conducting some type of demonstration project of FDG-PET for suspected dementia. The NIH panel analysis concluded that FDG-PET was a promising diagnostic tool but recommended that additional evidence be developed before broad adoption of the technology. In September 2004, a revised NCD was issued providing limited coverage of FDG-PET for suspected dementia when the differential diagnosis included frontotemporal dementia (FTD) and Alzheimer's disease (AD). The NCD also allowed for broad coverage of FDG-PET in the context of a large community-based practical clinical trial designed to evaluate the clinical utility of this test.

Since this NCD was issued in September 2004, a group at the University of California-Los Angeles (UCLA) has designed such a PCT. The proposed study would enroll 710 patients with diminished cognitive function at nine academic centers that specialize in the evaluation and management of AD. Every patient enrolled in the study would undergo an FDG-PET scan, but would be randomized as to whether the results of the scan are made available at the time of the scan or whether they are sealed and available only at the end of the two-year trial. The outcomes to be measured include initial or working diagnosis, initial management plan, measures of cognitive decline, utilization of other imaging studies, functional status, and percentage of patients admitted to nursing homes within two years. CMS has reviewed this study, approved the trial design, and agreed to cover the costs of PET scans for all patients enrolled in the study. However, as of late 2006, funding had not been approved for the research costs of this study. Efforts are still under way to secure this funding, but more than two years have passed since the coverage decision was issued. Some of the questions that the case study poses are the following:

Is it a good idea or is it necessary to do a pragmatic trial of PET for AD? Such a trial would require substantial resources to organize and implement, and it would be necessary to ensure that the value of the information would be sufficient to justify the effort and expense. Some experts have proposed an approach called "value of information analysis," and this type of careful consideration would be essential to ensuring that the proposed question was worth answering, that the optimal method would be a PCT, and that this topic would be a high priority in the context of the range of questions that might be addressed.

Is it necessary to conduct a study prior to adoption widely into practice; are there alternative methodologies to the method developed; could this be better evaluated through a quasi-experimental study design? Would observational methods possibly provide sufficiently reliable information? For the most part, such questions have not been addressed prior to the design and funding of clinical research, probably because decision makers have not taken a prominent role in the selection and design of clinical research studies.

Then, for whatever study is proposed and necessary, how is it going to happen? Who will design, fund, and implement the study? While Medicare now has coverage in place for the use of FDG-PET in cases of suspected dementia and at least two reasonable trial protocols have been developed, funding of the studies has not yet been secured, and there is still currently no access for Medicare patients to PET scanning for AD. Conversations are now under way to discuss how best to expand the infrastructure to support comparative effectiveness research, including PCTs such as the one envisioned by Medicare.

Where and how would it best be implemented? How could you actually connect the efforts of the UCLA group with test beds such as AHRQ's Developing Evidence to Inform Decisions about Effectiveness (DEcIDE) network, the HMO research network, practice-based research networks, the American College of Radiology Imaging Network, et cetera? With adequate funding, existing research networks could be engaged to conduct these studies, and new networks would likely be established as demand increases.

Although there are groups willing to design and implement PCTs, an important limitation faced by these groups is the lack of current organizational capacity to focus on their design and implementation. One effort underway to address this need is a project recently initiated at Center for Medical Technology Policy (CMTP). CMTP is based in San Francisco and funded by California Health Care Foundation and Blue Shield of California Foundation. It provides a neutral forum for decision makers—payers, purchasers, patients, and clinicians—to take leadership in creating evidence about comparative clinical effectiveness, with an emphasis on those questions for which prospective, experimental studies may be required. The CMTP will focus on identifying critical knowledge gaps and priority setting of studies from the perspective of decision makers; study design from a pragmatic perspective (i.e., focused on information important to decision makers); and implementation that is rapid, affordable, and still provides reliable evidence for decision making. The work of CMTP is intended to be complementary to the work of the Institute of Medicine (IOM) Roundtable on Evidence-Based Medicine, since its focus is to develop pilot projects around evidence gaps and on promising technologies of high demand or with a major health impact. Some examples include CT angiography, molecular diagnostic tests, intensity-modulated radiation therapy (IMRT), tele-ICU (intensive care unit), and bariatric surgery (minimally invasive). Each of these examples is a technology that is promising, important, and unlikely to be evaluated through the current structure and funding mechanism of the current clinical research enterprises.

COMPUTERIZED PROTOCOLS TO ASSIST CLINICAL RESEARCH

Alan H. Morris, M.D.
Latter Day Saints Hospital and University of Utah

Adequately explicit methods and computerized protocols could allow researchers to efficiently conduct large-scale complex clinical studies and enable translation of research methods into clinical practice. Additionally, they could formalize experiential learning and provide an innovative means of enhancing education for clinicians and clinical researchers. These tools should be embraced by the nation's clinical research infrastructure.

Clinicians and clinical investigators do not have tools that enable uniform decision making. As a result, currently conducted clinical trials, especially non-blinded trials, do not use replicable experimental and clinical care methods. This may explain why many critical care clinical trials have failed to produce evidence of clinical benefit, in spite of large investments of resources (Marshall 2000). The disappointingly low quality of critical care clinical trials (Cronin et al. 1995; Lefering and Neugebauer 1995; Cook et al. 1996) could, in part, be due to the widespread use of suboptimal methods. Meta-analyses cannot overcome this low clinical trial quality since meta-analyses can generate credible conclusions only if the analyzed clinical trial data are credible and representative (Morris and Cook 1998; LeLorier et al. 1997). Meta-analyses focus on methodology at the trial design scale (e.g., were true randomization and effective blinding employed?) but do not deal with the methodologic details of the patient-clinician encounter for either outpatient (Johnson 2004) or critical care (Cronin et al. 1995; Lefering and Neugebauer 1995; Cook et al. 1996) clinical trials. The medical community is thus challenged to develop replicable clinical trial methods and to use them to produce more rigorous clinical experiments and results.

Similar challenges exist in the translation of findings to practice. Two major problem areas impede effective healthcare responses and healthcare learning: information overload and absence of effective tools to aid decision-makers at the point and time of decision. Human decision-makers are limited by short-term memory constraints, making them able to deal effectively with only about four individual constructs when making a decision (Morris 2006). This contrasts, strikingly, with the hundreds of patient variables, thousands of constructs, and tens to hundreds of thousands of published documents faced by clinical decision-makers. The recent introduction of genomics and proteomics into medicine has only compounded the problem and will likely increase the information overload by orders of magnitude. Nevertheless, we still depend on a four-year medical school model for learning, influenced by the early twentieth century Flexner Report. Even with current extended postgraduate medical training, we need a new approach to learning in medicine.

Clinician Performance and Clinical Trial Reproducibility

These issues are highlighted by the unnecessary variation in clinical practice that was brought to the healthcare community's attention in the 1970s (Wennberg and Gittelsohn 1973) and appears to be an unavoidable feature of modern medicine (Senn 2004; Lake 2004; Wennberg and Gittelsohn 1973; Wennberg 2002; Morris 2004). The argument that variability is desirable because of individual patient needs incorporates two assumptions. First is the assumption that clinicians can consistently tailor treatment to a patient's specific needs, particularly when reliable evidence for preferable therapies is absent. However, clinicians cannot easily predict who will respond to a specific intervention (Senn 2004; Lake 2004) and frequently fail to deal correctly with the individualized needs of patients and thereby cause harm (Silverman 1993; IOM 2001; Horwitz et al. 1996; Redelmeier et al. 2001; Berwick 2003; Runciman et al. 2003; Barach and Berwick 2003; Sox 2003; Senn 2004; Lake 2004; Corke et al. 2005; Berwick 2005; Redelmeier 2005; Warren and Mosteller 1993; IOM 1999). In general, variability is fostered by incorrect perceptions (Morris 2006; Arkes and Hammond 1986; Arkes 1986; Morris 1998, 2000a) and is associated with unwanted and widespread error (IOM 1999; IOM 2001; Runciman et al. 2003; Leape et al. 2002; Kozer et al. 2004; Schiff et al. 2003; Lamb et al. 2003; Zhang et al. 2002). For many, if not most medical interventions, the medical community and the community of patients can only draw conclusions about the balance between potential good and harm through examination of the results of systematic investigations. Second is the assumption that nonuniformity is itself desirable because it fosters insight and innovation. However, many questions addressed in modern medicine frequently involve small improvements (odds ratios of 3 or less) that will escape the attention of most observers if not examined within systematic studies (Hulley and Cummings 1988). The mismatch between human decision-making ability (Redelmeier et al. 2001; Redelmeier 2005; Kahneman et al. 1982) and the excess information clinicians routinely encounter probably contributes to both the variability of performance and the high error rate of clinical decisions (Tversky and Kahneman 1982; Jennings et al. 1982; McDonald 1976; Abramson et al. 1980; Morris et al. 1984; Morris 1985; Morris et al. 1985; Iberti et al. 1990; Iberti et al. 1994; Leape 1994; Gnaegi et al. 1997; Wu et al. 1991). The clinical process improvement movement has successfully adopted a standardization approach (Berwick 2003; James and Hammond 2000; Berwick 1994; Horn and Hopkins 1994; James et al. 1994). Without standardization, our chances of detecting promising elements of clinical management are reduced and frequently low.

It is not enough that the medical community develops standards—clinicians must also follow standards. There is a chasm between perception and practice as well as between healthcare delivery goals and their achievement (IOM 2001). These lead to error and reduce the quality of medical care (IOM 1999). This, in part, has led to the NIH Roadmap call for strategies and tools for translation of research results into clinical practice. This effort should involve a serious engagement with clinical trials. Even with compelling clinical trial results, compliance of physicians with evidence-based treatments or guidelines is low across a broad range of healthcare topics (Evans et al. 1998; Nelson et al. 1998; Schacker et al. 1996; Kiernan et al. 1998; Galuska et al. 1999; Dickerson et al. 1999) and persists even when guidelines based on reputable evidence are available (Akhtar et al. 2003; Rubenfeld et al. 2004; Safran et al. 1996; Redman 1996). Many factors, including cultural issues and health beliefs, influence compliance (Cochrane 1998; Jones 1998). Widespread distribution of evidence-based guidelines (Schultz 1996; Lomas et al. 1989; Greco and Eisenberg 1993) and education programs (Singer et al. 1998; Pritchard et al. 1998; Teno et al. 1997a; Teno et al. 1997b; Lo 1995) have had only limited impact on this low compliance. However, both paper-based and computerized decision support tools that provide explicit, point-of-care (point-of-decision making) instructions to clinicians have overcome many of these problems and have achieved clinician compliance rates of 90-95 percent (Morris 2000a; East et al. 1999; Acute Respiratory Distress Syndrome Network 2000a, 2006b). There is no threshold beyond which protocols are adequately explicit. Our current operational definition of adequate clinician compliance is: clinicians adequately comply when they accept and carry out at least 90 percent of protocol instructions (Morris 2006, 1998, 2003).

Adequately Explicit Methods

Replication of an experimental result requires a detailed experimental method. This is a challenge for clinical trials for two reasons. First, editorial policies severely restrict methodologic detail in publications. Second and more important, most clinical trials are not conducted with adequately explicit methods. For example, high-frequency ventilation studies in neonates (Courtney et al. 2002; Johnson et al. 2002) were described (Stark 2002) as "rigorously controlled conditions with well-defined protocols" (Courtney et al. 2002) with a method that includes "aggressive weaning if blood gases . . . remained . . . in range." This method statement will not lead different clinicians to the same interpretations and actions. Thus the method is not adequately explicit. Adequately explicit methods include detailed and specific rules such as "if (last PaO_2 – current PaO_2) < 10, and (current PaO_2 time – last PaO_2 time) < 2 hours and > 10 minutes, and FIO_2 > 0.8, and PEEP > 15 cm H_2O), then decrease PEEP by 1 cm H_2O." A rule such as this can lead multiple clinicians to the same decision.

Explicitness

The explicitness of protocols varies continuously. An adequately explicit protocol has detail adequate to generate specific instructions (patient-specific orders). An adequately explicit protocol can elicit the same decision from different clinicians when faced with the same clinical information. Inadequately explicit protocols omit important details (Armstrong et al. 1991; Don 1985; Karlinsky et al. 1991) and elicit different clinical decisions from different clinicians because clinical decision-makers must fill in gaps in the logic of inadequately explicit protocols or guidelines. Judgment, background, and experience vary among clinicians and so will their choices of the rules and variables they use to fill in the gaps of inadequately explicit guidelines and protocols. In addition, because humans are inconsistent, any single clinician may produce different choices at different times, even though faced with the same patient data (Morris 2006; Morris 1998; Morris 2003).

Computerized adequately explicit protocols can contain the greatest detail (East et al. 1992) and may lead to the upper limit of achievable uniformity of clinician decision making with open-loop control (East et al. 1999; Henderson et al. 1992; Morris et al. 1994; Morris 2000b) (closed-loop controllers automate processes and automatically implement decisions; (Sheppard et al. 1968; Blesser 1969; Sheppard 1980; Sheppard et al. 1974). Paper-based versions can also contain enough detail to be adequately explicit (Acute Respiratory Distress Syndrome Network 2000a, 2000b). Adequately explicit protocols, unlike general guidelines, can serve as physician orders and can function as dynamic standing orders since they can respond to changes in patient state. In continuous quality improvement terms, an adequately explicit method is part of the "stabilization of process" necessary to improve quality (Deming 1986; Shewart 1931; Walton 1986; Deming 1982).

Performance

In manuscripts currently being prepared, computerized protocol decision support provides exportable and replicable adequately explicit methods for clinical investigation and clinical care. These computerized protocols enable replicable clinician decisions in single or multiple clinical sites. They thus enable a rigorous scientific laboratory at the holistic clinical investigation scale. We have, during the past two decades (Morris 2006; East et al. 1999; East et al. 1992; Henderson et al. 1992; Morris et al. 1994; Morris 2000b), used computerized protocols for more than 1 million hours in thousands of patients in multiple hospitals with support from NIH (Extracorporeal CO_2 Removal in ARDS, Acute Respiratory Distress Syndrome Network, Reengineering Clinical Research in Critical Care) and AHRQ (Computerized Protocols for Mechanical Ventilation in ARDS).

Our current work with a computerized protocol to control blood glucose with intravenous (IV) insulin (eProtocol-insulin) provides a case study. We compared three 80-110 mg/dL blood glucose target decision support strategies with different detail and process control: (1) a simple guideline (without a bedside tool), (2) a bedside paper-based protocol, and (3) a bedside computerized protocol (eProtocol-insulin). The distributions of blood glucose were significantly different ($P < .001$) as were the mean blood glucose values and fractions of measurements within the 80-110 mg/dL target range. Thereafter, eProtocol-insulin was introduced and used at these multiple clinical sites, located in different cultures, after which the blood glucose distributions became almost superimposable. We conclude that eProtocol-insulin provides a replicable and exportable experimental method in different cultures (southeastern and western United States, Asian). eProtocol-insulin has also been used, with similar results, in pediatric ICUs, leading to the conclusion that a common set of rules can operate successfully in both pediatric and adult medicine.

The rules and knowledge base of eProtocol-insulin were embedded in a clinical care electronic medical record in Intermountain Health Care, Inc. Multiple ICUs in different hospitals used eProtocol-insulin for blood glucose management in the usual clinical care of thousands of patients. Instructions for patient-tailored treatment with insulin were generated for more than 100,000 blood glucose measurements with high clinician bedside acceptance (>90 percent of the instructions) and adequate safety. This is a direct approach with computerized decision support tools (eProtocol-insulin) to rapidly translate research results (eProtocol-insulin developed for clinical investigation) into usual clinical practice.

In addition, in studies of computerized protocols for mechanical ventilation of patients with lung failure, the performance of the computerized protocols exceeds that of clinicians who adopt the same goals and meta-rules as those in the computerized protocol. This suggests that computerized adequately explicit protocols can function as enabling tools that lead clinician decision-makers to more consistently produce the clinical decisions they desire.

Adequately Explicit Methods and Scientific Experimental Requirements

Guidelines and protocols can reduce variation and increase compliance with evidence-based interventions, can effectively support clinical decision making (Grimshaw and Russell 1993), and can influence favorably both clinician performance and patient outcome (Safran et al. 1996; East et al. 1999; Grimm et al. 1975; Wirtschafter et al. 1981; Johnston et al. 1994; Mullett et al. 2001). They likely reduce error (Morris 2002), but this has not been formally studied. Simple protocols, such as physician reminders for a serum potassium measurement when a diuretic is ordered, are commonly employed (Hoch et al. 2003) and have an intuitive appeal to clinicians. More complex protocols have the same potential to aid clinicians and reduce error, but they are more difficult to comprehend. Decision support tools such as guidelines and protocols (Miller and Goodman 1998) are intended to standardize some aspect of clinical care and thereby help lead to uniform implementation of clinical interventions (IOM 1990; Tierney et al. 1995; Fridsma et al. 1996; Ely et al. 2001; MacIntyre 2001). However, many guidelines and protocols lack specific instructions and are useful only in a conceptual sense (Tierney et al. 1995; Fridsma 1996; Audet, Greenfield, and Field 1990; Fletcher and Fletcher 1990; Hadorn et al. 1992; Miller and Frawly 1995; Tierney et al. 1996). They neither standardize clinical decisions nor lead to uniform implementation of clinical interventions. Guidelines are general statements with little instruction for making specific decisions (Guidelines Committee Society of Critical Care Medicine 1992). In contrast, protocols are more detailed and can provide specific instructions. Unfortunately, even systematic and scholarly collections of flow diagrams commonly lack the detail necessary to standardize clinical decisions (Armstrong et al. 1991; Don 1985; Karlinsky et al. 1991). The distinction between guidelines and protocols, particularly adequately explicit protocols, is crucial (Morris 1998, 2000a; Holcomb et al. 2001). Most clinical investigators do not seem to recognize the difference between common ordinary protocols and guidelines and the uncommon adequately explicit methods that satisfy the scientific requirement of replicability (Morris 1998, 2000a; Hulley and Cummings 1988; Morris 2003; Pocock 1983; Atkins 1958).

Replicability of experimental results (confirmation of an observation) is a fundamental requirement for general acceptance of new knowledge in scientific circles (Campbell and Stanley 1966; Guyatt et al. 1993, 1994; Justice et al. 1999; Emanuel et al. 2000; Babbie 1986; Barrow 2000; Hawe et al. 2004). Actual or potential replicability of results is a basic requirement of all rigorous scientific investigation, regardless of scale (Campbell and Stanley 1966; Barrow 2000; Giancoli 1995; Pocock 1983; Bailey 1996; Piantadosi 1997; Brook et al. 2000; Hulley et al. 2001; Sackett et al. 1991; Babbie 1990). It applies equally to reductionist research in cell biology and to holisitic research in the integrated clinical environment. Recognition of the scale of inquiry (investigation) is important because results at one scale may be inapplicable at another (Morris 1998; Mandelbrot 1983). The Cardiac Arrhythmia Suppression Trial provides one example. While the test drugs effectively suppressed premature ventricular contractions (at the electrophysiologic scale) they were associated with an excess death rate in the treatment group at the holistic clinical care scale (Cardiac Arrhythmia Suppression Trial [CAST] Investigators 1989; Greene et al. 1992). The disparity between the results at the electrophysiologic scale and those at the holistic clinical care scale is a sobering example of emergent properties of complex systems (Schultz 1996) and a striking reminder of the need for replicable holistic clinical outcome data from rigorously conducted clinical studies.

Evidence-based clinician decision-making information emanates from the holistic clinical environment and comes from two major sources: clinical studies and clinical experience. Advances at lower scales of inquiry cannot replace the study of sick patients in the holistic clinical environment (Morris 1998; Schultz 1996). Clinical studies include observational studies and the more scientifically rigorous clinical trials (experiments). Usual experiential learning by clinicians can lead to important sentinel observations, but it also contributes to unnecessary variation in practice. Experiential learning is achieved within local contexts that contribute local bias. Since local contexts vary, this leads to highly variable, although strongly held, clinical opinions. Adequately explicit methods can also formalize experiential learning by enabling common methods among multiple users, sites, and disciplines (e.g., pediatrics, internal medicine). Interactions between different users of a common computerized protocol in an extended (distributed) development laboratory permit greater refinement of protocol rules than is likely to be realized in a single clinical development site. This reduces local bias and contributes to generalizability.

Attention to sources of nonuniformity between experimental groups is an essential part of experimental design (Pocock 1983; Hulley et al. 2001; Hennekens and Buring 1987; Rothman and Greenland 1998; Friedman et al. 1998; Chow and Liu 2004; Piantadosi 1997). Confounding variables (confounders) exist among the multiple variables that may determine subject outcome and can alter or reverse the results of clinical trials (Pocock 1983; Hulley et al. 2001; Hennekens and Buring 1987; Rothman and Greenland 1998; Cochrane-Collaboration 2001). Confounders can be present both before and after random allocation of subjects to the experimental groups of a clinical trial (Rothman and Greenland 1998). Those confounders present before allocation, commonly recognized in epidemiology texts (Hennekens and Buring 1987; Rothman and Greenland 1998), are usually adequately addressed by randomization and by restriction of randomized subjects. However, confounders introduced after subject assignment to the experimental groups include cointerventions (Hulley et al. 2001; Cochrane-Collaboration 2001; Sackett et al. 1991). Like the experimental intervention, cointerventions result from the interaction of the subject with the clinical environment (e.g., mechanical ventilation strategy, drug therapy for hypotension, intravenous fluid therapy, diagnostic strategies for suspected infection, monitoring intervals, laboratory tests, antibiotic therapy, sedation). They are easily overlooked but can alter or invalidate the results of clinical trials. Unlike the experimental intervention, cointerventions rarely receive adequate attention in the protocols of RCTs.

The Potential for Adequately Explicit Methods

Large-Scale Distributed Research Laboratories

Consider the difference in the number (N) of units of analysis for a chemical experiment involving 10 mL of 1M HCl and that of units of analysis for a clinical trial. The chemical experiment engages 6.02×10^{21}

interactions (0.01 × Avogadro's number). A clinical trial usually involves no more than 1,000 patients. Because of the constraints of small N, clinical trials require sophisticated, and frequently difficult to understand, statistical analyses. To overcome this serious clinical experimental limitation, the medical community should, in my opinion, develop large-scale distributed human outcomes research laboratories. These laboratories could be developed within the clinical care environment on multiple continents if we had easily distributable, replicable clinical experimental and clinical care methods. Such laboratories could, for example, deliver 200,000 ICU experimental subjects with a few months. They could enable the experimental definition of dose-response curves, rather than the common current goal of comparing two experimental groups. They could avoid the onerous attributes of current clinical trial techniques, including loss of enthusiasm among investigative teams, and pernicious secular changes.

Adequately explicit computerized protocols have already been implemented for continuous quality improvement, for clinical trials, and for clinical care. Work for the past two decades has been focused on the ICU, because of two enabling ICU attributes: a highly quantified environment and rapid evolution of clinical problems. Many clinical environments do not posses these attributes. However, certain clinical problems in non-ICU environments seem good targets for application of computerized protocols as well. These include the clinical care (e.g., medication titration) of outpatients with congestive heart failure and outpatients with insulin-dependent diabetes mellitus. Both of these problems could benefit from titration in the home with capture of only a few clinically important data elements. Other clinical problems such as psychiatric disorders seem less obvious targets for application of adequately explicit protocols. However, even early work suggests that this domain of clinical practice is also appropriate for application of rule-based decision-support systems (Meehl and Rosen 1955).

Emergency situations may preclude clinician keyboard-based interactions, such as those we have been using. However, voice recognition, handheld wireless communication devices, and other technologies will likely be widely available in the future and will enable more efficient and less distracting interactions with adequately explicit protocols. Future developments will likely reduce or remove the barrier that keyboard data entry now represents for emergency and other urgent clinician decisions that require immediate and repeated interactions. We believe that our work with adequately explicit computerized protocols has just scratched the surface. Much more exploration will be necessary before appropriate, and certainly before comprehensive, answers to these questions can be offered.

At this early stage of application and evaluation, it likely that many, but not all, clinical problems will be appropriate targets for adequately explicit protocols (computerized or not). This seems a reasonable conclusion if only because of the extensive literature indicating favorable outcome changes when decision support tools of many kinds are employed to aid clinician decision makers. It has seemed to my colleagues and to me that application of adequately explicit computerized treatment protocols for titration of clinical problems is more easily achieved than application of protocols for diagnosis. The diagnostic challenges frequently seem broader and more encompassing than the treatment challenges once a diagnosis has been made. Furthermore, many clinical decisions should embrace the wishes of patients or their surrogates. Capturing patient or surrogate assessments of outcome utilities and incorporating them in the rules of adequately explicit protocols seems a daunting but surmountable challenge. More systematic work is needed to define the roles of adequately explicit computerized protocols in many diagnostic and therapeutic arenas.

The evaluation of a potential target includes assessment of the reliability of available measurements and other replicable data. A measurement-rich and quantified clinical setting increases the likelihood of driving adequately explicit rules with patient-specific data. However, even difficult-to-define constructs such as "restlessness" can be made more replicable by listing the specific observations a clinician might use to identify the construct. We all have only five senses through which we receive information from the world about us. The challenge of knowledge engineering is to specify the few elements received by these senses that drive specific decisions. Our experience during the past two decades indicates that this is manageable.

Formalizing Experiential Learning as a Means of Enabling a Learning Healthcare System

Adequately explicit computerized protocols could supplement traditional peer-reviewed publication with direct electronic communication between research investigators and thereafter between investigators and clinical care users. This could introduce a new way of developing and distributing knowledge. Evidence-based knowledge for clinical decision making comes from two sources: first, from formal studies that include observational and experimental work (RCTs provide the most compelling results); second, from experiential knowledge. Currently, this experiential knowledge is derived primarily from individual experience and thus is influenced by local factors and bias. This individual experience contributes to strongly held but variable opinions that lead to unnecessary variation in clinical practice (Wennberg 2002). Adequately explicit computerized protocols could formalize this experiential learning in two sequential stages.

In the first stage, knowledge could be captured through multiple investigator and center participation in development and refinement of protocol rules. We have used this process successfully in our current NIH Roadmap contract work with blood glucose management. Our current computerized protocol for blood glucose management with IV insulin (eProtocol-insulin) was developed and refined by collaborators who include multiple pediatric and adult intensivists in more than 14 U.S. and Canadian clinical sites. This diminishes local factor and bias concerns; they become smaller as the number of different participants and institutions increase.

In the second stage, education of practitioners could occur during utilization of a protocol for clinical care. Adequately explicit computerized protocols could take advantage of an electronic infrastructure and translate research experience into clinical practice by adopting a direct electronic education strategy at the point of care or point of decision making. For example, the adequately explicit instructions of eProtocol-insulin could be linked to a new on-demand explanatory educational representation of the protocol logic. A user could question the specific eProtocol-insulin instruction at whatever level of detail the user wishes. The knowledge captured by the protocol developers during the first stage could thus be presented at the time, and within the context, of a specific clinical care question, but only when demanded and without requiring the user to address the published literature. This new educational strategy could complement traditional knowledge transfer through education based on reading and coursework and through published work. For some activities this new educational strategy could become the dominant learning strategy for clinicians. For example, when protocols are modified to incorporate new knowledge, the updated electronic protocol, once validated appropriately, could become the expected and most direct route for transferring this new knowledge to the clinical practitioner.

REFERENCES

Abramson, N, K Wald, A Grenvik, D Robinson, and J Snyder. 1980. Adverse occurrences in intensive care units. *Journal of the American Medical Association* 244:1582-1584.

Acute Respiratory Distress Syndrome Network. 2000a. *Mechanical Ventilation Protocol.* Available from www.ardsnet.org or NAPS Document No 05542 (Microfiche Publications, 248 Hempstead Turnpike, West Hempstead, NY).

———. 2000b. Ventilation with lower tidal volumes as compared with traditional tidal volumes for acute lung injury and the Acute Respiratory Distress Syndrome. *New England Journal of Medicine* 342(18):1301-1308.

Akhtar, S, J Weaver, D Pierson, and G Rubenfeld. 2003. Practice variation in respiratory therapy documentation during mechanical ventilation. *Chest* 124(6):2275-2282.

American Psychiatric Association (APA). 1998. *Practice Guideline for the Treatment of Patients with Bipolar Disorder.* Washington, DC: APA.

Arkes, H. 1986. Impediments to accurate clinical judgment and possible ways to minimize their impact. In *Judgment and Decision Making: An Interdisciplinary Reader*, edited by H Arkes and K Hammond. Cambridge, UK: Cambridge University Press.

Arkes, H, and K Hammond, eds. 1986. *Judgment and Decision Making: An Interdisciplinary Reader.* Cambridge, UK: Cambridge University Press.

Armstrong, R, C Bullen, S Cohen, M Singer, and A Webb. 1991. *Critical Care Algorithms.* New York: Oxford University Press.

Atkins, H. 1958 (December). The three pillars of clinical research. *British Medical Journal* 2(27):1547-1553.

Audet, A-M, S Greenfield, and M Field. 1990. Medical practice guidelines: current activities and future directions. *Annals of Internal Medicine* 113:709-714.

Babbie, E. 1986. *Observing Ourselves: Essays in Social Research.* Belmont, CA: Wadsworth Publishing Co.

———. 1990. *Survey Research Methods.* Belmont, CA: Wadsworth Publishing Co.

Bailey, R. 1996. *Human Performance Engineering.* 3rd ed. Upper Saddle River: Prentice Hall.

Barach, P, and D Berwick. 2003. Patient safety and the reliability of health care systems. *Annals of Internal Medicine* 138(12):997-998.

Barrow, J. 2000. *The Book of Nothing.* New York: Pantheon Books.

Bazil, C, and T Pedley. 1998. Advances in the medical treatment of epilepsy. *Annual Review of Medicine* 49:135-162.

Berwick, D. 1994. Eleven worthy aims for clinical leadership of health system reform. *Journal of the American Medical Association* 272(10):797-802.

———. 2003. Disseminating innovations in health care. *Journal of the American Medical Association* 289(15):1969-1975.

———. 2005. My right knee. *Annals of Internal Medicine* 142(2):121-125.

Blesser, W. 1969. *A Systems Approach to Biomedicine.* New York: McGraw-Hill Book Company.

Brook, R, E McGlynn, and P Shekelle. 2000. Defining and measuring quality of care: a perspective from U.S. researchers. *International Journal of Quality Health Care* 12(4):281-295.

Bull, S, C Conell, and D Campen. 2002. Relationship of clinical factors to the use of Cox-2 selective NSAIDs within an arthritis population in a large HMO. *Journal of Managed Care Pharmacy* 8(4):252-258.

Campbell, D, and J Stanley. 1966. *Experimental and Quasi-Experimental Designs for Research* (reprinted from Handbook of Research on Teaching, 1963). Boston, MA: Houghton Mifflin Co.

Cardiac Arrhythmia Suppression Trial (CAST) Investigators. 1989. Preliminary report: effect of encainide and flecainide on mortality in a randomized trial of arrhythmia suppression after myocardial infarction. *New England Journal of Medicine* 321:406-412.

Chow, S-C, and J-P Liu. 2004. *Design and Analysis of Clinical Trials.* Hoboken, NJ: John Wiley & Sons, Inc.

Clancy, C. 2006 (July 20-21) *Session 1: Hints of a Different Way—Case Studies in Practice-Based Evidence, Opening Remarks.* Presentation at the Roundtable on Evidence-Based Medicine Workshop, The Learning Health Care System. Washington, DC: Institute of Medicine, Roundtable on Evidence-Based Medicine.

Cochrane, G. 1998. Compliance in asthma. *European Respiratory Review* 8(56):239-242.

Cochrane-Collaboration. 2001. *The Cochrane Reviewer's Handbook Glossary.* Version 4.1.4. M Clarke and A Oxman, eds. In The Cochrane Library, Issue 4, 2001. Oxford: Update Software.

Cook, D, B Reeve, G Guyatt, D Heyland, L Griffith, L Buckingham, and M Tryba. 1996. Stress ulcer prophylaxis in critically ill patients. Resolving discordant meta-analyses. *Journal of the American Medical Association* 275(4):308-314.

Cook, T, D Campbell. 1979. *Quasi-Experimentation: Design and Analyses Issues for Field Settings*. Boston, MA: Houghton Mifflin Co.

Corke, C, P Stow, D Green, J Agar, and M Henry. 2005. How doctors discuss major interventions with high risk patients: an observational study. *British Medical Journal* 330(7484):182.

Courtney, S, D Durand, J Asselin, M Hudak, J Aschner, and C Shoemaker. 2002. High-frequency oscillatory ventilation versus conventional mechanical ventilation for very-low-birth-weight infants. *New England Journal of Medicine* 347(9):643-652.

Cronin, L, D Cook, J Carlet, D Heyland, D King, M Lansang, and C Fisher, Jr. 1995. Corticosteroid treatment for sepsis: a critical appraisal and meta-analysis of the literature. *Critical Care Medicine* 23(8):1430-1439.

Deming, W. 1982. *Quality, Productivity, and Competitive Position*. Cambridge, MA: Massachusetts Institute of Technology, Center for Advanced Engineering Study.

———. 1986. *Out of the Crisis*. Cambridge: Massachusetts Institute of Technology, Center for Advanced Engineering Study.

Dickerson, J, A Hingorani, M Ashby, C Palmer, and M Brown. 1999. Optimisation of antihypertensive treatment by crossover rotation of four major classes. *Lancet* 353(9169):2008-2013.

Don, H, ed. 1985. *Decision Making in Critical Care, Clinical Decision Making Series*. Philadelphia, PA: BC Decker Inc.

East, T, S Böhm, C Wallace, T Clemmer, L Weaver, J Orme Jr., and A Morris. 1992. A successful computerized protocol for clinical management of pressure control inverse ratio ventilation in ARDS patients. *Chest* 101(3):697-710.

East, T, L Heermann, R Bradshaw, A Lugo, R Sailors, L Ershler, C Wallace, A Morris, G McKinley, A Marquez, A Tonnesen, L Parmley, W Shoemaker, P Meade, P Taut, T Hill, M Young, J Baughman, M Olterman, V Gooder, B Quinnj, W Summer, V Valentine, J Carlson, B Bonnell, B deBoisblanc, Z McClarity, J Cachere, K Kovitz, E Gallagher, M Pinsky, D Angus, M Cohenj, L Hudson, and K Steinberg. 1999. Efficacy of computerized decision support for mechanical ventilation: results of a prospective multi-center randomized trial. *Proceedings of the American Medical Informatics Association Symposium* 251-255.

Ely, E, M Meade, E Haponik, M Kollef, D Cook, G Guyatt, and J Stoller. 2001. Mechanical ventilator weaning protocols driven by nonphysician health-care professionals: evidence-based clinical practice guidelines. *Chest* 120(90060):454S-463S.

Emanuel, E, D Wendler, and C Grady. 2000. What makes clinical research ethical? *Journal of the American Medical Association* 283(20):2701-2711.

Evans, R, S Pestotnik, D Classen, T Clemmer, L Weaver, J Orme Jr., J Lloyd, and J Burke. 1998. A computer-assisted management program for antibiotics and other anti-infective agents. *New England Journal of Medicine* 338(4):232-238.

Fletcher, R, and S Fletcher. 1990. Clinical practice guidelines. *Annals of Internal Medicine* 113:645-646.

Fridsma, D, J Gennari, and M Musen. 1996. *Making Generic Guidelines Site-Specific*. Paper read at Proceedings 1996 AMIA Annual Fall Symposium (Formerly SCAMC), at Washington, DC.

Friedman, G, M Collen, L Harris, E Van Brunt, and L Davis. 1971. Experience in monitoring drug reactions in outpatients. The Kaiser-Permanente Drug Monitoring System. *Journal of the American Medical Association* 217(5):567-572.

Friedman, L, C Furberg, and D DeMets. 1998. *Fundamentals of Clinical Trials*. 3rd ed. New York: Springer-Verlag.

Galuska, D, J Will, M Serdula, and E Ford. 1999. Are health care professionals advising obese patients to lose weight? *Journal of the American Medical Association* 282(16): 1576-1578.

Garrido, T, L Jamieson, Y Zhou, A Wiesenthal, and L Liang. 2005. Effect of electronic health records in ambulatory care: retrospective, serial, cross sectional study. *British Medical Journal* 330(7491):581.

Giancoli, D. 1995. *Physics.* 3rd ed. Englewood Cliffs, NJ: Prentice Hall.

Gnaegi, A, F Feihl, and C Perret. 1997. Intensive care physicians' insufficient knowledge of right-heart catheterization at the bedside: time to act?. *Critical Care Medicine* 25(2): 213-220.

Graham, D, D Campen, R Hui, M Spence, C Cheetham, G Levy, S Shoor, and W Ray. 2005. Risk of acute myocardial infarction and sudden cardiac death in patients treated with cyclo-oxygenase 2 selective and non-selective non-steroidal anti-inflammatory drugs: nested case-control study. *Lancet* 365(9458):475-481.

Greco, P, and J Eisenberg. 1993. Changing physicians' practices. *New England Journal of Medicine* 329(17):1271-1274.

Greene, H, D Roden, R Katz, R Woosley, D Salerno, R Henthorn, and CASTinvestigators. 1992. The Cardiac Arrythmia Suppression Trial: First CAST . . . Then CAST-II. *Journal of the American College of Cardiology* 19:894-898.

Greene, S, and A Geiger. 2006. A review finds that multicenter studies face substantial challenges but strategies exist to achieve Institutional Review Board approval. *Journal of Clinical Epidemiology* 59(8):784-790.

Grimm, R, K Shimoni, W Harlan, and E Estes. 1975. Evaluation of patient-care protocol use by various providers. *New England Journal of Medicine* 292:507-511.

Grimshaw, J, and I Russell. 1993. Effect of clinical guidelines on medical practice: a systematic review of rigorous evaluations. *Lancet* 342:1317-1322.

Guidelines Committee Society of Critical Care Medicine. 1992. Guidelines for the care of patients with hemodynamic instability associated with sepsis. *Critical Care Medicine* 20(7):1057-1059.

Guyatt, G, D Sackett, and D Cook. 1993. User's guide to the medical literature: II. How to use an article about therapy or prevention: A. Are the results of the study valid? *Journal of the American Medical Association* 270(21):2598-2601.

———. 1994. User's guide to the medical literature: II. How to use and article about therapy or prevention; B. What were the results and will they help me in caring for my patient? *Journal of the American Medical Association* 271(1):59-63.

Hadorn, D, K McCormick, and A Diokno. 1992. An annotated algorithm approach to clinical guideline development. *Journal of the American Medical Association* 267(24): 3311-3314.

Hawe, P, A Shiell, and T Riley. 2004. Complex interventions: how "out of control" can a randomised controlled trial be? *British Medical Journal* 328(7455):1561-1563.

Henderson, S, R Crapo, C Wallace, T East, A Morris, and R Gardner. 1992. Performance of computerized protocols for the management of arterial oxygenation in an intensive care unit. *International Journal of Clininical Monitoring and Computing* 8:271-280.

Hennekens, C, and J Buring. 1987. *Epidemiology in Medicine.* Edited by S Mayrent. 1st ed. 1 volume. Boston, MA: Little, Brown and Company.

Henriksen, O. 1998. An overview of benzodiazepines in seizure management. *Epilepsia* 39 (Suppl. 1):S2-S6.

Hoch, I, A Heymann, I Kurman, L Valinsky, G Chodick, and V Shalev. 2003. Countrywide computer alerts to community physicians improve potassium testing in patients receiving diuretics. *Journal of the American Medical Informatics Association* 10(6):541-546.

Holcomb, B, A Wheeler, and E Ely. 2001. New ways to reduce unnecessary variation and improve outcomes in the intensive care unit. *Current Opinion in Critical Care* 7(4):304-311.

Horn, S, and D Hopkins, eds. 1994. *Clinical Practice Improvement: A New Technology for Developing Cost-Effective Quality Health Care.* Vol. 1, Faulkner & Gray's Medical Outcomes and Practice and Guidelines Library. New York: Faulkner & Gray, Inc.

Horwitz, R, B Singer, R Makuch, and C Viscoli. 1996. Can treatment that is helpful on average be harmful to some patients? A study of the conflicting information needs of clinical inquiry and drug regulation. *Journal of Clinical Epidemiology* 49(4):395-400.

Hulley, S, and S Cummings. 1988. *Designing Clinical Research.* Baltimore, MD: Williams and Wilkins.

Hulley, S, S Cummings, S Warren, D Grady, N Hearst, and T Newman. 2001. *Designing Clinical Research.* 2nd ed. Philadelphia, PA: Lippincott Williams and Wilkins.

Iberti, T, E Fischer, M Leibowitz, E Panacek, J Silverstein, T Albertson, and PACS Group. 1990. A multicenter study of physician's knowledge of the pulmonary artery catheter. *Journal of the American Medical Association* 264:2928-2932.

Iberti, T, E Daily, A Leibowitz, C Schecter, E Fischer, and J Silverstein. 1994. Assessment of critical care nurses' knowledge of the pulmonary artery catheter. The Pulmonary Artery Catheter Study Group. *Critical Care Medicine* 22:1674-1678.

IOM (Institute of Medicine). 1990. *Clinical Practice Guidelines: Directions for a New Program.* Washington, DC: National Academy Press.

———. 1999. *To Err Is Human: Building a Safer Health System.* Washington, DC: National Academy Press.

———. 2001. *Crossing the Quality Chasm: A New Health System for the 21st Century.* Washington, DC: National Academy Press.

James, B, and M Hammond. 2000. The challenge of variation in medical practice. *Archives of Pathology & Laboratory Medicine* 124(7):1001-1003.

James, B, S Horn, and R Stephenson. 1994. Management by fact: What is CPI and how is it used? In *Clinical Practice Improvement: A New Technology for Developing Cost-Effective Quality Health Care,* edited by S Horn and D Hopkins. New York: Faulkner & Gray, Inc.

Jennings, D, T Amabile, and L Ross. 1982. Informal covariation assessment: data-based versus theory-based judgments. In *Judgment Under Uncertainty: Heuristics and Biases,* edited by D Kahneman, P Slovic, and A Tversky. Cambridge, UK: Cambridge University Press.

Johnson, A, J Peacock, A Greenough, N Marlow, E Limb, L Marston, and S Calvert. 2002. High-frequency oscillatory ventilation for the prevention of chronic lung disease of prematurity. *New England Journal of Medicine* 347(9):633-642.

Johnson, B. 2004. Review: prophylactic use of vitamin D reduces falls in older persons. *Evidence Based Medicine* 9(6):169.

Johnston, M, K Langton, B Haynes, and A Mathieu. 1994. Effects of computer-based clinical decision support systems on clinician performance and patient outcome. *Annals of Internal Medicine* 120:135-142.

Jones, P. 1998. Health status, quality of life and compliance. *European Respiratory Review* 8(56):243-246.

Justice, A, K Covinsky, and J Berlin. 1999. Assessing the generalizability of prognostic information. *Annals of Internal Medicine* 130(6):515-524.

Kahneman, D, P Slovik, and A Tversky. 1982. *Judgment Under Uncertainty: Heuristics and Biases.* Cambridge, UK: Cambridge University Press.

Karlinsky, J, J Lau, and R Goldstein. 1991. *Decision Making in Pulmonary Medicine.* Philadelphia, PA: BC Decker.

Kiernan, M, A King, H Kraemer, M Stefanick, and J Killen. 1998. Characteristics of successful and unsuccessful dieters: an application of signal detection methodology. *Annals of Behavioral Medicine* 20(1):1-6.

Kolata, G. 2006. Medicare says it will pay, but patients say 'no thanks'. *New York Times*, March 3.

Kozer, E, W Seto, Z Verjee, C Parshuram, S Khattak, G Koren, and D Jarvis. 2004. Prospective observational study on the incidence of medication errors during simulated resuscitation in a paediatric emergency department. *British Medical Journal* 329(7478):1321.

Lake, A. 2004. Every prescription is a clinical trial. *British Medical Journal* 329(7478):1346.

Lamb, R, D Studdert, R Bohmer, D Berwick, and T Brennan. 2003. Hospital disclosure practices: results of a national survey. *Health Affairs* 22(2):73-83.

Leape, L. 1994. Error in medicine. *Journal of the American Medical Association* 272: 1851-1857.

Leape, L, D Berwick, and D Bates. 2002. What practices will most improve safety? Evidence-based medicine meets patient safety. *Journal of the American Medical Association* 288(4):501-507.

Lefering, R, and E Neugebauer. 1995. Steroid controversy in sepsis and septic shock: a meta-analysis. *Critical Care Medicine* 23(7):1294-1303.

LeLorier, J, G Gregoire, A Benhaddad, J Lapierre, and F Derderian. 1997. Discrepancies between meta-analyses and subsequent large randomized, controlled trials. *New England Journal of Medicine* 337(8):536-542.

Lo, B. 1995. Improving care near the end of life: why is it so hard? *Journal of the American Medical Association* 274:1634-1636.

Lomas, J, G Anderson, K Domnick-Pierre, E Vayda, M Enkin, and W Hannah. 1989. Do practice guidelines guide practice? The effect of a consensus statement on the practice of physicians. *New England Journal of Medicine* 321(19):1306-1311.

MacIntyre, N. 2001. Evidence-based guidelines for weaning and discontinuing ventilatory support: a collective task force facilitated by the American College of Chest Physicians; the American Association for Respiratory Care; and the American College of Critical Care Medicine. *Chest* 120 (90060):375S-396S.

Mandelbrot, B. 1983. *The Fractal Geometry of Nature*. New York: W. H. Freeman and Company.

Marshall, J. 2000. Clinical trials of mediator-directed therapy in sepsis: what have we learned? *Intensive Care Medicine* 26(6 Suppl. 1):S75-S83.

McDonald, C. 1976. Protocol-based computer reminders, the quality of care and the non-perfectability of man. *New England Journal of Medicine* 295:1351-1355.

Meehl, P, and A Rosen. 1955. Antecedent probability and the efficiency of psychometric signs, patterns, or cutting scores. *Psychological Bulletin* 52(3):194-216.

Miller, P, and S Frawly. 1995. Trade-offs in producing patient-specific recommendations from a computer-based clinical guideline: a case study. *Journal of the American Medical Informatics Association* 2:238-242.

Miller, R, and K Goodman. 1998. Ethical challenges in the use of decision-support software in clinical practice. In *Ethics, Computing, and Medicine: Informatics and the Transformation of Health Care*, edited by K Goodman. Cambridge, UK: Cambridge University Press.

Morris, A. 1985. Elimination of pulmonary wedge pressure errors commonly encountered in the ICU. *Cardiologia (Italy)* 30(10):941-943.

———. 1998. Algorithm-based decision making. In *Principles and Practice of Intensive Care Monitoring*, edited by M Tobin. New York: McGraw-Hill, Inc.

———. 2000a. Developing and implementing computerized protocols for standardization of clinical decisions. *Annals of Internal Medicine* 132:373-383.

————. 2000b. Evaluating and Refining a Hemodynamic Protocol for use in a multicenter ARDS clinical trial. *American Journal of Respiratory and Critical Care Medicine (ATS Proceedings Abstracts)* 161(3 Suppl.):A378.

————. 2002. Decision support and safety of clinical environments. *Quality and Safety in Health Care* 11:69-75.

————. 2003. Treatment algorithms and protocolized care. *Current Opinions in Critical Care* 9 (3):236-240.

————. 2004. Iatrogenic illness: a call for decision support tools to reduce unnecessary variation. *Quality and Safety in Health Care* 13(1):80-81.

————. 2006. The importance of protocol-directed patient management for research on lung-protective ventilation. In *Ventilator-Induced Lung Injury*, edited by D Dereyfuss, G Saumon, and R Hubamyr. New York: Taylor & Francis Group.

Morris, A, and D Cook. 1998. Clinical trial issues in mechanical ventilation. In *Physiologic Basis of Ventilatory Support*, edited by J Marini and A Slutsky. New York: Marcel Dekker, Inc.

Morris, A, R Chapman, and R Gardner. 1984. Frequency of technical problems encountered in the measurement of pulmonary artery wedge pressure. *Critical Care Medicine* 12(3):164-170.

————. 1985. Frequency of wedge pressure errors in the ICU. *Critical Care Medicine* 13:705-708.

Morris, A, C Wallace, R Menlove, T Clemmer, J Orme, L Weaver, N Dean, F Thomas, T East, M Suchyta, E Beck, M Bombino, D Sittig, S Böhm, B Hoffmann, H Becks, N Pace, S Butler, J Pearl, and B Rasmusson. 1994. Randomized clinical trial of pressure-controlled inverse ratio ventilation and extracorporeal CO_2 removal for ARDS [erratum 1994;149(3, Pt 1):838, Letters to the editor 1995;151(1):255-256, 1995;151(3):1269-1270, and 1997;156(3):1016-1017]. *American Journal of Respiratory Critical Care Medicine* 149(2):295-305.

Mullett, C, R Evans, J Christenson, and J Dean. 2001. Development and impact of a computerized pediatric antiinfective decision support program. *Pediatrics* 108(4):E75.

Nelson, E, M Splaine, P Batalden, and S Plume. 1998. Building measurement and data collection into medical practice. *Annals of Internal Medicine* 128:460-466.

Newhouse, J, W Manning, C Morris, L Orr, N Duan, E Keeler, A Leibowitz, K Marquis, M Marquis, C Phelps, and R Brook. 1981. Some interim results from a controlled trial of cost sharing in health insurance. *New England Journal of Medicine* 305(25):1501-1507.

Park, S, D Ross-Degnan, A Adams, J Sabin, and S Soumerai. 2005. A population-based study of the effect of switching from typical to atypical antipsychotics on extrapyramidal symptoms among patients with schizophrenia. *British Journal of Psychiatry* 187:137-142.

Pearson, S, S Soumerai, C Mah, F Zhang, L Simoni-Wastila, C Salzman, L Cosler, T Fanning, P Gallagher, and D Ross-Degnan. 2006. Racial disparities in access following regulatory surveillance of benzodiazepines. *Archives of Internal Medicine* 166:572-579.

Persell, S, J Wright, J Thompson, K Kmetik, and D Baker. 2006. Assessing the validity of national quality measures for coronary artery disease using an electronic health record. *Archives of Internal Medicine* 166(20):2272-2272.

Piantadosi, S. 1997. *Clinical Trials: A Methodologic Perspective.* New York: John Wiley & Sons, Inc.

Platt, R, R Davis, J Finkelstein, A Go, J Gurwitz, D Roblin, S Soumerai, D Ross-Degnan, S Andrade, M Goodman, B Martinson, M Raebel, D Smith, M Ulcickas-Yood, and K Chan. 2001. Multicenter epidemiologic and health services research on therapeutics in the HMO Research Network Center for Education and Research on Therapeutics. *Pharmacoepidemiology and Drug Safety* 10(5):373-377.

Pocock, S. 1983. *Clinical Trials: A Practical Approach.* Original edition. New York: John Wiley & Sons, Inc.

Pritchard, R, E Fisher, J Teno, S Sharp, D Reding, W Knaus, J Wennberg, and J Lynn. 1998. Influence of patient preferences and local health system characteristics on the place of death. SUPPORT Investigators. Study to Understand Prognoses and Preferences for Outcomes and Risks of Treatment. *Journal of the American Geriatrics Society* 46(10):1242-1250.

Ray, W, J Daugherty, and K Meador. 2003. Effect of a mental health "carve-out" program on the continuity of antipsychotic therapy. *New England Journal of Medicine* 348(19):1885-1894.

Redelmeier, D. 2005. The cognitive psychology of missed diagnoses. *Annals of Internal Medicine* 142(2):115-120.

Redelmeier, D, L Ferris, J Tu, J Hux, and M Schull. 2001. Problems for clinical judgment: introducing cognitive psychology as one more basic science. *Canadian Medical Association Journal* 164(3):358-360.

Redman, B. 1996. Clinical practice guidelines as tools of public policy: conflicts of purpose, issues of autonomy, and justice. *Journal of Clinical Ethics* 5(4):303-309.

Ries, A, B Make, S Lee, M Krasna, M Bartels, R Crouch, and A Fishman. 2005. The effects of pulmonary rehabilitation in the national emphysema treatment trial. *Chest* 128(6):3799-3809.

Roblin, D, R Platt, M Goodman, J Hsu, W Nelson, D Smith, S Andrade, and S Soumerai. 2005. Effect of increased cost-sharing on oral hypoglycemic use in five managed care organizations: how much is too much? *Medical Care* 43 (10):951-959.

Ross-Degnan, D, L Simoni-Wastila, J Brown, X Gao, C Mah, L Cosler, T Fanning, P Gallagher, C Salzman, R Shader, T Inui, and S Soumerai. 2004. A controlled study of the effects of state surveillance on indicators of problematic and non-problematic benzodiazepine use in a Medicaid population. *International Journal of Psychiatry in Medicine* 34(2):103-123.

Rothman, K, and S Greenland. 1998. *Modern Epidemiology.* 2nd ed. Philadelphia, PA: Lippincott-Raven.

Roundtable on Evidence-Based Medicine. 2006. *Institute of Medicine Roundtable on Evidence-Based Medicine Charter and Vision Statement.* Available from http://www.iom.edu/CMS/28312/RT-EBM/33544.aspx (accessed April 27, 2007).

Rubenfeld, G, C Cooper, G Carter, T Thompson, and L Hudson. 2004. Barriers to providing lung-protective ventilation to patients with acute lung injury. *Critical Care Medicine* 32(6):1289-1293.

Runciman, W, A Merry, and F Tito. 2003. Error, blame and the law in health care: an antipodean perspective. *Annals of Internal Medicine* 138(12):974-979.

Sackett, D, R Haynes, G Guyatt, and P Tugwell. 1991. *Clinical Epidemiology: A Basic Science for Clinical Medicine.* 2nd ed. Boston, MA: Little, Brown and Company.

Safran, C, D Rind, R Davis, D Ives, D Sands, J Currier, W Slack, D Cotton, and H Makadon. 1996. Effects of a knowledge-based electronic patient record on adherence to practice guidelines. *MD Computing* 13(1):55-63.

Schacker, T, A Collier, J Hughes, T Shea, and L Corey. 1996. Clinical and epidemiologic features of primary HIV infection [published erratum appears in *Ann Intern Med* 1997 Jan 15;126(2):174]. *Annals of Internal Medicine* 125(4):257-264.

Schiff, G, D Klass, J Peterson, G Shah, and D Bates. 2003. Linking laboratory and pharmacy: opportunities for reducing errors and improving care. *Archives of Internal Medicine* 163(8):893-900.

Schultz, S. 1996. Homeostasis, humpty dumpty, and integrative biology. *News in Physiological Science* 11:238-246.

Schwartz, D, and J Lellouch. 1967. Explanatory and pragmatic attitudes in therapeutical trials. *Journal of Chronic Diseases* 20(8):637-648.

Selby, J. 1997. Linking automated databases for research in managed care settings. *Annals of Internal Medicine* 127(8 Pt 2):719-724.

Senn, S. 2004. Individual response to treatment: is it a valid assumption? *British Medical Journal* 329(7472):966-968.

Sheppard, L. 1980. Computer control of the infusion of vasoactive drugs. *Annals of Biomedical Engineering* 8(4-6):431-434.

Sheppard, L, N Kouchoukos, and M Kurtis. 1968. Automated treatment of critically ill patients following operation. *Annals of Surgery* 168:596-604.

Sheppard, L, J Kirklin, and N Kouchoukos. 1974. Chapter 6: computer-controlled interventions for the acutely ill patient. *Computers in Biomedical Research.* New York: Academic Press.

Shewart, W. 1931. *Economic control of quality of manufactured product.* New York: D. Van Nostrand Co., Inc. (republished in 1980, American Society for Quality Control, Milwaukee, WI).

Silverman, W. 1993. Doing more good than harm. *Annals of the New York Academies of Science* 703:5-11.

Singer, M, R Haft, T Barlam, M Aronson, A Shafer, and K Sands. 1998. Vancomycin control measures at a tertiary-care hospital: impact of interventions on volume and patterns of use. *Infection Control and Hospital Epidemiology* 19(4):248-253.

Smalley, W, M Griffin, R Fought, L Sullivan, and W Ray. 1995. Effect of a prior authorization requirement on the use of nonsteroidal anti-inflammatory drugs by Medicaid patient. *New England Journal of Medicine* 332:1641-1645.

Soumerai, S. 2004. Benefits and risks of increasing restrictions on access to costly drugs in Medicaid. *Health Affairs* 23(1):135-146.

Soumerai, S, J Avorn, D Ross-Degnan, and S Gortmaker. 1987. Payment restrictions for prescription drugs under Medicaid. Effects on therapy, cost, and equity. *New England Journal of Medicine* 317(9):550-556.

Soumerai, S, D Ross-Degnan, J Avorn, T McLaughlin, and I Choodnovskiy. 1991. Effects of Medicaid drug-payment limits on admission to hospitals and nursing homes. *New England Journal of Medicine* 325(15):1072-1077.

Soumerai, S, D Ross-Degnan, E Fortess, and J Abelson. 1993. A critical analysis of studies of state drug reimbursement policies: research in need of discipline. *Milbank Quarterly* 71(2):217-252.

Soumerai, S, T McLaughlin, D Ross-Degnan, C Casteris, and P Bollini. 1994. Effects of a limit on Medicaid drug-reimbursement benefits on the use of psychotropic agents and acute mental health services by patients with schizophrenia. *New England Journal of Medicine* 331(10):650-655.

Soumerai, S, D Ross-Degnan, E Fortess, and B Walser. 1997. Determinants of change in Medicaid pharmaceutical cost sharing: does evidence affect policy? *Milbank Quarterly* 75(1):11-34.

Sox, H. 2003. Improving patient care. *Annals of Internal Medicine* 138(12):996.

Stark, A. 2002. High-frequency oscillatory ventilation to prevent bronchopulmonary dysplasia—are we there yet? *New England Journal of Medicine* 347(9):682-684.

Tamblyn, R, R Laprise, J Hanley, M Abrahamowicz, S Scott, N Mayo, J Hurley, R Grad, E Latimer, R Perreault, P McLeod, A Huang, P Larochelle, and L Mallet. 2001. Adverse events associated with prescription drug cost-sharing among poor and elderly persons. *Journal of the American Medical Association* 285(4):421-429.

Teno, J, J Lynn, A Connors, N Wenger, R Phillips, C Alzola, D Murphy, N Desbiens, and W Knaus. 1997a. The illusion of end-of-life resource savings with advance directives. SUPPORT Investigators. Study to Understand Prognoses and Preferences for Outcomes and Risks of Treatment. *Journal of the American Geriatrics Society* 45(4):513-518.

Teno, J, S Licks, J Lynn, N Wenger, A Connors, R Phillips, M O'Connor, D Murphy, W Fulkerson, N Desbiens, and W Knaus. 1997b. Do advance directives provide instructions that direct care? SUPPORT Investigators. Study to Understand Prognoses and Preferences for Outcomes and Risks of Treatment. *Journal of The American Geriatrics Society* 45(4):508-512.

Tierney, W, J Overhage, B Takesue, L Harris, M Murray, D Vargo, and C McDonald. 1995. Computerizing guidelines to improve care and patient outcomes: the example of heart failure. *Journal of the American Medical Informatics Association* 2(5):316-322.

Tierney, W, J Overhage, and C McDonald. 1996. *Computerizing Guidelines: Factors for Success.* Paper read at Proceedings of the 1996 American Medical Informatics Association Annual Fall Symposium (formerly SCAMC), Washington, DC.

Trontell, A. 2004. Expecting the unexpected—drug safety, pharmacovigilance, and the prepared mind. *New England Journal of Medicine* 351(14):1385-1387.

Tunis, S. Chief Medical Officer, Centers for Medicare and Medicaid Services, Office of Clinical Standards and Quality. February 25, 2005, letter.

Tunis, S, D Stryer, and C Clancy. 2003. Practical clinical trials: increasing the value of clinical research for decision making in clinical and health policy. *Journal of the American Medical Association* 290(12):1624-1632.

Tversky, A, and D Kahneman. 1982. Availability: a heuristic for judging frequency and probability. In *Judgment Under Uncertainty: Heuristics and Biases*, edited by D Kahneman, P Slovic and A Tversky. Cambridge, UK: Cambridge University Press.

Vogt, T, J Elston-Lafata, D Tolsma, and S Greene. 2004. The role of research in integrated healthcare systems: the HMO Research Network. *American Journal of Managed Care* 10(9):643-648.

Wagner, A, S Soumerai, F Zhang, and D Ross-Degnan. 2002. Segmented regression analysis of interrupted time series studies in medication use research. *Journal of Clinical Pharmacy and Therapeutics* 27(4):299-309.

Wagner, A, D Ross-Degnan, J Gurwitz, F Zhang, D Gilden, L Cosler, S Soumerai. 2007 (in press). Restrictions on benzodiazepine prescribing and rates of hip fracture New York state regulation of benzodiazepine prescribing is associated with fewer prescriptions but no reduction in rates of hip fracture. *Annals of Internal Medicine.*

Walton, M. 1986. *The Deming Management Method.* New York: Putnam publishing group (Perigee books).

Warren, K, and F Mosteller, eds. 1993. *Doing More Good than Harm: The Evaluation of Health Care Interventions.* Vol. 703, Annals of the New York Academies of Science. New York: The New York Academy of Sciences.

Wennberg, J. 2002. Unwarranted variations in healthcare delivery: implications for academic medical centres. *British Medical Journal* 325(7370):961-964.

Wennberg, J, and A Gittelsohn. 1973. Small area variation analysis in health care delivery. *Science* 142:1102-1108.

Wirtschafter, D, M Scalise, C Henke, and R Gams. 1981. Do information systems improve the quality of clinical research? Results of a randomized trial in a cooperative multi-institutional cancer group. *Compututers and Biomedical Research* 14:78-90.

Wu, A, S Folkman, S McPhee, and B Lo. 1991. Do house officers learn from their mistakes? *Journal of the American Medical Association* 265:2089-2094.

Zhang, J, V Patel, and T Johnson. 2002. Medical error: is the solution medical or cognitive? *Journal of the American Medical Informatics Association* 9(6 Suppl.):S75-S77.

2

The Evolving Evidence Base—
Methodologic and Policy Challenges

OVERVIEW

An essential component of the learning healthcare system is the capacity to continually improve approaches to gathering and evaluating evidence, taking advantage of new tools and methods. As technology advances and our ability to accumulate large quantities of clinical data increases, new challenges and opportunities to develop evidence on the effectiveness of interventions will emerge. With these expansions comes the possibility of significant improvements in multiple facets of the information that underlies healthcare decision making, including the potential to develop additional insights on risk and effectiveness; an improved understanding of increasingly complex patterns of comorbidity; insights on the effect of genetic variation and heterogeneity on diagnosis and treatment outcomes; and evaluation of interventions in a rapid state of flux such as devices and procedures. A significant challenge will be in piecing together evidence from the full scope of this information to determine what is best for individual patients. This chapter offers an overview of some of the key methodologic and policy challenges that must be addressed as evidence evolves.

In the first paper in this chapter, Robert M. Califf presents an overview of the alternatives to large randomized controlled trials (RCTs), and Telba Irony and David Eddy present three methods that have been developed to augment and improve current approaches to generating evidence. Califf suggests that, while the RCT is a valuable tool, the sheer volume of clinical decisions requires that we understand the best alternative methods to use when RCTs are inapplicable, infeasible, or impractical. He outlines the potential benefits and pitfalls of practical clinical trials (PCTs), cluster randomized trials, observational treatment comparisons, interrupted time series, and instrumental variables analysis, noting that advancements in methodologies are important; but increasing the evidence base will also require expanding our capacity to do clinical research—which can be exemplified by the need for increased organization, clinical trials that are embedded in a nodal network of health systems with electronic health records, and development of a critical mass of experts to guide us through study methodologies.

Another issue complicating evaluation of medical devices is their rapid rate of turnover and improvement, which makes their appraisal especially complicated. Telba Irony discusses the work of the Food and Drug Administration (FDA) in this area through the agency's Critical Path Initiative and its Medical Device Innovation Initiative. The latter emphasizes the need for improved statistical approaches and techniques to learn about the safety and effectiveness of medical device interventions in an efficient way, which can also adapt to changes in technology during evaluation periods. Several examples were discussed of the utilization of Bayesian analysis to accelerate the approval process of medical devices. David M. Eddy presented his work with Archimedes to demonstrate how the use of mathematical models is a promising approach to help answer clinical questions, particularly to fill the gaps in empirical evidence. Many current gaps in evidence relate to unresolved questions posed at the conclusion of clinical trials; however most of these unanswered questions do not get specifically addressed in subsequent trials, due to a number of factors including cost, feasibility, and clinical interest. Eddy suggests that models can be particularly useful in utilizing the existing clinical trial data to address issues such as head-to-head comparisons, combination therapy or dosing, extension of trial results to different settings, longer follow-up times, and heterogeneous populations. Recent work on diabetes prevention in high-risk patients illustrates how the mathematical modeling approach allowed investigators to extend trials in directions that were otherwise not feasible and provided much needed evidence for truly informed decision making. Access to needed data will increase with the spread of electronic health records (EHRs) as long as person-specific data from existing trials are widely accessible.

As we accumulate increasing amounts of data and pioneer new ways to utilize information for patient benefit, we are also developing an improved understanding of increasingly complex patterns of comorbidity and insights into the effect of genetic variation and heterogeneity on diagnosis and treatment outcomes. Sheldon Greenfield outlines the many factors that lead to heterogeneity of treatment effects (HTE)—variations in results produced by the same treatment in different patients—including genetic, environmental, adherence, polypharmacy, and competing risk. To improve the specificity of treatment recommendations, Greenfield suggests that prevailing approaches to study design and data analysis in clinical research must change. The authors propose two major strategies to decrease the impact of HTE in clinical research: (1) the use of composite risk scores derived from multivariate models should be considered in both the design of a priori risk stratification groups and data analysis of clinical research studies; and (2) the full range of sources of HTE, many of which arise for members of the general population not eligible for trails, should be addressed by integrating the multiple existing phases of clinical research, both before and after an RCT.

In a related paper, David Goldstein gives several examples that illustrate the mounting challenges and opportunities posed by genomics in tailoring treatment appropriately. He highlights recent work on the Clinical Antipsychotic Trials of Intervention Effectiveness (CATIE), which compared the effectiveness of atypical antipsychotics and one typical antipsychotic in the treatment of schizophrenia and Alzheimer's disease. While results indicated that, with respect to discontinuation of treatment, there was no difference between typical and atypical antipsychotics, in terms of adverse reactions, such as increased body weight or development of the irreversible condition known as tardive dyskinesia, these medications were actually quite distinct. Pharmacogenetics thus offers the potential ability to identify subpopulations of risk or benefit through the development of clinically useful diagnostics, but only if we begin to amass the data, methods, and resources needed to support pharmacogenetics research.

The final cluster of papers in this chapter engage some of the policy issues in expanding sources of evidence, such as those related to the interoperability of electronic health records, expanding post-market surveillance and the use of registries, and mediating an appropriate balance between patient privacy and access to clinical data. Weisman et al. comment on the rich opportunities presented by interoperable EHRs for post-marketing surveillance data and the development of additional insights on risk and effectiveness. Again, methodologies outside of the RCT will be increasingly instrumental in filling gaps in evidence that arise from the use of data related to interventions in clinical practice because the full value of an intervention cannot truly be appreciated without real-world usage. Expanded systems for post-marketing surveillance offer substantial opportunities to generate evidence; and in defining the approach, we also have an opportunity to align the interests of many healthcare stakeholders. Consumers will have access to technologies as well as information on appropriate use; manufacturers and regulatory agencies might recognize significant benefit from streamlined or harmonized data collection requirements; and decision makers might acquire means to accumulate much-needed data for comparative effectiveness studies or recognition of safety signals. Steve Teutsch and Mark Berger comment on the obvious utility of clinical studies, particularly comparative effectiveness studies—to demonstrate which technology is more effective, safer, or beneficial for subpopulations or clinical situation—for informing the decisions of patients, providers, and policy makers. However they also note several of the inherent difficulties of our current approach to generating needed information, including a lack of consensus on evidence standards and how they might vary depending on circumstance, and a needed advancement in the utilization, improvement, and validation of study methodologies.

An underlying theme in many of the workshop papers is the effect of HIPAA (Health Insurance Portability and Accountability Act) regulation on current research and the possible implications for utilizing data collected at the point of care for generation of evidence on effectiveness of interventions. In light of the substantial gains in quality of care and advances in research possible by linking health information systems and aggregating and sharing data, consideration must be given to how to provide access while maintaining appropriate levels of privacy and security for personal health information. Janlori Goldman and Beth Tossell give an overview of some of the issues that have emerged in response to privacy concerns about shared medical information. While linking medical information offers clear benefits for improving health care, public participation is necessary and will hinge on privacy and security being built in from the outset. The authors suggest a set of first principles regarding identifiers, access, data integrity, and participation that help move the discussion toward a workable solution. This issue has been central to many discussions of how to better streamline the healthcare system and facilitate the process of clinical research, while maximizing the ability to provide privacy and security for patients. A recent Institute of Medicine (IOM) workshop, sponsored by the National Cancer Policy Forum, examined some of the issues surrounding HIPAA and its effect on research, and a formal IOM study on the topic is anticipated in the near future.

EVOLVING METHODS: ALTERNATIVES TO LARGE RANDOMIZED CONTROLLED TRIALS

Robert M. Califf, M.D.
Duke Translational Medicine Institute and the Duke University Medical Center

Researchers and policy makers have used observational analyses to support medical decision making since the beginning of organized medical practice. However, recent advances in information technology have allowed researchers access to huge amounts of tantalizing data in the form of administrative and clinical databases, fueling increased interest in the question of whether alternative analytical methods might offer sufficient validity to elevate observational analysis in the hierarchy of medical knowledge. In fact, 25 years ago, my academic career was initiated with access to one of the first prospective clinical databases, an experience that led to several papers on the use of data from practice and the application of clinical experience to the evaluation and treatment of patients with coronary artery disease (Califf et al. 1983). However, this experience led me to conclude that no amount of statistical analysis can substitute for randomization in ensuring internal validity when comparing alternative approaches to diagnosis or treatment.

Nevertheless, the sheer volume of clinical decisions made in the absence of support from randomized controlled trials requires that we understand the best alternative methods when classical RCTs are unavailable, impractical, or inapplicable. This discussion elaborates upon some of the alternatives to large RCTs, including practical clinical trials, cluster randomized trials, observational treatment comparisons, interrupted time series, and instrumental variables analysis, and reviews some of the potential benefits and pitfalls of each approach.

Practical Clinical Trials

The term "large clinical trial" or "megatrial" conjures an image of a gargantuan undertaking capable of addressing only a few critical questions. The term "practical clinical trial" is greatly preferred because the size of a PCT need be no larger than that required to answer the question posed in terms of health outcomes—whether patients live longer, feel better, or incur fewer medical costs. Such issues are the relevant outcomes that drive patients to use a medical intervention.

Unfortunately, not enough RCTs employ the large knowledge base that was used in developing the principles relevant to conducting a PCT (Tunis et al. 2003). A PCT must include the comparison or alternative therapy that is relevant to the choices that patients and providers will make; all too often, RCTs pick a "weak" comparator or placebo. The populations studied should be representative; that is, they should include patients who would be likely to receive the treatment, rather than including low-risk or narrow populations selected in hopes of optimizing the efficacy or safety profile of the experimental therapy. The time period of the study should include the period relevant to the treatment decision, unlike short-term studies that require hypothetical extrapolation to justify continuous use.

Also, the background therapy should be appropriate for the disease, an issue increasingly relevant in the setting of international trials that include populations from developing countries. Such populations may be comprised of "treatment-naïve" patients, who will not offer the kind of therapeutic challenge presented by patients awaiting the new therapy in countries where active treatments are already available. Moreover, patients in developing countries usually do not have access to the treatment after it is marketed. Well-designed PCTs offer a solution to the "outsourcing" of clinical trials to populations of questionable relevance to therapeutic questions better addressed in settings where the treatments are intended to be used. Of course, the growth of clinical trials remains important for therapies that will actually be used in developing countries, and appropriate trials in these countries should be encouraged (Califf 2006a).

Therefore, the first alternative to a "classical" RCT is a properly designed and executed PCT. Research questions should be framed by the clinicians who will use the resulting information, rather than by companies aiming to create an advantage for their products through clever design. Similarly, a common fundamental mistake occurs when scientific experts without current knowledge of clinical circumstances are allowed to design trials. Instead, we need to involve clinical decision makers in the design of trials to ensure they are feasible and attractive to practice, as well as making certain that they include elements critical to providing generalizable knowledge for decision making.

Another fundamental problem is the clinical research enterprise's lack of organization. In many ways, the venue for the conduct of clinical trials is hardly a system at all, but rather a series of singular experiences in which researchers must deal with hundreds of clinics, health systems, and companies (and their respective data systems). Infrastructure for performing trials should be supported by the both the clinical care system and the National Institutes of Health (NIH), with continuous learning about the conduct of trials and constant improvements in their efficiency. However, the way trials are currently conducted is an engineering disaster. We hope that eventually trials will be embedded in a nodal network of health systems with electronic health records combined with specialty registries that cut across health systems (Califf et al. [in press]). Before this can happen, however, not only must EHRs be in place, but common data standards and nomenclature must be developed, and there must be coordination among numerous federal agencies (FDA, NIH, the Centers for Disease Control and Prevention [CDC], the Centers for Medicare and Medicaid Services [CMS]) and private industry to develop regulations that will not only allow, but encourage, use of interoperable data.

Alternatives to Randomized Comparisons

The fundamental need for randomization arises from the existence of treatment biases in practice. Recognizing that random assignment is essential to ensuring the internal validity of a study when the likely effects of an intervention are modest (and therefore subject to confounding by indication), we cannot escape the fact that nonrandomized comparisons will have less internal validity. However, nonrandomized analyses are nonetheless needed, because not every question can be answered by a classical RCT or a PCT, and a high-quality observational study is likely to be more informative than relying solely on clinical experience. For example, interventions come in many forms—drugs, devices, behavioral interventions, and organizational changes. All interventions carry a balance of potential benefit and potential risk; gathering important information on these interventions through an RCT or PCT might not always be feasible.

As an example of organizational changes requiring evaluation, consider the question: How many nurses, attendants, and doctors are needed for an inpatient unit in a hospital? Although standards for staffing have been developed for some environments relatively recently, in the era of computerized entry, EHRs, double-checking for medical errors, and bar coding, the proper allocation of personnel remains uncertain. Yet every day, executives make decisions based on data and trends, usually without a sophisticated understanding of their multivariable and time-oriented nature.

In other words, there is a disassociation between the experts in analysis of observational clinical data and the decision makers. There are also an increasing number of sources of data for decision making, with more and more healthcare systems and multispecialty practices developing data repositories. Instruments to extract data from such systems are also readily available. While these data are potentially useful, questionable data analyses and gluts of information (not all of it necessarily valid or useful) may create problems for decision makers.

Since PCTs are not feasible for answering the questions that underlie a good portion of the decisions made every day by administrators and clinicians, the question is not really whether we should look beyond the PCT. Instead, we should examine how best to integrate various modes of decision making, including both PCTs and other approaches to data analysis, in addition to opinion based on personal experience. We must ask ourselves: Is it better to combine evidence from PCTs with opinion, or is it better to use a layered approach using PCTs for critical questions and nonrandomized analyses to fill in gaps between clear evidence and opinion?

For the latter approach, we must think carefully about the levels of decision making that we must inform every day, the speed required for this, how to adapt the methodology to the level of certainty needed, and ways to organize growing data repositories and the researchers who will analyze them to better develop evidence to support these decisions. Much of the work in this arena is being conducted by the Centers for Education and Research in Therapeutics (CERTs) (Califf 2006b). The Agency for Healthcare Research and Quality (AHRQ) is a primary source of funding for these efforts, although significant increases in support will be needed to permit adequate progress in overcoming methodological and logistical hurdles.

Cluster Randomized Trials

If a PCT is not practical, the second alternative to large RCTs is cluster randomized trials. There is growing interest in this approach among trialists, because health systems increasingly provide venues in which practices vary and large numbers of patients are seen in environments that have good data collection capabilities. A cluster randomized trial performs randomization on the level of a practice rather than the individual patient. For example, certain sites are assigned to intervention A, others use intervention B, and a third group serves as a control. In large regional quality improvement projects, factorial designs can be used to test more than one intervention. This type of approach can yield clear and pragmatic answers, but as with any method, there are limitations that must be considered. Although methods have been developed to adjust for the nonindependence of observations within a practice, these methods are poorly understood and difficult to explain to clinical audiences. Another persistent problem is contamination that occurs when practices are aware of the experiment and alter their practices regardless of the randomized assignment. A further practical issue is obtaining informed consent from patients entering a health system where the practice has been randomized, recognizing that individual patient choice for interventions often enters the equation.

There are many examples of well-conducted cluster randomized trials. The Society of Thoracic Surgeons (STS), one of the premier learning organizations in the United States, has a single database containing data on more than 80 percent of all operations performed (Welke et al. 2004). Ferguson and colleagues (Ferguson et al. 2002) performed randomization at the level of surgical practices to test a behavioral intervention to improve use of postoperative beta blockers and the use of the internal thoracic artery as the main conduit for myocardial revascularization. Embedding this study into the ongoing STS registry proved advantageous, because investigators could examine what happened before and what happened after the experiment. They were able to show that both interventions work, that the use of this practice improved surgical outcomes, and that national practice improved after the study was completed.

Variations of this methodologic approach have also been quite successful, such as the amalgamation of different methods described in a recent study by (Schneeweiss et al. 2004). This study used both cluster randomization and time sequencing embedded in a single trial to examine nebulized respiratory therapy in adults and the effects of a policy change. Both approaches were found to yield similar results with regard to healthcare utilization, cost, and outcomes.

Observational Treatment Comparisons

A third alternative to RCTs is the observational treatment comparison. This is a potentially powerful technique requiring extensive experience with multiple methodological issues. Unfortunately, the somewhat delicate art of observational treatment comparison is mostly in the hands of naïve practitioners, administrators, and academic investigators who obtain access to databases without the skills to analyze them properly. The underlying assumption of the observational treatment comparison is that if the record includes information on which patients received which treatment, and outcomes have been measured, a simple analysis can evaluate which treatment is better. However in using observational treatment comparisons, one must always consider not only the possibility of confounding by indication and inception time bias, but also the possibility of missing data at baseline to adjust for differences, missing follow-up data, and poor characterization of outcomes due to a lack of prespecification. In order to deal with confounding, observational treatment comparisons must include adjustment for known prognostic factors, adjustment for propensity (including consideration of inverse weighted probability estimators for chronic treatments), and employment of time-adjusted covariates when inception time is variable.

Resolving some of these issues with definitions of outcomes and missing data will be greatly aided by development of interoperable clinical research networks that work together over time with support from government agencies. One example is the National Electronic Clinical Trials and Research (NECTAR) network—a planned NIH network that will link practices in the United States to academic medical centers by means of interoperable data systems. Unfortunately, NECTAR remains years away from actual implementation.

Despite the promise of observational studies, there are limitations that cannot be overcome even by the most experienced of researchers. For example, SUPPORT (Study to Understand Prognoses and Preferences for Outcomes and Risks of Treatment) (Connors et al. 1996; Cowley and Hager 1996) examined use of a right heart catheter (RHC) using prospectively collected data, so there were almost no missing data. After adjusting for all known prognostic factors and using a carefully developed propensity score, this study found an association between use of RHC in critically ill patients and an increased risk of death. Thirty other observational studies came to the same conclusion, even when looking within patient subgroups to ensure that comparisons were being made between comparable groups.

None of the credible observational studies showed a benefit associated with RHC, yet more than a billion dollars' worth of RHCs were being inserted in the United States every year.

Eventually, five years after publication of the SUPPORT RHC study, the NIH funded a pair of RCTs. One focused on heart disease and the other on medical intensive care. The heart disease study (Binanay et al. 2005; Shah et al. 2005) was a very simple trial in which patients were selected on the basis of admission to a hospital with acute decompensated heart failure. These patients were randomly assigned to receive either an RHC or standard care without an RHC. This trial found no evidence of harm or of benefit attributable to RHC. Moreover, other trials were being conducted around the world; when all the randomized data were in, the point estimate comparing the two treatments was 1.003: as close to "no effect" as we are likely ever to see. In this instance, even with some of the most skillful and experienced researchers in the world working to address the question of whether RHC is a harmful intervention, the observational data clearly pointed to harm, whereas RCTs indicated no particular harm or benefit.

Another example is drawn from the question of the association between hemoglobin and renal dysfunction. It is known that as renal function declines, there is a corresponding decrease in hemoglobin levels; therefore, worse renal function is associated with anemia. Patients with renal dysfunction and anemia have a significantly higher risk of dying, compared to patients with the same degree of renal dysfunction but without anemia. Dozens of different databases all showed the same relationship: the greater the decrease in hemoglobin level, the worse the outcome.

Based on these findings, many clinicians and policy makers assumed that by giving a drug to manage the anemia and improve hematocrit levels, outcomes would also be improved. Thus, erythropoietin treatment was developed and, on the basis of observational studies and very short term RCTs, has become a national practice standard. There are performance indicators that identify aggressive hemoglobin correction as a best practice; CMS pays for it; and nephrologists have responded by giving billions of dollars worth of erythropoietin to individuals with renal failure, with resulting measurable increases in average hemoglobin.

To investigate effects on outcome, the Duke Clinical Research Institute (DCRI) coordinated a PCT in patients who had renal dysfunction but did not require dialysis (Singh et al. 2006). Subjects were randomly assigned to one of two different target levels of hematocrit, normal or below normal. We could not use placebo, because most nephrologists were absolutely convinced of the benefit of erythropoietin therapy. However, when an independent data monitoring committee stopped the study for futility, a trend toward *worse* outcomes (death, stroke, heart attack, or heart failure) was seen in patients randomized to the more "normal" hematocrit target; when the final data were tallied, patients randomized to the more aggressive target had a *significant increase in the composite of death, heart attack, stroke and heart failure.* Thus the conclusions drawn from observational comparisons were simply incorrect.

These examples of highly touted observational studies that were ultimately seen to have provided incorrect answers (both positive and negative for different interventions) highlight the need to improve methods aimed at mitigating these methodological pitfalls. We must also consider how best to develop a critical mass of experts to guide us through these study methodologies, and what criteria should be applied to different types of decisions to ensure that the appropriate methods have been used.

Interrupted Time Series and Instrumental Variables

A fourth alternative to large RCTs is the interrupted time series. This study design requires significant expertise because it includes all the potential difficulties of observational treatment comparisons, plus uncertainties about temporal trends. However, one example is drawn from an analysis of administrative data, in which data were used to assess retrospective drug utilization review and effects on the rate of prescribing errors and on clinical outcomes (Hennessy et al. 2003). This study concluded that, although retrospective drug utilization review is required of all state Medicaid programs, the authors were unable to identify an effect on the rate of exceptions or on clinical outcomes.

The final alternative to RCTs is the use of instrumental variables, which are variables unrelated to biology that produce a contrast in treatment that can be characterized. A national quality improvement registry of patients with acute coronary syndromes evaluated the outcomes of use of early versus delayed cardiac catheterization using instrumental variable analysis (Ryan et al. 2005). The instrumental variable in this case was whether the patient was admitted to the hospital on the weekend (when catheterization delays were longer) or on a weekday (when time to catheterization is shorter). Results indicated a trend toward greater benefit of early invasive intervention in this high-risk condition. One benefit of this approach is that variables can be embedded in an ongoing registry (e.g., population characteristics in a particular zip code can be used to create an approximation of the socioeconomic status of a group of patients). However, results often are not definitive, and it is common for this type of study design to raise many more questions than it answers.

Future Directions: Analytical Synthesis

A national network funded by the AHRQ demonstrates a concerted, systematic approach to addressing all these issues in the context of clinical questions that require a synthesis of many types of analysis. The Developing Evidence to Inform Decisions about Effectiveness (DEcIDE) network seeks to inform the decisions that patients, healthcare providers, and administrators make about therapeutic choices. The DCRI's first project as part of the DEcIDE Network examines the issue of choice of coronary stents. This is a particularly interesting study because, while there are dozens of RCTs addressing this question, new evidence continues to emerge. Briefly, when drug-eluting stents (DES) first became available to clinicians, there was a radical shift in practice from bare metal stents (BMS) to DES. Observational data from our database—now covering about 30 years of practice—are very similar to those reported in RCTs and indicate reduced need for repeat procedures with DES, because they prevent restenosis in the stented area.

The problem, however, is that only one trial has examined long-term outcomes among patients who were systematically instructed to discontinue dual platelet aggregation inhibitors (i.e., aspirin and clopidogrel). This study (Pfisterer et al. In press; Harrington and Califf 2006) was funded by the Swiss government and shows a dramatic increase in abrupt thrombosis in people with DES compared with BMS when clopidogrel was discontinued per the package insert instructions, leaving the patients receiving only aspirin to prevent platelet aggregation. In the year following discontinuation of clopidogrel therapy, the primary composite end point of cardiac death or myocardial infarction occurred significantly more frequently among patients with DES than in the BMS group. This was a small study, but it raises an interesting question: If you could prevent restenosis in 10 out of 100 patients but had 1 case of acute heart attack per 100, how would you make that trade-off? This is precisely the question we are addressing with the DEcIDE project.

Despite all these complex issues, the bottom line is that when evidence is applied systematically to practice improvement, there is a continuous improvement in patient outcomes (Mehta et al. 2002; Bhatt et al. 2004). Thus the application of clinical practice guidelines and performance measures seems to be working, but all of us continue to dream about improving the available evidence base and using this evidence on a continuous basis. However, this can only come to pass when we use informatics to integrate networks, not just within health systems but across the nation. We will need continuous national registries (of which we now have examples), but we also need to link existing networks so that clinical studies can be conducted more effectively. This will help ensure that patients, physicians, and scientists form true "communities of research" as we move from typical networks of academic health center sites linked only by a single data coordinating center to networks where interoperable sites can share data.

A promising example of this kind of integration exists in the developing network for child psychiatry. This is a field that historically has lacked evidence to guide treatments; however, there are currently 200 psychiatrists participating in the continuous collection of data that will help answer important questions, using both randomized and nonrandomized trials (March et al. 2004).

The classical RCT remains an important component of our evidence-generating system. However, it needs to be replaced in many situations by the PCT, which has a distinctly different methodology but includes the critical element of randomization. Given the enormous number of decisions that could be improved by appropriate decision support however, alternative methods for assessing the relationships between input variables and clinical outcomes must be used. We now have the technology in place in many health systems and government agencies to incorporate decision support into practice, and methods will evolve with use. An appreciation of both the pitfalls and the advantages of these methods, together with the contributions of experienced analysts, will be critical to avoiding errant conclusions drawn from these complex datasets, in which confounding and nonintuitive answers are the rule rather than the exception.

EVOLVING METHODS: EVALUATING MEDICAL DEVICE INTERVENTIONS IN A RAPID STATE OF FLUX

Telba Irony, Ph.D.
Center for Devices and Radiological Health, Food and Drug Administration

Methodological obstacles slow down the straightforward use of clinical data and experience to assess the safety and effectiveness of new medical device interventions in a rapid state of flux. This paper discusses current and future technology trends, the FDA's Critical Path Initiative, the Center for Devices and Radiological Health (CDRH), Medical Device Innovation Initiative and, in particular, statistical methodology being currently implemented by CDRH to take better advantage of data generated by clinical studies designed to assess safety and effectiveness of medical device interventions.

The Critical Path is the FDA's premier initiative aiming to identify and prioritize the most pressing medical product development problems and the greatest opportunities for rapid improvement in public health benefits. As a major source of breakthrough technology, medical devices are becoming more critical to the delivery of health care in the United States. In addition, they are becoming more and more diverse and complex as improvements are seen in devices ranging from surgical sutures and contact lenses to prosthetic heart valves and diagnostic imaging systems.

There are exciting emerging technology trends on the horizon and our objective is to obtain evidence on the safety and effectiveness of new medical device products as soon as possible to ensure their quick approval and time to market. New trends comprise computer-related technology and molecular medicine including genomics, proteomics, gene therapy, bioinformatics, and personalized medicine. We will also see new developments in wireless systems and robotics to be applied in superhigh-spatial-precision surgery, in vitro sample handling, and prosthetics. We foresee an increase in the development and use of minimally invasive technologies, nanotechnology (extreme miniaturization), new diagnostic procedures (genetic, in vitro, or superhigh-resolution sensors), artificial organ replacements, decentralized health care (home or self-care, closed-loop home systems, and telemedicine), and products that are a combination of devices and drugs.

CDRH's mission is to establish a reasonable assurance of the safety and effectiveness of medical devices and the safety of radiation-emitting electronic products marketed in the United States. It also includes monitoring medical devices and radiological products for continued safety after they are in use, as well as helping the public receive accurate, evidence-based information needed to improve health. To accomplish its mission, CDRH must perform a balancing act to get safe and effective devices to the market as quickly as possible while ensuring that devices currently on the market remain safe and effective. To better maintain this balance and confront the challenge of evaluating new medical device interventions in a rapid state of flux, CDRH is promoting the Medical Device Innovation Initiative. Through this initiative, CDRH is expanding current efforts to promote scientific innovation in product development, focusing device research on cutting-edge science, modernizing the review of innovative devices, and facilitating a least burdensome approach to clinical trials. Ongoing efforts include the development of guidance documents to improve clinical trials and to maximize the information gathered by such trials, the expansion of laboratory research, a program to improve the quality of the review of submissions to the CDRH, and expansion of the clinical and scientific expertise at the FDA. The Medical Device Critical Path Opportunities report (FDA 2004) identified key opportunities in the development of biomarkers, improvement in clinical trial design, and advances in bioinformatics, device manufacturing, public health needs, and pediatrics.

The "virtual family" is an example of a project encompassed by this initiative. It consists of the development of anatomic and physiologically accurate adult and pediatric virtual circulatory systems to help assess the safety and effectiveness of new stent designs prior to fabrication, physical testing, animal testing, and human trials. This project is based on a computer simulation model which is designed to mimic all physical and physiological responses of a human being to a medical device. It is the first step toward a virtual clinical trial subject. Another example is the development of a new statistical model for predicting the effectiveness of implanted cardiac stents through surrogate outcomes, to measure and improve the long-term safety of these products.

To better generate evidence on which to base clinical decisions, the Medical Device Innovation Initiative emphasizes the need for improved statistical approaches and techniques to learn about the safety and effectiveness of medical device interventions in an efficient way. It seeks to conduct smaller and possibly shorter trials, and to create a better decision-making process.

Well-designed and conducted clinical trials are at the center of clinical decision making today and the clinical trial gold standard is the prospectively planned, randomized, controlled clinical trial. However, it is not always feasible to conduct such a trial, and in many cases, conclusions and decisions must be based on controlled, but not randomized, clinical trials, comparisons of an intervention to a historical control or registry, observational studies, meta-analyses based on publications, and post-market surveillance. There is a crucial need to improve assessment and inference methods to extract as much information as possible from such studies and to deal with different types of evidence.

Statistical methods are evolving as we move to an era of large volumes of data on platforms conducive to analyses. However, being able to easily analyze data can also be dangerous because it can lead to false discoveries, resources wasted chasing false positives, wrong conclusions, and suboptimal or even bad decisions. CDRH is therefore investigating new statistical technology that can help avoid misleading conclusions, provide efficient and faster ways to learn from evidence, and enable better and faster medical decision making. Examples include new methods to adjust for multiplicity to ensure that study findings will be reproduced in practice as well as new methods to deal with subgroup analysis.

A relatively new statistical method that is being used to reduce bias in the comparison of an intervention to a nonrandomized control group is propensity score analysis. It is a method to match patients by finding patients that are equivalent in the treatment and control groups. This statistical method may be used in nonrandomized controlled trials and the control group may be a registry or a historical control. The use of this technique in observational studies attempts to balance the observed covariates. However, unlike trials in which there is random assignment of treatments, this technique cannot balance the unobserved covariates.

One of the new statistical methods being used to design and analyze clinical trials is the Bayesian approach, which has been implemented and used at CDRH for the last seven years, giving excellent results. The Bayesian approach is a statistical theory and approach to data analysis that provides a coherent method for learning from evidence as it accumulates. Traditional (also called frequentist) statistical methods formally use prior information only in the design of a clinical trial. In the data analysis stage, prior information is not part of the analysis. In contrast, the Bayesian approach uses a consistent, mathematically formal method called Bayes' Theorem for combining prior information with current information on a quantity of interest. When good prior information on a clinical use of a medical device exists, the Bayesian approach may enable the FDA to reach the same decision on a device with a smaller-sized or shorter-duration pivotal trial. Good prior information is often available for medical devices. The sources of prior information include the company's own previous studies, previous generations of the same device, data registries, data on similar products that are available to the public, pilot studies, literature controls, and legally available previous experience using performance characteristics of similar products. The payoff of this approach is the ability to conduct smaller and shorter trials, and to use more information for decision making. Medical device trials are amenable to the use of prior information because the mechanism of action of medical devices is typically physical, making the effects local and not systemic. Local effects are often predictable from prior information when modifications to a device are minor.

Bayesian methods may be controversial when the prior information is based mainly on personal opinion (often derived by elicitation methods). They are often not controversial when the prior information is based on empirical evidence such as prior clinical trials. Since sample sizes are typically small for device trials, good prior information can have greater impact on the analysis of the trial and thus on the FDA decision process.

The Bayesian approach may also be useful in the absence of informative prior information. First, the approach can provide flexible methods for handling interim analyses and other modifications to trials in midcourse (e.g., changes to the sample size). Conducting an interim analysis during a Bayesian clinical trial and being able to predict the outcome at midcourse enables early stopping either for early success or for futility. Another advantage of the Bayesian approach is that it allows for changing the randomization ratio at mid-trial. This can ensure that more patients in the trial receive the intervention with the highest probability of success, and it is not only ethically preferable but also encourages clinical trial participation. Finally, the Bayesian approach can be useful in complex modeling situations where a frequentist analysis is difficult to implement or does not exist.

Several devices have been approved through the use of the Bayesian approach. The first example was the INTER FIX™ Threaded Fusion Device by Medtronic Sofamor Danek, which was approved in 1999. That device is indicated for spinal fusion in patients with degenerative disc disease. In that case, a Bayesian predictive analysis was used in order to stop the trial early. The statistical plan used data of 12-month visits combined with partial data of 24-month visits to predict the results of patients who had not reached 24 months in the study (later these results were confirmed). Later (after approval) the sponsor completed the follow-up requirements for the patients enrolled in the study. The final results validated the Bayesian predictive analysis, which significantly reduced the time that was needed for completion of the trial (FDA 1999).

Another example is the clinical trial designed to assess the safety and effectiveness of the LT-CAGE™ Tapered Fusion Device, by Medtronic Sofamor Danek, approved in September 2000. This device is also indicated for spinal fusion in patients with degenerative disc disease. The trial to assess safety and effectiveness of the device was planned as Bayesian, and Bayesian statistical methods were used to analyze the results. Data from patients that were evaluated at 12 and 24 months were used combined with data from patients evaluated only at 12 months in order to make predictions and comparisons for success rates at 24 months. The Bayesian predictions performed during the interim analyses significantly reduced the sample size and the time that was needed for completion of the trial. Again, the results were later confirmed (Lipscomb et al. 2005; FDA 2002).

A third example, where prior information was used along with interim analyses is the Bayesian trial for the St. Jude Medical Regent heart valve, which was a modification of the previously approved St. Jude Standard heart valve. The objective of this trial was to assess the safety and effectiveness of the Regent heart valve. The trial used prior information from the St. Jude Standard heart valve by borrowing the information via Bayesian hierarchical models. In addition, the Bayesian experimental design provided a method to determine the stopping time based on the amount of information gathered during the trial and the prediction of what future results would be. The trial stopped early for success (FDA 2006).

In 2006, the FDA issued a draft guidance for industry and FDA staff that elaborates on the use of Bayesian methods. It covers Bayesian statistics, planning a Bayesian clinical trial, analyzing a Bayesian clinical trial, and post-market surveillance. A public meeting for discussion of the guidance took place in July 2006; this can be found at http://www.fda.gov/cdrh/meetings/072706-bayesian.html.

In general, adaptive trial designs, either Bayesian or frequentist, constitute an emerging field that seems to hold promise for more ethical and efficient development of medical interventions by allowing fuller integration of available knowledge as trials proceed. However, all aspects and trade-offs of such design need to be understood before they are widely used. Clearly there are major logistic, procedural, and operational challenges in using adaptive clinical trial designs, not all of them as yet resolved. However, they have the potential to play a large role and be beneficial in the future. The Pharmaceutical Research and Manufacturers of America (PhRMA) and the FDA organized a workshop that took place on November 13 and 14, 2006, in Bethesda, Maryland, to discuss challenges, opportunities and scope of adaptive trial designs in the development of medical interventions. PhRMA has formed a working group on adaptive designs that aims to facilitate a constructive dialogue on the topic by engaging statisticians, clinicians, and other stakeholders in academia, regulatory agencies, and industry to facilitate broader consideration and implementation of such designs. PhRMA produced a series of articles that have been published in the *Drug Information Journal*, Volume 40, 2006.

Finally, formal decision analysis is a mathematical tool that should be used when making decisions on whether or not to approve a device. This methodology has the potential to enhance the decision-making process and make it more transparent by better accounting for the magnitude of the benefits as compared with the risks of a medical intervention.

CDRH is also committed to achieving a seamless approach to regulation of medical devices in which the pre-market activities are integrated with continued post-market surveillance and enforcement. In addition, appropriate and timely information is fed back to the public. This regulatory approach encompasses the entire life cycle of a medical device. The "total product life cycle" enhances CDRH's ability to fulfill its mission to protect and promote public health. CDRH's pre-market review program cannot guarantee that all legally marketed devices will function perfectly in the post-market setting. Pre-market data provide a reasonable estimate of device performance but may not be large enough to detect the occurrence of rare adverse events. Moreover, device performance can render unanticipated outcomes in post-market use, when the environment is not as controlled as in the pre-market setting. Efforts are made to forecast post-market performance based on pre-market data, but the dynamics of the post-market environment create unpredictable conditions that are impossible to investigate during the pre-market phase. As a consequence, CDRH is committed to a Post-market Transformation Initiative and recently published two documents on the post-market safety of medical devices. One describes CDRH's post-market tools and the approaches used to monitor and address adverse events and risks associated with the use of medical devices that are currently on the market (see "Ensuring the Safety of Marketed Medical Devices: CDRH's Medical Device Post-market Safety Framework"). The second document provides a number of recommendations for improving the post-market program (see "Report of the Post-market Transformation Leadership Team: Strengthening FDA's Post-market Program for Medical Devices"). Both of these documents are available at http://www.fda.gov/cdrh/postmarket/mdpi.html. It is important to mention that one of the recommended actions to transform the way CDRH handles post-market information to assess the performance of marketed medical device products is to design a pilot study to investigate quantitative decision-making techniques to evaluate medical devices throughout the "total product life cycle."

In conclusion, as the world of medical devices becomes more complex, the Center for Devices and Radiological Health is developing tools to collect information, make decisions, and manage risk in the twenty-first century. Emerging medical device technology will fundamentally transform the healthcare and delivery system, provide new and cutting-edge solutions, challenge existing paradigms, and revolutionize the way treatments are administered.

EVOLVING METHODS: MATHEMATICAL MODELS TO HELP FILL THE GAPS IN EVIDENCE

David M. Eddy, M.D., Ph.D., and David C. Kendrick, M.D., M.P.H.
Archimedes, Inc.

A commitment to evidence-based medicine makes excellent sense. It helps ensure that decisions are founded on empirical observations. It helps ensure that recommended treatments are in fact effective and that ineffective treatments are not recommended. It also helps reduce the burden, uncertainty, and variations that plague decisions based on subjective judgments. Ideally, we would answer every important question with a clinical trial or other equally valid source of empirical observations.

Unfortunately, this is not feasible. Reasons include high costs, long durations, large sample sizes, difficulty getting physicians and patients to participate, large number of options to be studied, speed of technological innovation, and the fact that the questions can change before the trials are completed. For these reasons we need to find alternative ways to answer questions—to fill the gaps in the empirical evidence.

One of these is to use mathematical models. The concept is straightforward. Mathematical models use observations of real events (data) to derive equations that represent the relationships between variables. These equations can then be used to calculate events that have never been directly observed. For a simple example, data on the distances traveled when moving at particular speeds for particular lengths of time can be used to derive the equation "distance = rate × time" ($D = RT$). Then, that equation can be used to calculate the distance traveled at any other speeds for any other times. Mathematical models have proven themselves enormously valuable in other fields, from calculating mortgage payments, to designing budgets, to flying airplanes, to taking photos of Mars, to e-mail. They have also been successful in medicine, examples being computed tomography (CT) scans and magnetic resonance imaging (MRI), radiation therapy, and electronic health records. Surely there must be a way they can help us improve the evidence base for clinical medicine.

There is very good reason to believe they can, provided some conditions are met. First, we must understand that models will never be able to completely replace clinical trials. There are several reasons. Most fundamentally, trials are our anchor to reality—they are observations of real events. Models are not directly connected to reality. Indeed, models are built from trials and other sources of empirical observations. They are simplified representations of reality, filtered by observations and constrained by equations and will never be as accurate as reality. Not only are they one step removed from empirical observations, but they cannot exist without them. Thus, if it is feasible to answer a question with a clinical trial, then that is the preferred approach. Models should be used to fill the gaps in evidence only when clinical trials are not feasible.

The second condition is that the model should be validated against the clinical trials that do exist. More specifically, before we rely on a model to answer a question we should ensure that it accurately reproduces or predicts the most important clinical trials that are adjacent to or surround that question. The terms "adjacent to" and "surround" are intended to identify the trials that involve similar populations, interventions, and outcomes. For example, suppose we want to compare the effects of atorvastatin, simvastatin, and pravastatin on the 10-year rate of myocardial infarctions (MIs) in people with coronary artery disease (previous MI, angina, history of percutaneous transluminal coronary angioplasty [PTCA], or bypass). These head-to-head comparisons have never been performed, and it would be extraordinarily difficult to do so, given the long time period (10 years), very large sample sizes required (tens of thousands), and very high costs (hundreds of millions of dollars). However a mathematical model could help answer these questions if it had already been shown to reproduce or predict the existing trials of these drugs versus placebos in similar populations. In this case the major adjacent trials would include 4S, the Scandinavian Simvastatin Survival Study (Randomised trial of cholesterol lowering in 4,444 patients with coronary heart disease [4S] 1994); WOSCOPS (Shepherd et al. 1995); CARE (Flaker et al. 1999), LIPID (Prevention of cardiovascular events and death with pravastatin in patients with coronary heart disease and a broad range of initial cholesterol levels [LIPID] 1998), PROSPER (Shepherd et al. 2002), CARDS (Colhoun et al. 2004), TNT (LaRosa et al. 2005), and IDEAL (Pedersen et al. 2005).

The methods for selecting the surrounding trials and performing the validations are beyond the scope of this paper, but four important elements are that (1) the trials should be identified or at least reviewed by a third party, (2) the validations should be performed at the highest level of clinical detail of which the model is capable, (3) all the validations should be performed with the same version of the model, and (4) to the greatest extent possible, the validations should be independent in the sense that they were not used to help build the model. On the third point, it would be meaningless if a model were tweaked or parameters were refitted to match the results of each trial. On the fourth point, it is almost inevitable that some trials will have been used to help build a model. In those cases we say that the validation is "dependent"; these validations ensure that the model can faithfully reproduce the assumptions used to build it. If no information from a trial was used to help build the model, we say that a validation against that trial is "independent." These validations provide insights into the model's ability to simulate events in new areas, such as new settings, target populations, interventions, outcomes, and durations.

If these conditions are met for a question, it is not feasible to conduct a new trial to answer the question, and there is a model that can reproduce or predict the major trials that are most pertinent to the question, then it is reasonable to use the model to fill in the gaps between the existing trials. While that approach will not be as desirable as conducting a new clinical trial, one can certainly argue that it is better than the alternative, which is clinical or expert judgment.

If a model *is* used, then the degree of confidence we can place in its results will depend on the number of adjacent trials against which it has been validated, on the "distance" between the questions being asked and the real trials, and on how well the model's results matched the real results. For example, one could have a fairly high degree of confidence in a model's results if the question is about a subpopulation of an existing trial whose overall results the model has already predicted. Other examples of analyses about which we could be fairly confident are the following:

- Head-to head comparisons of different drugs, all of which have been studied in their own placebo-controlled trials, such as comparing atorvastatin, simvastatin, and pravastatin;
- Extension of a trial's results to settings with different levels of physician performance and patient compliance;
- Studies of different doses of drugs, or combinations of drugs, for which there are good data from phase II trials on biomarkers, and there are other trials connecting the biomarkers to clinical outcomes;
- Extensions of a trial's results to longer follow-up times; and
- Analyses of different mixtures of patients, such as different proportions of people with CAD, particular race/ethnicities, comorbidities,

or use of tobacco, provided the model's accuracy for these groups has been tested in other trials.

As one moves further from the existing trials and validations, the degree of confidence in the model's results will decrease. At the extreme, a model that is well validated for, say Type 2 diabetes, cannot be considered valid for a different disease, such as coronary artery disease (CAD), congestive heart failure (CHF), cancer, or even Type 1 diabetes. A corollary of this is that a model is never "validated" in a general sense, as though that were a property of the model that carries with it to every new question. Models are validated for specific purposes, and as each new question is raised, their accuracy in predicting the trials that surround that question needs to be examined.

Example: Prevention of Diabetes in High-Risk People

We can illustrate these concepts with an example. Several studies have indicated that individuals at high risk for developing diabetes can be identified from the general population and that with proper management the onset of diabetes can be delayed, or perhaps even prevented altogether (Tuomilehto et al. 2001; Knowler et al. 2002; Snitker et al. 2004; Chiasson et al. 1998; Gerstein et al. 2006). Although these results indicate the potential value of treating high-risk people, the short durations and limited number of interventions studied in these trials leave many important questions unanswered.

Taking the Diabetes Prevention Program (DPP) as an example, it showed that in people at high risk of developing diabetes, over a follow-up period of four years about 35 percent developed diabetes (the control arm). Metformin decreased this to about 29 percent, for a relative reduction of about 17 percent. Lifestyle modification decreased it to about 18 percent, for a relative reduction of about 48 percent. Over the mean follow-up period of 2.8 years the relative reduction was about 58 percent. This is certainly an encouraging finding and is sufficient to stimulate interest in diabetes prevention. However 2.8 years or even 4 years is far too short to determine the effects of these interventions on the long term progression of diabetes or any of its complications; for example:

- Do the prevention programs just postpone diabetes or do they prevent it altogether?
- What are the long-term effects of the prevention programs on the probabilities of micro- and macrovascular complications of diabetes, such as cardiovascular disease, retinopathy, and nephropathy?

- What are the effects on long-term costs, and what are the cost-effectiveness ratios of the prevention programs?
- Are there any other programs that might be more cost effective?
- What would a program have to cost in order to break even—no increase in net cost?

These new questions need to be answered if we are to plan diabetes prevention programs rationally. Ideally, we would answer them by continuing the DPP for another 20 to 30 years. But that is not possible for obvious reasons. The only possible method is to use a mathematical model to extend the trial. Specifically, if a model contains all the important variables and can demonstrate that it is capable of reproducing the DPP, along with other trials that document the outcomes of diabetes, then we could use it to run a simulated version of the DPP for a much longer period of time. This approach would also enable us to explore other types of prevention activities and see how they compare with metformin and the lifestyle modification program used in the DPP.

An example of such a model is the Archimedes model. Descriptions of the model have been published elsewhere (Schlessinger and Eddy 2002; Eddy and Schlessinger 2003a, 2003b). Basically, the core of the model is a set of ordinary and differential equations that represent human physiology at roughly the level of detail found in general medical textbooks, patient charts, and clinical trials. It is continuous in time, with clinical events occurring at any time. Biological variables are continuous and relate to one another in ways that they are understood to interact in vivo. Building out from this core, the Archimedes model includes the development of signs and symptoms, patient behaviors in seeking care, clinical events such as visits and admissions, protocols, provider behaviors and performance, patient compliance, logistics and utilization, health outcomes, quality of life, and costs. Thus the model simulates a comprehensive health system in which virtual people get virtual diseases, seek care at virtual hospitals and clinics, are seen by virtual healthcare providers, who have virtual behaviors, use virtual equipments and supplies, generate virtual costs, and so forth. An analogy is Electronic Arts' SimCity game, but starting at the level of detail of the underlying physiologies of each of the people in the simulation rather than city streets and utility systems. This relatively high level of physiological detail enables the model to simulate diseases such as diabetes and their treatments. For example, in the model people have livers, which produce glucose, which is affected by insulin resistance and can be affected by metformin. Similarly, people in the model can change their lifestyles and lose weight, which affects the progression of many things including insulin resistance, blood pressure, cholesterol levels, and so forth. Thus the Archimedes model is well positioned to study the effects of activities to prevent diabetes.

The Archimedes model is validated by using the simulated healthcare system to conduct simulated clinical trials that correspond to real clinical trials (Eddy et al. 2005). This provides the opportunity to compare the outcomes calculated in the model with outcomes seen in the real trials. Thus far the model has been validated against more than 30 trials. The first 18 trials, with seventy-four separate treatment arms and outcomes, were selected by an independent committee appointed by the American Diabetes Association (ADA) and have been published (Eddy et al. 2005). The overall correlation coefficient between the model's results and those of the actual trials is 0.98. Ten of the eighteen trials in the ADA-chosen validations provided independent validations; they were not used to build the model itself. The correlation coefficient for these independent validations was 0.96. An example of an independent validation that is particularly important for this application is a prospective, independent validation of the DPP trial itself; the published results matched the predicted results quite closely (Figure 2-1). The Archimedes model also accurately simulated several trials that

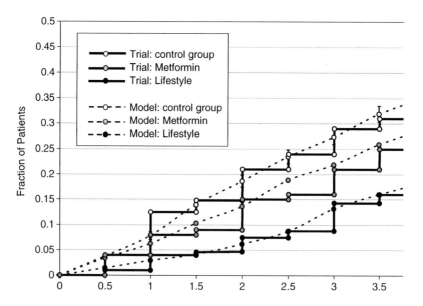

FIGURE 2-1 Model's predictions of outcomes in Diabetes Prevention Program. Comparison of proportions of people progressing to diabetes in the control group observed in the real Diabetes Prevention Program (DPP) (solid lines) and in the simulation of the DPP by the Archimedes model (dashed lines).
SOURCE: Eddy et al. *Annals of Internal Medicine* 2005; 143:251-264.

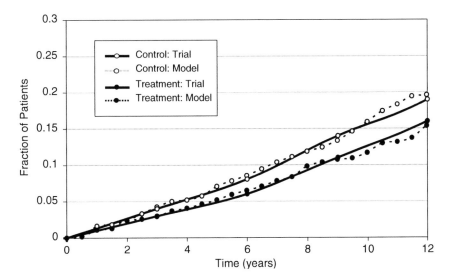

FIGURE 2-2 Comparison of model's calculations and results of the United Kingdom Prospective Diabetes Study (UKPDS): Rates of myocardial infarctions in control and treated groups.
SOURCE: Eddy et al. *Annals of Internal Medicine* 2005; 143:251-264.

observed the progression of diabetes, development of complications, and effects of treatment.

An important example is the progression of diabetes and development of coronary artery disease in the United Kingdom Prospective Diabetes Study (Figure 2-2). The ability of the model to simulate or predict a large number of trials relating to diabetes and its complications builds confidence in its results.

Thus the prevention of diabetes in high-risk people meets the criteria outlined above—it is impractical or impossible to answer the important questions with real clinical trials, there is a model capable of addressing the questions at the appropriate level of physiological detail, and the model has been successfully validated against a wide range of adjacent clinical trials.

Methods

Use of the Archimedes model to analyze the prevention of diabetes in high risk people has been reported in detail elsewhere (Eddy et al. 2005). To summarize, the first step was to create a simulated population that corresponds to the population used in the DPP trial. This was done by starting with a representative sample of the U.S. population, from the National Health and Nutrition Examination Survey (NHANES (National Health and Nutrition Evaluation Survey 1998-2002), and then applying the inclusion and exclusion criteria for the DPP to select a sample that matched the DPP population. Specifically, the DPP defined individuals to be at high risk for developing diabetes and included them in the trial if they had all of the following: body mass index (BMI) > 24, fasting plasma glucose (FPG) 90-125 mg/dL, and oral glucose tolerance test (OGTT) of 140-199 mg/dL. We then created copies or clones of the selected people from NHANES, by matching them on approximately 35 variables. A total of 10,000 people were selected and copied. This group was then exposed to three different interventions, corresponding to the arms of the real trial (baseline or control, metformin begun immediately, and the DPP lifestyle program begun immediately). The three groups were then followed for 30 years and observed for progression of diabetes and development of major complications such as myocardial infarction, stroke, end-stage renal disease, and retinopathy. Cost-generating events as well as symptoms and outcomes that affect the quality of life were also measured. The results could then be used to answer the questions about the long-term effects of diabetes prevention.

Do the Prevention Programs Just Postpone Diabetes or Do They Prevent It Altogether?

This can be answered by comparing the effects of metformin and lifestyle on the proportion of people who developed diabetes over the 30-year period. The results are shown in Figure 2-3. The natural rate of progression to diabetes, seen in the control group, was 72 percent over the 30-year follow-up period. Lifestyle modification, as offered in the DPP and continued until a person develops diabetes, would reduce the incidence of diabetes to about 61 percent, for a relative reduction of 15 percent. Thus, over a 30-year horizon the DPP lifestyle modification would actually prevent diabetes in about 11 percent of cases, while delaying it in the remaining 61 percent. In the metformin arm, about 4 percent of cases of diabetes would be prevented, for a 5.5 percent relative reduction in the 30-year incidence of diabetes.

What Are the Long-Term Effects of the Prevention Programs on the Probabilities of Micro- and Macrovascular Complications of Diabetes, like Cardiovascular Disease, Retinopathy, and Nephropathy?

This question is also readily answered, in this case by counting the number of clinical outcomes that occur in the control and lifestyle groups. The effects of the DPP lifestyle program on long-term complications of dia-

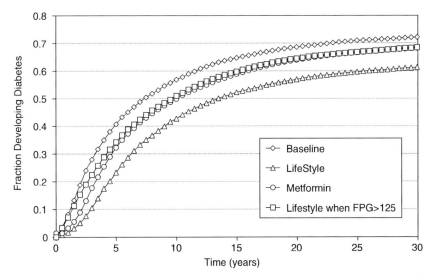

FIGURE 2-3 Model's calculation of progression to diabetes in four programs. SOURCE: Eddy et al. *Annals of Internal Medicine* 2005; 143:251-264.

betes are shown in Table 2-1. The 30-year rate of serious complications (including myocardial infarctions, congestive heart failure, retinopathy, stroke, nephropathy, and neuropathy) was reduced by an absolute 8.4 percent, from about 38.2 percent to about 29.8 percent, or a relative decrease of about 22 percent. The effects on other outcomes are shown in Table 2-1.

What Are the Effects on Long-Term Costs, and What Are the Cost-Effectiveness Ratios of the Prevention Programs?

The effects of the prevention activities on these outcomes can be determined by tracking all the clinical events and conditions that affect quality of life or that generate costs. Over 30 years, the aggregate per-person cost of providing care for diabetes and its complications in the control group was $37,171. The analogous costs in the metformin and lifestyle groups were $4,081 and $9,969 higher, respectively. The average cost-effectiveness ratios for the metformin and lifestyle groups (both compared to no intervention, or the control group), measured in terms of dollars per quality adjusted life year (QALY) gained, were $35,523 and $62,602, respectively.

TABLE 2-1 Expected Outcomes Over Various Time Horizons for Typical Person with DPP Characteristics

Years of Follow-Up	Without Lifestyle Program (baseline)			Difference made by Lifestyle Program		
	10	20	30	10	20	30
Diabetes	56.91%	68.55%	72.18%	–14.26%	–11.58%	–10.84%
CAD/CHF						
Have an MI	3.98%	8.53%	12.02%	–0.39%	–1.07%	–1.65%
Develop CHF (systolic or diastolic)	0.23%	0.67%	1.19%	–0.07%	–0.07%	–0.08%
Retinopathy						
Develop "Blindness" (legal)	0.71%	2.16%	3.02%	–0.39%	–1.04%	–1.44%
Develop prolific diabetic retinopathy	1.38%	3.15%	4.33%	–0.68%	–1.36%	–1.40%
Develop retinopathy	1.11%	2.57%	3.39%	–0.53%	–1.15%	–1.21%
Total serious eye complication	3.20%	7.89%	10.74%	–1.60%	–3.55%	–4.05%
Stroke (ischemic or hemorrhagic)	2.89%	6.99%	11.61%	–0.46%	–0.97%	–1.42%
Nephropathy						
Develop ESRD	0.00%	0.00%	0.07%	0.00%	0.00%	–0.04%
Need Dialysis	0.00%	0.00%	0.05%	0.00%	0.00%	–0.03%
Need a kidney transplant	0.00%	0.00%	0.02%	0.00%	0.00%	–0.01%
Total serious kidney complication	0.00%	0.00%	0.15%	0.00%	0.00%	–0.08%
Neuropathy (symptomatic)						
Develop foot ulcers	0.68%	1.43%	1.78%	–0.38%	–0.65%	–0.74%

Are There Any Other Programs That Might Be More Cost-Effective?

The DPP had three arms: control, metformin begun immediately (i.e., when the patient is at risk of developing diabetes, but has not yet developed diabetes), and lifestyle modification begun immediately. Given the high cost of the lifestyle intervention as it was implemented in the DPP, it is reasonable to ask what the effect would be of waiting until a person progressed to diabetes and then beginning the lifestyle intervention. It is clearly not possible to go back and restart the DPP with this new treatment arm, but it is fairly easy to add it to a simulated trial. The results are summarized in Table 2-2. Compared to beginning the lifestyle modification immediately, waiting until a person develops diabetes gives up about 0.034 QALY, or about 21 percent of the effectiveness seen with immediate lifestyle modifica-

TABLE 2-1 Continued

Years of Follow-Up	Without Lifestyle Program (baseline)			Difference made by Lifestyle Program		
	10	20	30	10	20	30
Need a Partial foot amputation	0.17%	0.58%	0.74%	−0.04%	−0.31%	−0.37%
Need an Amputation	0.00%	0.00%	0.03%	0.01%	0.02%	−0.01%
Total serious foot complication	0.84%	2.01%	2.55%	−0.41%	−0.94%	−1.12%
Total for all complications	11.15%	26.08%	38.24%	−2.94%	−6.60%	−8.40%
Deaths						
CHD	2.22%	6.65%	11.90%	−0.61%	−1.07%	−2.01%
Stroke	0.37%	0.94%	1.48%	−0.08%	−0.25%	−0.26%
Renal disease	0.00%	0.02%	0.09%	0.00%	−0.01%	−0.04%
Death from any complication	2.59%	7.61%	13.47%	−0.70%	−1.32%	−2.31%
Life Years			24.032			0.288
QALYs (undiscounted)			16.125			0.276
QALYs (discounted 3%)			11.319			0.159

ABBREVIATIONS:
DPP – Diabetes Prevention Program; CAD – coronary artery disease; CHF – congestive heart failure; MI – myocardial infarction; ESRD – end-stage renal disease; CHD – coronary heart disease; QALY – quality-adjusted life-year
NOTE: For each time horizon, the entries are the chance of having a complication or the decrease in chance of a complication, up to the end of that time horizon. The columns labeled "Baseline" give the chances that would apply with the Baseline program; "Difference" gives the increase or decrease in chance of a complication caused by the DPP lifestyle program. The chances that would occur with the DPP lifestyle program can be determined from the table by subtracting the "Difference" from the "Baseline" figures.
SOURCE: Eddy et al. *Annals of Internal Medicine* 2005; 143:251-264.

tion. However, the delayed lifestyle program increases costs about $3,066, or about one-third as much as the immediate lifestyle program. Thus the delayed program is more cost-effective in the sense that it delivers a quality-adjusted life year at a lower cost than beginning the lifestyle modification immediately—$24,523 versus $62,602. If the immediate lifestyle program is compared to the delayed lifestyle program, the marginal cost per QALY of the immediate program is about $201,818.

What Would a Program Have to Cost in Order to Break Even—No Increase in Net Cost?

This can be addressed by conducting a sensitivity analysis on the cost of the intervention. Figure 2-4 shows the relationship between the cost of the

TABLE 2-2 30-Year Costs, QALYs, and Incremental Costs/QALY for Four Programs from Societal Perspective (Discounted 3%)

	Cost per person	QALY per person	Average cost/ QALY[a]	Incremental increase in cost	Incremental increase in QALYs	Incremental cost/QALY
Baseline	$37,171	11.319				
Lifestyle when FPG>125[b]	$40,237	11.444	$24,523	$3,066	0.125	$24,523
DPP Lifestyle[c]	$47,140	11.478	$62,602	$6,903	0.034	$201,818
Metformin	$41,189	11.432	$35,523	dominated	dominated	dominated

[a]Compared to Baseline.
[b]Incremental values are compared to Baseline.
[c]Incremental values are compared to Lifestyle when >125.
ABBREVIATIONS: QALY – quality-adjusted life-year, FPG – fasting plasma glucose, DPP – Diabetes Prevention Program.
SOURCE: Eddy et al. *Annals of Internal Medicine* 2005; 143:251-264.

DPP lifestyle program and the net financial costs. In order to break even, the DPP lifestyle program would have to cost $100 if begun immediately and about $225 if delayed until after a person develops diabetes. In the DPP trial itself, the lifestyle modification program cost $1,356 in the first year and about $672 in subsequent years.

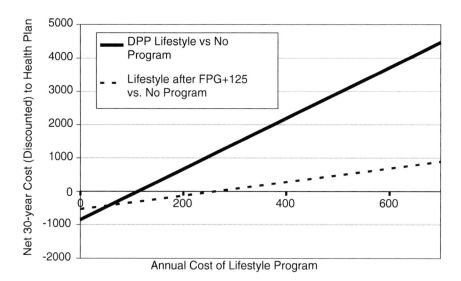

FIGURE 2-4 Costs of two programs for diabetes prevention.
SOURCE: Eddy et al. *Annals of Internal Medicine* 2005; 143:251-264.

Discussion and Conclusions

This example illustrates how models can be used to help fill the gaps in the evidence provided by clinical trials and other well-designed empirical studies. Each of the questions addressed above is undeniably important, but each is also impossible to answer empirically. One way or another we are going to have to develop methods for filling the gaps between trials. The solution we describe here is to use trials to establish the effectiveness of interventions, but then use models to extend the trials in directions that are otherwise not feasible. In this case the DPP established that both metformin and intensive lifestyle modification decrease the rate of progression to diabetes in high-risk people. Its results suggest that either of those interventions, plus variations on them such as different doses or timing, should reduce downstream events such as the complications of diabetes and their costs. However they are incapable of determining the actual magnitudes of the downstream effects—the actual probabilities of the complications with and without the interventions, and the actual effects on costs. The DPP trial itself is reported to have cost on the order of $175 million. Continuing it for another 30 years, or even another 10 years, is clearly not possible. Furthermore, once the beneficial effects of the interventions have been established it would be unethical to continue the trial as originally designed. Thus, if we are limited to the clinical trial by itself, we will never know the long-term heath and economic outcomes that are crucially needed for rational planning.

There are three main ways to proceed. One is to ignore the lack of information about the magnitudes of the effects and promote the prevention activities on the general principle that their benefits have been shown. Since this option is not deterred by a lack of information about actual health or economic effects, it might as well promote the most expensive and effective intervention—in this case intensive lifestyle modification begun immediately. This type of nonquantitative reasoning has been the mainstay of medical decision making for decades and might still be considered viable except for two facts. First, it provides no basis for truly informed decision making; if a patient or physician wants to know what can be expected to occur or wants to consider other options, this approach is useless. Second, this approach almost uniformly drives up costs. While that might have been acceptable in the past, it is not acceptable or maintainable today.

The second approach is to rely on expert opinion to estimate the long-term effects. The difficulty here is that the size of the problem far exceeds the capacity of the human mind. When we can barely multiply 17×23 in our heads, there is no hope that we can mentally process all the variables that affect the outcomes of preventing diabetes with any degree of accuracy.

As a result, different experts come up with different estimates, and there is no way to determine if any of them is even close to being correct.

The third approach is the one taken here—to use mathematical models to keep all the variables straight and perform all the calculations. In a sense, this is the logical extension of using expert opinion; use the human mind for what it is best at—storing and retrieving information, finding patterns, raising hypotheses, designing trials—and then call on formal analytical methods and the power of computers (all human-made, by the way) to perform the quantitative parts of the analysis. This approach can also be viewed as the logical extension of the clinical trial and other empirical research. Trials produce raw data. We already use quantitative methods to interpret the data—classical statistics if nothing else. The types of models we are talking about here are in the same vein, but they extend the methods to encompass information from a wider range of clinical trials and other types of research (to build and validate the models) and then extend the analyses in time to estimate long-term outcomes.

With all this said, however, it is also important to note that in the same ways that not all experts are equal and not all trial designs are equal, not all models are equal. Our proposal that models can be used to help fill the gaps in trials carries a qualification that this should be done only if the ability of the model to simulate real trials has been demonstrated. One way to put this is that if a model is to be used to fill a gap in the existing evidence, it should first be shown to accurately simulate the evidence that exists on either side of the gap. In this example, the model should be shown to accurately simulate (or as in this case, prospectively predict) the DPP trial of the prevention of diabetes (Figure 2-4) as well as other trials of outcomes that have studied the development of complications and their treatments (e.g., Figure 2-2). The demonstration of a model's ability to simulate existing trials, as well as the condition that additional trials are not feasible, form the conditions we would propose for using models to fill the gaps in evidence.

This example has demonstrated that there are problems, and models, that meet these conditions today. In addition there are good reasons to believe that the power and accuracy of models will improve considerably in the near future. The main factor that will determine the pace of improvement is the availability of person-specific data. Access to such data should increase with the spread of EHRs, as more clinical trials are conducted, as the person-specific data from existing trials are made more widely accessible, as models push deeper into the underlying physiology, and as modelers focus more on validating their models against the data that do exist.

HETEROGENEITY OF TREATMENT EFFECTS:
SUBGROUP ANALYSIS

Sheldon Greenfield, M.D., University of California at Irvine, and
Richard L. Kravitz, M.D., M.S.P.H., University of California at Davis

Three evolving phenomena indicate that results generated by randomized controlled trials are increasingly inadequate for the development of guidelines, for payment, and for creating quality-of-care measures. First, patients now eligible for trials have a broader spectrum of illness severity than previously. Patients at the lower end of disease severity, who are less likely to benefit from a drug or intervention, are now being included in RCTs. The recent null results from trials of calcium and of clopidogrel are examples of this phenomenon. Second, due to the changing nature of chronic disease along with increased patient longevity, more patients now suffer from multiple comorbidities. These patients are frequently excluded from clinical trials. Both of these phenomena make the results from RCTs generalizable to an increasingly small percentage of patients. Third, powerful new genetic and phenotypic markers that can predict patients' responsiveness to therapy and vulnerability to adverse effects of treatment are now being discovered. Within clinical trials, these markers have the potential for identifying patients' potential for responsiveness to the treatment to be investigated.

The current research paradigm underlying evidence-based medicine, and therefore guideline development and quality assessment, is consequently flawed in two ways. The "evidence" includes patients who may benefit only minimally from the treatment being tested, resulting in negative trials and potential undertreatment. Secondly, attempts to generalize the results from positive trials to patients who have been excluded from those trials (e.g., for presence of multiple comorbidities) have resulted in potential over- or ineffective treatment.

The major concern for clinical/health services researchers and policy makers is the identification of appropriate "inference groups." To whom are the results of trials being applied and for what purpose? Patients with multiple comorbidities are commonly excluded from clinical trials. Some of these conditions can mediate the effects of treatment and increase heterogeneity of response through (1) altered metabolism or excretion of treatment; (2) polypharmacy leading to drug interactions; (3) nonadherence resulting from polypharmcy; or (4) increasing overall morbidity and reducing life expectancy. Research in Type 2 diabetes has shown that comorbidities producing early mortality or poor health status reduce the effectiveness of long-term reduction of plasma glucose. In the United Kingdom Prospective Diabetes Study (UKPDS), reducing the level of coexistent hypertension had considerably greater impact on subsequent morbidity and mortality than did reducing hyperglycemia to near-normal levels. Two decision analytic models have shown that there is very little reduction in microvascular complications based on reductions in hyperglycemia among older patients with diabetes. Similarly, the effectiveness of aggressive treatment for early prostate cancer is much reduced among patients with moderate to major amounts of coexistent disease. This decreased effectiveness must be balanced against mortality from and complications of aggressive therapy to inform patient choice, to improve guidelines for treatment, and to develop measures of quality of care. Several recent national meetings have focused on how guidelines and quality measures need to be altered in "complex" patients, those with more than one major medical condition for whom attention to the heterogeneity of treatment effects (HTE) is so important.

Although the problem of HTE is increasingly recognized, solutions have been slow to appear. Proposed strategies have included exploratory subgroup analysis followed by trials that stratify on promising subgroups. Some have argued for expanded use of experimental designs (n of 1 trials, multiple time series crossover studies, matched pair analyses) that, unlike parallel group clinical trials, can examine individual treatment effects directly. Still others have championed observational studies prior to trials to form relevant subgroups and after trials, as has been done in prostate cancer, to assess the prognosis in subgroups of patients excluded from trials. These strategies could lead to less overtreatment and less undertreatment, and to the tailoring of treatment for maximum effectiveness and minimum cost. The following paper, by the Heterogeneity of Treatment Effects Research Agenda Consortium,[1] reviews these issues in greater detail.

Heterogeneity of Treatment Effects

Heterogeneity of Treatment Effects (HTE) has been defined by Kravitz et al. (Kravitz 2004) as variation in results produced by the same treatment in different patients. HTE has always been present; however, two contemporary trends have created an urgency to address the implications of HTE. One is the inclusion of a broader spectrum of illness or risk of outcome in some clinical trials. The other is mounting pressure from payers and patients to follow guidelines, pay according to evidence, and identify indicators of quality of care not only for patients in trials, but for the majority of the population that was not eligible for trials and to which the results

---

[1]Naihua Duan, Ph.D., Sheldon Greenfield, M.D., Sherrie H. Kaplan, Ph.D., M.P.H., David Kent, M.D., Richard Kravitz, M.D., M.S.P.H., Sharon-Lise Normand, Ph.D., Jose Selby, M.D., M.P.H., Paul Shekelle, M.D., Ph.D., Hal Stern, Ph.D., Thomas R. Tenhave, Ph.D., M.P.H.; paper developed for a research conference sponsored by Pfizer.

of trials may not apply. This latter problem has been exacerbated in recent years by large proportions of the patient population living longer and acquiring other medical conditions that have an impact on the effectiveness of the treatment under study.

With respect to clinical trials, the literature and clinical experience suggest that the problem of identifying subgroups that may be differentially affected by the same treatment is critical, both when the trial results are small or negative and when the trials demonstrate a positive average treatment effect. It has been assumed in devising guidelines, paying for treatments, and setting up quality measures that subgroups behave similarly to the population average. After a trial showing a negative average treatment effect, guideline recommendations may not call for introducing a treatment to a subgroup that would benefit from it. Similarly, when a trial demonstrates a positive average treatment effect across the population, this assumption may encourage the introduction of the added costs, risks, and burdens of a treatment to individuals who may receive no or only a small benefit from it.

The causes of HTE, such as genetic disposition, ethnicity, site differences in care, adherence, polypharmacy, and competing risk (Kravitz 2004), can be classified according to four distinct categories of risk: (1) baseline outcome risk, (2) responsiveness to treatment, (3) iatrogenic risk, and (4) competing risk.

Baseline outcome risk is the rate of occurrence of unfavorable outcomes in a patient population in the absence of the study treatment. Responsiveness to treatment reflects the change in patient outcome risk attributable to the treatment under study. If a sample's baseline outcome risk of myocardial infarction without treatment is 10 percent and the treatment was 20 percent effective, there would be a 2 percent absolute treatment effect, whereas the same level of effectiveness (20 percent) in a patient sample with a baseline outcome risk of 40 percent would yield an 8 percent absolute decrease in myocardial infarction.

The third type of risk, iatrogenic risk, is the likelihood of experiencing an adverse event related to the treatment under study. Finally, competing risk is the likelihood of experiencing unfavorable outcomes unrelated to the disease and treatment under study, such as death or disability due to comorbid conditions. The causes and implications of each of these sources of HTE are summarized below.

Baseline Outcome Risk

Variation in outcome risk is the best understood source of HTE. Figure 2-5, adapted from Kent and Hayward (Kent 2007), demonstrates how, even if the relative benefit of a treatment (responsiveness) and the risk of

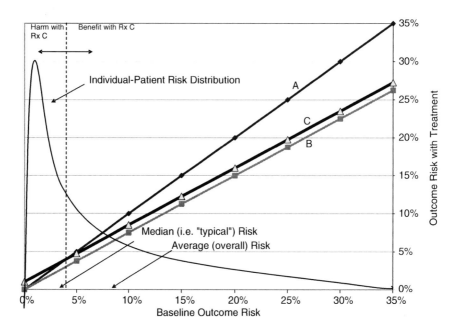

FIGURE 2-5 Wide variation of patients' baseline risk (their risk of suffering a bad outcome in the absence of treatment) is one reason trial results don't apply equally to all patients.
SOURCE: Adapted from Kent, D, and R Hayward, When averages hid individual differences in clinical trials, American Scientist, 2007, vol. 95 (Kent 2007).

adverse events (iatrogenic risk) are constant across a population, patients with the highest risk for the outcome targeted by a treatment often enjoy the greatest absolute benefit, while low-outcome risk patients derive little or no absolute benefit. The lines A, B, and C in this figure depict the expected outcomes with treatment (Y-axis) for a given baseline risk. Line A shows the expected result when the treatment has no effect of outcome. Line B shows the expected result if the treatment reduces the risk of the outcome by 25 percent. Line C shows the expected outcome if the treatment reduces the risk of the outcome by 25 percent but also causes a treatment-related harm independent of baseline risk of 1 percent (i.e., this line is parallel to B, but 1 percent higher). By comparing lines A and C, it is clear that for patients with baseline risks of less than 4 percent, the risks of Treatment C would outweigh its benefits (albeit slightly). The curve shows a hypothetical, unitless baseline risk distribution. High-outcome-risk patients (right of the dashed line in Figure 2-5) may derive sufficient treatment benefit to offset possible harmful side effects, but patients with lower baseline outcome risk, who may be the majority of the sample (left of the dashed line), may fail to derive sufficient benefit from the treatment to justify exposure to possible treatment-related harm. Therefore with a skewed distribution of this kind, it is possible to have an average risk that yields overall an overall positive trial with Treatment C, even though most patients in the trial have a risk profile that makes Treatment C unattractive. This phenomenon occurred in the PROWESS trial examining the use of drotrecogin alfa (activated) (Xigris) in sepsis (Vincent et al. 2003) where the overall treatment effect was positive but driven solely by its effect on the sickest patients (APACHE[2] > 25). A second RCT focusing on patients with low baseline outcome risk (APACHE < 25) showed no net benefit for this subpopulation (Abraham et al. 2005), demonstrating the wide possible variations due to HTE. A similar phenomenon may have occurred in a clopidogrel-aspirin trial (Bhatt 2006) where the sickest patients benefited and the least sick patients showed a trend toward harm. In this case, there was an overall null effect. In both sets of studies, the overall effect was misleading.

Iatrogenic Risk

The causes of side effects include both genetic and environmental components. An environmental example would be a hospital's failure to recognize and promptly treat side effects (Kravitz 2004).

Responsiveness to Treatment

Responsiveness describes the probability of clinical benefit for the individual from the treatment based on drug absorption, distribution, metabolism or elimination, drug concentration at the target site, or number and functionality of target receptors. Most of the reasons for variations in responsiveness are of genetic origin. Other causes of different trial responses in individual patients include behavioral and environmental variables (Kravitz 2004).

Competing Risk

The demographics of the majority of the population (or the average patient) are changing. The aging of the population, along with the advent of life-prolonging therapies, has caused an increase in the proportion of the patients within a diagnostic category who have multiple comorbidities, are treated with multiple medications, and therefore, have multiple competing

---

[2]Acute Physiology and Chronic Health Evaluation (APACHE) scores are often utilized to stratify patients according to risk.

sources of mortality. Compared with 20 years ago, patients with prostate cancer are much more likely to have coexisting congestive heart failure, chronic obstructive pulmonary disease (COPD), and diabetes and are much more likely to die from these conditions than from prostate cancer over the next few years. These patients are therefore much less likely to be able to benefit from arduous, long-term treatment. Two decision analyses have shown that intensive treatment of blood sugar in patients with diabetes who are older than 65 years has little impact on the reductions of complications in such patients (Vijan et al. 1997; CDC Diabetes Cost-Effectiveness Group 2002). Therefore, in these patients the effectiveness of aggressive treatment is substantially lower than that observed in clinical trials because these trials were conducted with younger patients without such comorbidities (Greenfield et al. [unpublished]).

Current Study Design and Analytical Approaches

Hayward and colleagues have noted that attention to HTE and its impact has been limited and focused almost exclusively on outcome risk (Hayward et al. 2005). In most trials only one subgroup was investigated at a time. These subgroups were usually not a priori specified.

A priori risk stratification, especially with multivariate risk groups, is almost never done. Comparisons of treatment effects across patients with varying outcome risk or illness severity usually involve post hoc subgroup analyses, which are not well suited for identifying the often multiple patient characteristics associated with differential treatment effects (Lagakos 2006).

The usefulness of multiple subgroup analyses is limited by at least two shortcomings. First, many subgroup analyses with multiple subgroup comparisons are performed using one variable at a time, increasing the likelihood of type I error (false positives), and requiring the allowable error rate (alpha) of each comparison to be set below 0.05 to ensure the overall alpha does not exceed 0.05. This reduces the likelihood of detecting significant differences between subgroups. This problem is compounded when subgroup analyses are conducted post hoc because subgroups are often underpowered when not prespecified in the study design. Even when subgroups are prespecified, however, one-variable-at-a-time analyses are still problematic. Secondly, one-at-a-time subgroup analysis treats risk categories dichotomously, which constrains the power of the analysis and increases the likelihood of type II error (false negatives).

To understand the distribution and impact of HTE in a way that improves the specificity of treatment recommendations, prevailing approaches to study design and data analysis in clinical research must change.

Recommendations and a New Research Agenda

Two major strategies can decrease the negative impact of HTE in clinical research: (1) The use of composite risk scores derived from multivariate models should be considered in both the design of a priori risk stratification groups and data analysis of clinical research studies; and (2) the full range of sources of HTE, many of which arise for members of the general population not eligible for trials, should be addressed by integrating multiple phases of clinical research, both before and after an RCT.

Addressing Power Limitations in Trials Using Composite Risk Scores

Multivariate risk models address the issues of both multiple comparisons and reliance on dichotomous subgroup definitions by combining multiple, hypothesized risk factors into a single continuous independent variable. A simulation study by Hayward et al. (Hayward et al. 2006) demonstrated that a composite risk score derived from a multivariate model predicting outcome risk alone significantly increased statistical power when assessing HTE compared to doing individual comparisons.

Despite these analytic advantages, using continuous risk scores derived from multivariate models may have drawbacks. One challenge of using continuous composite risk scores, for example, is that they do not provide a definitive cut point to determine when a treatment should or should not be applied. Because the decision to apply a specific treatment regimen is dichotomous, a specific cutoff distinguishing good versus bad candidates for a treatment must be determined. Relative unfamiliarity of the medical community with these multivariate approaches coupled with potential ambiguity in treatment recommendations from these methods are barriers to acceptance of their use.

The confusion introduced by ambiguous cut points for continuous risk scores is compounded by the methods used to develop risk models. Different risk models may predict different levels of risk for the same patient. That is, a patient with a given set of risk factors may be placed in different risk categories depending on the model used. Even continuous risk scores that correlate very highly may put the same patient in different risk groups. For patients at the highest and lowest levels of risk, there should be little ambiguity in treatment decisions regardless of the risk model used. Many other patients, however, will fall in a "gray area" where risk models with small differences in model may generate different categories of risk assignment.

To help promote understanding and acceptance of these methods by the medical community, demonstrations comparing the performance of different types of continuous composite risk scores to the performance of traditional one-at-a-time risk factor assessment in informing treatment decisions would be beneficial (Rothwell and Warlow 1999; Zimmerman et al. 1998; Kent et al. 2002; Selker et al. 1997; Fiaccadori et al. 2000; Teno et al. 2000; Slotman 2000; Stier et al. 1999; Pocock et al. 2001).

A final important point is that current multivariate approaches focus exclusively on targeted-outcome risk, but other sources of HTE remain unaddressed. Risk, in the context of a treatment decision, was defined as the sum of targeted-outcome risk, iatrogenic risk, and competing risk. If iatrogenic risk and competing risk are distributed heterogeneously in a patient population, methods to account for them alongside targeted-outcome risk should also be incorporated in the analysis of trial results. The advantages, drawbacks, and methodologic complexities of composite measures have recently been reviewed (Kaplan and Normand 2006).

Integrating Multiple Phases of Research

Clinical researchers can address the various sources of HTE across at least six phases of research: (1) observational studies performed before RCT and aimed at the trial outcome, (2) the primary RCT itself, (3) post-trial analysis, (4) Phase IV clinical studies, (5) observational studies following trials, and (6) focused RCTs. The recommended applications of these phases for studying each of the four sources of HTE are outlined in Table 2-3 and described below.

Baseline outcome risk in clinical trials. To address both design-related and analysis-related issues, outcome risk variation as a source of HTE should be addressed in two phases: (1) *risk stratification* of the trial sample based on data from pre-trial observational studies (cell a) and (2) *risk adjustment* in the analysis of treatment effects based on pre-trial observational studies when available, or post hoc analysis of the trial control group data when observational studies are not feasible (cells a and b in Table 2-3).

As noted in the paper by Hayward et al. (Hayward et al. 2006), modeling HTE requires that risk groups, continuous or discrete, must be pre-specified and powered in the study design. Data from prior observational

TABLE 2-3 Studying Sources of HTE Across Multiple Phases of Research

	Pre-trial Observational Study	RCT	Post Hoc Trial Analysis	Phase IV Clinical Study	Post-trial Observational Study	Focused RCT
Baseline risk	X(a)		X(b)			
Responsiveness		X(c)		X(d)		X(e)
Iatrogenic risk		X(f)		X(g)		
Competing risk					X(h)	

research such as those collected in the PROWESS trial (Vincent et al. 2003) can be modeled to identify predictors of baseline outcome risk for pre-trial subgroup specification at a much lower cost per subject than a second RCT. To date, however, prespecifying risk groups is not common practice outside of cardiology and a small number of studies in other fields.

Even in studies where comparisons across risk factors are prespecified, those risk factors are seldom collapsed into a small number of continuous composite risk scores to maximize power and minimize the number of multiple comparisons needed. In the clopidogrel trial (Bhatt et al. 2006), for example, a possibly meaningful difference in treatment effects between symptomatic and asymptomatic cardiac patients may have been masked by looking at these groups (those with and without symptoms) dichotomously and alongside 11 subgroup comparisons.

A priori risk stratification may not be supported by clinical researchers because it either delays the primary RCT while pre-trial observational data are collected or requires that a second, expensive, focused RCT be conducted after a model for baseline outcome risk is developed from the primary trial and follow-up studies. Because of the additional time and costs required, a priori risk stratification cannot become a viable component of clinical research unless the stakeholders that fund, conduct, and use clinical research sufficiently value its benefits. A comprehensive demonstration of the costs and benefits of this approach is needed to stimulate discussion of this possibility.

Post hoc analysis of control group data from the trial itself may also be used to identify risk factors when observational studies are not feasible. By identifying characteristics predicting positive and negative outcomes in the absence of treatment, control group analysis works as a small-scale observational study to produce a composite risk score to adjust estimates of treatment effectiveness from primary RCT. Even though the results from a model of one group's risk may not necessarily apply to another group such as the treatment group, these same data provide a reasonable starting point to select and risk-stratify a clinically meaningful subsample for a future focused RCT.

To maximize the statistical power of treatment effectiveness models for a given RCT sample size, composite risk scores generated from multivariate analysis of observational or control group data should be introduced when feasible. Introducing composite risk scores generated from multivariate analysis of observational or control group data would maximize the statistical power of models of treatment effectiveness for a given RCT sample size. Whether or not a priori risk stratification is feasible, continuous composite risk scores should be generated from observational data or trial control group analysis to provide a risk-adjusted estimate of treatment effectiveness.

In exploratory cases where stratification factors that lead to treatment heterogeneity are not known, the latent class trajectory models of Muthen and Shedden (Muthen and Shedden 1999) may be used to identify latent subgroups or classes of patients by which treatments vary. Predictors of these classes can then be identified and form the basis of composite risk scores for future studies of treatment heterogeneity. Leiby et al. (in review) have applied such an approach to a randomized trial for a medical intervention of interstitial cystitis. Overall, the treatment was not effective. However, latent class trajectory models did identify a subgroup of responder patients for whom the treatment was effective in improving the primary end point, the Global Response Assessment. Additional work is needed on identifying baseline factors that are associated with this treatment heterogeneity and can form the basis of a composite score for a future trial.

Responsiveness. Responsiveness to an agent or procedure is studied in the trial and also needs to be studied in a Phase IV study for those not included in the trial to see how the agent responds in unselected populations, where side effects or preference-driven adherence, polypharmacy, competing risk, or disease modifying effects are in play (cells c, d), or in a focused second trial (cell e).

Iatrogenic risk. Vulnerability to adverse effects needs to be studied in two phases, in the trials (cell f) and in Phase IV studies (cell g).

Competing risk. The effects of polypharmacy, adherence in the general population, and utility can be best studied in observational studies among populations that would not be included in trials, especially those who are elderly and/or have multiple comorbidities (cell h). The most critical issue for understanding competing risk is deciding when a clinical quality threshold measure shown to be "effective" in clinical trials (e.g., HbA1c < 7.0 percent for diabetes) is recommended for populations not studied in the trials. Cholesterol reduction, blood pressure control, and glucose control in diabetes are examples of measures with quality thresholds that are not required for all populations. Even when, as in the case of cholesterol, they have been studied in the elderly, they have not been studied in non-trial populations where the patients have other medical conditions, economic problems, polypharmacy, or genetics that may alter the effectiveness of the treatment. For glucose in patients with diabetes and for treatment of patients with prostate cancer, there is an additional issue, that of "competing comorbidities" or competing risk, where the other conditions may shorten life span such that years of treatment (in the case of diabetes) or aggressive treatment with serious complications (prostate cancer) may not allow the level of effectiveness achieved in the trials (Litwin et al. [in press]).

Clinicians intuitively decide how to address competing risk. For example, in a 90-year-old patient with diabetes and end-stage cancer, it is obvious to the clinician that blood pressures of 130/80 need not be achieved.

In most cases, however, the criteria by which clinical decisions are made should be based explicitly on research data. This evidence base should begin with observational studies to identify key patient subgroups that derive more or less net benefit from a treatment in the presence of competing risk. Failing to account for competing risks may overestimate the value of a treatment in certain subgroups. If 100 patients are treated, for example, and 90 die from causes unrelated to the treated condition, even if the treatment effect is 50 percent, only 5 people benefit (number needed to treat = 20). If the original 100 patients are not affected by other diseases, however, 50 will benefit from the treatment (number needed to treat = 2).

When treatment effects are underestimated for a subgroup, treatments that are arduous, have multiple side effects, or are burdensome over long periods of time may be rejected by doctors and patients, even if the patient belongs to a subgroup likely to benefit from treatment. For this reason, research methodologies supplemental to RCTs should be introduced to predict *likelihood to benefit* for key patient subgroups not included in trials.

Observational studies, because of their lower cost and less restrictive inclusion criteria, can include larger and more diverse samples of patients to address important research questions the RCTs cannot. Unlike RCTs, observational studies can include high-risk patients who would not be eligible for trials, such as elderly patients and individuals with multiple, complex medical conditions, and would provide insight in predicting likelihood to benefit for this large and rapidly growing fraction of chronic disease patients. The generalizability of RCTs can be addressed in observational studies if designed properly, based on principles for good observational studies (Mamdani et al. 2005; Normand et al. 2005; Rochon et al. 2005).

There are possible solutions to the problems of HTE, the principal one being multivariate pre-trial risk stratification based on observational studies. For patients not eligible for trials, mainly elderly patients with multiple comorbidities, observational studies are recommended to determine mortality risk from the competing comorbidities so that positive results could be applied judiciously to non-trial patients. Government and nongovernmental funders of research will have to be provided incentives to expand current research paradigms.

HETEROGENEITY OF TREATMENT EFFECTS: PHARMACOGENETICS

David Goldstein, Ph.D.
Duke Institute for Genome Sciences and Policy

Many clinical challenges remain in the treatment of most therapeutic areas. This paper discusses the potential role of pharmacogenetics in helping to address some of these challenges, focusing particular attention on the treatment of epilepsy and schizophrenia. Several points are emphasized: (1) progress in pharmacogenetics will likely require pathway-based approaches in which many variants can be combined to predict treatment response; (2) pharmacodynamic determinants of treatment response are likely of greater significance than pharmacokinetic; and (3) the allele frequency differences of functional variants among human populations will have to be taken into account in using sets of gene variants to predict treatment response.

Pharmacogenetics has previously focused on describing variation in a handful of proteins and genes but it is now possible to assess entire pathways that might be relevant to disease or to drug responses. The clinical relevance will come as we identify genetic predictors of a patient's response to treatment. Polymorphisms can have big effects on such responses, and identification of these effects can offer significant diagnostic value about how patients respond to medicine, to avoid rare adverse drug reactions (ADRs), or to select which of several alternative drugs has the highest efficacy.

The CATIE trial (Clinical Antipsychotic Trials of Intervention Effectiveness) compared the effectiveness of atypical antipsychotics (olanzapine, quetiapine, risperidone, ziprasidone) with a typical antipsychotic, perphenazine. The end point was discontinuation of treatment, and in this respect there is really no difference between typical and atypical antipsychotics. Results such as these signal an end to the blockbuster drug era, in that often no drug, or even drug class, is much better than the others. However certain drugs were better or worse for certain patients. For example, olanzapine increases body weight more than 7 percent in about 30 percent of patients, and for older medicines, with many of the typical antipsychotics a similar proportion of patients will develop tardive dyskinesia (TD) as an adverse reaction. TDs are involuntary movements of the tongue, lips, face, trunk, and extremities and are precisely the type of adverse reaction (AR) one would want to avoid, because when the medicine is removed the AR continues without much amelioration over time. So perhaps as many as 30 percent of patients exposed to a typical antipsychotic will develop this AR, whereas the majority will not.

This means that in deciding which medications to use at the level of the individual patient, these medications are quite different from each other. A significant problem is that there is very little information on which patients might experience an adverse reaction to a particular type of drug. In this particular case, there is virtually no information on who will get TD or who will suffer severe weight gain such that they would not continue medication. These types of results unambiguously constitute a call to arms to the genetics community because this is an area in which we can truly add value by helping clinicians to distinguish patients and guide clinical decision making.

Having a predictor for TD on typicals would be an unambiguous, clinically useful diagnostic. However currently, within the field of pharmacogenetics, we have very few examples of such utility. We have examples that may be of some relevance in some context, but you would have to do an RCT to determine how to utilize this information. In general, at the germline versus the somatic level, the current set of genetic differences among patients is not that clinically important, particularly when you contrast them with something like a predictor of weight gain or TD in the use of atypicals or typicals. These are the types of things we are working toward in the pharmacogenetics community, and it looks as though some of these problems are quite crackable and there will be genetic diagnostics of significant relevance and impact to clinical decisions.

The idea of moving toward doing more genetic studies in the context of a trial is quite exciting because the data will be quite rich. However there are real doubts that the amount of genetic information and the complexity of clinical data will allow the identification of any kind of association, and as a result the pharmacogenetics community is going to flood the literature with claims about a particular polymorphism's relevance to a specific disease or drug use within a specific subgroup. Therefore, as we move toward these types of analyses, it is very important to specify a hypothesis in advance and one will need to be quite careful about what results one wants to pay attention to. For CATIE, the project design included hypotheses that were specified in advance of any genetic analyses to allow appropriate correction for planned comparisons. This trial is ongoing, and preliminary results are discussed here to give a flavor of what kinds of information might be derived from these types of analyses in the future.

We have delineated two broad categories of analyses. One is to look at determinants of phamacokinetics (PK) to see if functional variation in dopaminergic genes related to dose and discontinuation has any effect. These analyses focus on how the drug is moved around the body and factors that influence how the drug is metabolized. The second category is on pharmaco-dynamic polymorphisms (PD) or the genetic differences and determinants among people that might affect how the drug works. Here we are looking at differences in the target of the drug, the target pathways, or genetic differences that influence the etiology of the condition as related to specified measures of responses and to adverse drug reactions. To perform a comprehensive pharmacogenetic analysis of drug effectiveness and adverse drug reactions, we looked at PK though dosing variation and asked whether genetic differences influence the eventual decision the clinician makes about what dosage to use. We looked at enzymes that metabolize the drug and common polymorphisms in these enzymes. Our early results indicated that in terms of PK variation, there were no impacts on dosing decisions by clinicians.

Pharmacodynamic analysis on the other hand looks more promising in terms of clinical utility. CATIE examined the relatively obvious pathways that might influence how the drug acts and how patients might respond to antipsychotics. All antipsychotics have dopinergic activities, so the dopinergic system is an obvious place to start. This pathway approach included looking at neurotransmitters—the synthesis, metabolism, transporters, receptors, et cetera—for dopamine, serotonin, glutamate, gamma-aminobutyric acid (GABA), acetylcholine, and histamine. In addition, memory and neuro-cognition related genes, and genes previously implicated in drug response were examined. We scanned through these pathways for polymorphisms and tried to relate these to key aspects of how patients respond to treatment. We also considered other classes of candidate genes, in particular those genes that might influence the cognitive impairments associated with schizophrenia that are not currently well treated by antipsychotics. Ultimately we selected about 118 candidate genes and a total of 3,072 single nucleotide poly-morphisms (SNPs) and looked at neurocognitive phenotypes, optimized dose, overall effectiveness, and occurrence of TD, weight gain, and anti-cholinergic adverse events. This study emphasizes the importance of clearly specifying the hypothesis in advance. If a study does not clearly articulate what the opportunity space for associations were prior to undertaking the study, ignore it, because there likely will have been arbitrary amounts of data mining and you cannot trust that approach. Both of these studies are in the process of being completed and submitted for publication along with collaborators from the CATIE study and others.

By helping to subgroup diseases genetically and providing pointers toward the genetic and physiological cause of variable and adverse reac-tions, pharmacogenetics will also have indirect benefits for future drug development. In addition, some drugs that work well generally are rejected, withdrawn, or limited in use because of rare but serious ADRs. Examples include the antiepileptic felbamate, the atypical antipsychotic clozapine, and most drug withdrawals owing to QT-interval-associate arrhythmias. If pharmacogenetic predictors of adverse events could prevent the exposure of genetically vulnerable patients and so preserve even a single drug, the costs of any large-scale research effort in pharmacogenetics could be fully recov-ered. An example of this is vigabatrin, which is a good antiepilepsy drug in terms of efficacy, and for some types of seizures (e.g., infantile spasms) it is clinically essential. Unfortunately, in some cases it also has a devastating effect on the visual field and can constrain the visual field to the point of almost eliminating peripheral vision. This adverse reaction has dramatically restricted the use of this medicine and, in fact, it was never licensed in the United States. We've done a study to try to identify genetic differences that might predict this and have potentially identified a polymorphism where the minor allele is the only place that we see severe reduction in visual field, which could be used to predict this reaction to vigabatrin. Again, this is the kind of pharmacogenetics result that provides an opportunity for improving clinical treatment of epilepsy in that this medication, which might not otherwise be used broadly, can be prescribed to the appropriate population. The wrinkle here is that we are using very large tertiary referral centers and we have used all of the vigabatrin-exposed patients for whom we have DNA samples. We think we see an association and would like to develop results like this but we need data. Our results with vigabatrin need to be confirmed in larger sample size. Since we do not have most of the exposure data available to study, it is possible that we will never be able to conclude either way.

The current work in the field gives grounds for real optimism that careful pharmacogenetic studies, in virtually all classes of medications, will identify genetic differences that are relevant to how patients respond to treatment and therefore impact clinical decision making. These will not be pharmacokinetic but rather pharmacodynamic. The examples presented illustrate several of the challenges and opportunities for pharmacogenetics. These types of information will be increasingly generated, but we need to think about how such information will be useful and utilized for clinical decision making. For example, despite the fact that we have no evidence that variation in the genes being studied actually influence decisions of clinicians in a useful way, devices such as Amplichip are being pushed as a useful diagnostic. Because variations will increasingly be investigated for use in clinical diagnostics, we need to think about how such diagnostics should be evaluated and what kinds of evidence are needed before they are widely utilized. The preliminary results of the vigabatrin study makes an extremely strong argument that what we want to be doing as we go forward is setting up the framework to do these types of studies, because it is entirely possible that once a medication is introduced and generates huge numbers of exposures, if it generates a rare adverse event and is withdrawn, a pharmacogenetics study could resurrect the use of that medication in the appropriate population.

Two overriding priorities in pharmacogenetics research are the establishment of appropriate cohorts to study the most important variable responses to medicines, both in terms of variable efficacy and in terms of common or more rare but severe adverse reactions. It must be appreciated that larger randomized trials are not always the most appropriate settings for specific pharmacogenetic questions and it will often be necessary to recruit patients specifically for pharmacogenetics projects. For example, in the case of weight gain and atypical antipsychotics, the ideal dataset would be to look at weight in patients not previously exposed to an atypical. Secondarily, it is important that a framework is developed for evaluating the clinical utility of pharmacogenetic diagnostics.

BROADER POST-MARKETING SURVEILLANCE FOR INSIGHTS ON RISK AND EFFECTIVENESS

Harlan Weisman, M.D., Christina Farup, M.D., Adrian Thomas, M.D., Peter Juhn, M.D., M.P.H., and Kathy Buto, M.P.A.
Johnson & Johnson

The establishment of electronic medical records linked to a learning healthcare system has enormous potential to accelerate the development of real-world data on the benefits and risks of new innovative therapies. When integrated appropriately with physician expertise and patient preferences and variation, data from novel sources of post-marketing surveillance will further enable various stakeholders to distinguish among clinical approaches on how much they improve care and their overall value to the healthcare system. To ensure these goals are achieved without jeopardizing patient benefit or medical innovation, it is necessary to establish a road map, charting a course toward a common framework for post-marketing surveillance, initial evidence evaluation, appropriate and timely reevaluations, and application to real-world use with all key stakeholders involved in the process. Continuous improvement requires policy makers to address accountability for decisions they make based on this common framework that impacts patient health. Where possible, post-marketing data requirements of different global agencies or authorities should be harmonized to enhance the efficiency and quality of safety data from these sources, and to reduce the burden on governments and industry due to costs of collection and unnecessary duplication of efforts. In addition, policy development should strive to find the right alignment of incentives and controls to accelerate adoption of evidence on medicine, technology, and services that advance the standard of care.

The current landscape of health care in the United States is one of organized chaos where providers, payers, employers, patients, and manufacturers often have different vantage points and objectives that can result in inadequate patient access, poor care delivery, inconsistent quality, and increasing costs. A recent study on the quality of health care in the United States found that adults receive only half of the recommended care for their conditions (McGlynn et al. 2003). It is important to remember that although these multiple stakeholders approach health care from different angles, they all share the same objective: to improve patient health. To move to a system that delivers effective and high-quality care, which optimally balances benefits and risks, health care must be transformed to a knowledge-based learning network, focused on the patient and aligned on data systems, evaluation, and treatment guidelines, without sacrificing the human elements of empathy, caring, and healing. An interoperable electronic health record that provides longitudinal, real-time, clinical and economic outcomes at the patient level will be a critical enabler to allow for a wealth of new information to drive fact-based treatment decisions that are transparent and shared between patients and physicians, as well as with other stakeholders including payers. The resultant improvement in efficiencies, cost savings, and most important, clinical outcomes should permit physicians and other healthcare providers to restore not only the scientific basis of modern medicine, but also the humanity of traditional medicine through active engagement and dialogue between patients and healthcare providers.

Post-marketing surveillance of new technologies will be a key component of this system because it will provide needed real-world information on unique populations not evaluated in clinical trials and a better characterization of the full benefit-risk profile over the life cycle of product use. Because the benefits and risks of a new technology are never fully known at launch, ongoing evaluation of a product based on real-world use in broader populations of patients, with comorbidities and concomitantly prescribed therapies, is important to new insights. In addition, the full value of innovative new therapies may only be appreciated with real-world usage and comparative economic evaluation based on observed outcomes; this information will enable decision makers to continue to assess the overall value and appropriate use of a product in the healthcare system. However, the scope of what we need to know to assess value in an era of information overload and complex healthcare systems changes rapidly and continuously. To properly evaluate new products we need to acknowledge the advantages and limitations of the methods we have historically used for regulatory approval. Randomized clinical trials with blinding are currently used in the approval of drugs and higher-risk devices to ensure high internal validity of findings. However, RCTs may have limited validity for broader use in diverse populations (e.g., old versus young, urban versus rural). Observational studies conducted within an interoperable electronic medical record can be utilized to lend additional insights beyond efficacy, including real-world effectiveness and long-term outcomes.

Methodological challenges for conducting real-world observational studies can be daunting, but the opportunities for evidence development are substantial. The study of an intervention within a dynamic healthcare system adds a level of significant complexity and raises many questions. How can we deal with confounding by indication and the increasing variation of health states? How can we apply comparative effectiveness studies conducted in broad populations and allow for individual variation in treatment outcomes? When an adverse event occurs, is it due to the progression of underlying patient pathology or therapeutic interventions? How do we apply comparative effectiveness (average patient) to individual patients, each of whom brings his or her own specific variability (whether due to genetics, nutrition, environment, or risk tolerance)?

Selection of research methods and decisions about the level of evidence required must also take into consideration the type of technology. For example, devices can vary from a simple gauze bandage to a complex implant with a drug component. For many devices used in surgical procedures, patient outcomes are highly dependent on operator skill and can also depend on the hospital's volume of procedures. In a review of the literature by the Institute of Medicine, more than two-thirds of published studies reported an association between hospital volume and patient outcomes for certain diagnoses and surgical procedures (IOM 2000). Randomized clinical trials with blinding are the gold standard for drug evaluations of safety and efficacy but may not be possible in device studies. For example, the comparators and procedures of the new device and control may be so different (e.g., open vs. minimally invasive) that it may not be possible to blind the trial. The timing of evidence in a device's development is also an important consideration because technical development often occurs in parallel to efficacy and safety evaluations. Evaluations that are premature can lead to inaccurate conclusions about the benefit-risk profile, and evaluations that are too late may be irrelevant because iterative improvements may have been introduced to the market in the interim. Moreover, we face an expanding universe of treatment opportunities. Regenerative medicine and stem cell therapies look promising and potentially revolutionary, but realizing their substantial benefits will depend on our ability to develop the capacity necessary to answer the kinds of questions that these new therapies raise at the appropriate level of detail.

Although all stakeholders seem to be aligned on the *need* to define evidence requirements, there is not alignment on *what* evidence is needed under specific circumstances. For every drug or device the number of potential questions to answer about appropriate use is limitless; thus there is a need to prioritize what new evidence is needed to close the critical gaps of knowledge so that quality decisions can be made. We also need to think carefully about what evidence we need to make good decisions for healthcare policy. Additional issues to consider include the level of certainty required for the evidence gaps and the urgency of the information. Once we determine that evidence is needed and has been generated, how will the evidence be reviewed and assessed? As outlined by Teutsch and Berger, the integration of evidence-based medicine into decision making requires a deliberative process with two key components: (1) evidence review and synthesis and 2) evidence-based decision making (Teutsch and Berger 2005). We need to develop transparent methods and guidelines to gather, analyze, and integrate evidence to get true alignment of the manufacturers, payers, and providers. One major consideration that needs to be anticipated and managed is how this new form of clinical data will be integrated into policies and treatment paradigms to ensure that sufficient evidence drives these changes and that inappropriate use of exploratory data does not lead to premature policy decisions, or to partially informed clinical decisions. Finally, an efficient process for new evidence to undergo a timely evaluation with peer review and synthesis into the existing evidence base needs to be further developed with appropriate perspective and communication for patients.

There are many issues to consider as we build toward this learning system. We have a unique opportunity to begin to align the many interests of healthcare stakeholders by not only providing consumers earlier access to these technologies but also generating the evidence necessary to make better decisions about the appropriate application of new technologies. It is critical that a nonproprietary (open source) approach be encouraged to ensure commonality of data structure and interoperability of EHRs, providing for the ability to appropriately combine data from different EHR populations and allow patients to be followed across treatment networks. Where possible, post-marketing data requirements of different global agencies or authorities should be harmonized to reduce costs of collection and unnecessary duplication. An example of where this seems particularly feasible is in meeting post-marketing requirements of the Centers for Medicare and Medicaid Services and the Food and Drug Administration. In some circumstances, CMS is requiring "real-world" data collection in order to assess the benefit and risk of technologies in the Medicare population, while FDA is requiring post-market surveillance studies to further evaluate the benefit-risk equation in broader populations than required for market entry. Having a single set of data used for both regulatory approval (i.e., FDA's "safe and effective") and coverage determination (i.e., CMS's "reasonable and necessary") has the potential to bring new innovations to market faster and may reduce costly data collection efforts. As coverage determinations become increasingly "dynamic" (i.e., contingent upon further evidence generation), this may create an opportunity to collect data that can be used for ongoing coverage determinations as well as for post-market safety surveillance. Multiple uses of common datasets would require the following: (1) agreement among the interested agencies (i.e., FDA and CMS) that a common dataset would qualify for both safety assessments and coverage determinations; (2) input from both agencies for specific data collection requirements to inform the design of the data collection tools and the management of the data; (3) clear accountabilities for funding the data collection and explicit rules for accessing the data; and (4) clarification of how collection of data on off-label use for coverage determinations will be reconciled with regulatory status. If these steps are taken, manufacturers may be able to bring innovative products to patients more quickly while continuing to fund and direct future innovations.

Establishing incentives for evidence generation by manufacturers within an integrated EHR will foster even greater acceleration. Examples of incentives for drug and device manufacturers should include those that reward evidence generation in the marketplace. In general, expansion of a drug's use with new indications or claims requires the provision of two RCTs to the FDA. With the acceleration of data from reliable sources such as EHRs and the enhancement of methods for retrospective analyses of these data sources, alternative levels of evidence could be considered for FDA review for expanded claims or promotional uses. Insurance coverage policies could support uses for which post-market surveillance studies are being done, rather than restrict coverage until the post-market data are collected and analyzed. It is a widely recognized fact that completion of post-approval commitment studies in the United States is problematic, often for pragmatic reasons related to willingness to participate by patients and physicians when products are available clinically. The potential for EHRs to provide information that could replace certain of these studies would be a major advance and would provide a framework to continue the collection of relevant real-world and high-quality information on benefits and risks. When real-world, comparative studies are required, shared funding of data collection should be considered; the CMS program of "coverage with evidence development" is one prototype of this approach. Alternative incentives include extension of patent protections for the period of post-marketing data collection.

Currently for device manufacturers, there are even fewer incentives for evidence due to their typically narrower patent claim scope and shorter life cycles. Often innovative devices that are breakthrough treatments generate substantial evidence on value only to be quickly followed by a cheaper "me-too" device (a device that creatively worked around intellectual property issues) with little or no evidence that is accepted in the marketplace. It is less likely that the manufacturer with the innovative breakthrough device as the first market entrant will develop all of the needed evidence before the next competitor enters the market because the competitor will likely capitalize on the same data with no investment. Providing device manufacturers with similar extensions of their exclusivity periods (as, for example, via patent term extensions) as pharmaceuticals during the period of data collection could help rectify this situation.

Opportunities for collaboration across pharmaceutical and device companies to advance development of electronic medical records and evidence generation as a whole should be encouraged. For example, the data contained within the placebo arm of randomized controlled trials could provide a wealth of information when pooled together and would provide a larger cohort of populations for comparative analyses. Another example of potential collaboration is in the design of these new EHR systems, especially for the identification of safety signals. The industry could play a role in working with payers, regulators, and healthcare delivery networks to explore ways to access EHR and claims databases to form a proactive longitudinal framework of automated surveillance within the context of ensuring patient and practitioner privacy. In addition, no current scientific standards exist for signal detection and surveillance of safety; industry could play an important role to develop these standards through a collaboration in which algorithms, methods, and best scientific practices are shared. Finally, in most cases, there is no unique identification of medical devices in EHRs. Industry and other stakeholders will have to collaborate to determine which devices need unique identification, the appropriate technology, and a reasonable strategy for investments in the necessary infrastructure.

Many manufacturers place great emphasis on the importance of the value added by their products. In our case (Johnson & Johnson) the company is guided by a set of core principles to ensure the safe use of medicines and devices: (1) patients and doctors need timely and accurate information about the benefits and risks of a product so they can make well-informed choices; (2) the FDA and other global authorities are, and should remain, the principal arbiters of benefits and risks, determining whether to approve and maintain availability of products through transparent and aligned regulations; and (3) the best government policies and actions are those that continue to enhance patient health and safety and to promote innovation.

With these principles in mind, we propose a model for benefit-risk evaluation characterized by early and continuous learning enabled by EHRs. In this model, once an indication is approved and the product moves into real-world use, high-quality data, infrastructure, and analysis capability will enable benefit-risk monitoring and lead to refinement of understanding elements underlying risk and expanding upon possible benefits either through appropriate application of an intervention or through further innovation based on qualities of benefit or risk. This should be a system that understands the need for and appropriate methods to generate the right evidence for the right questions. It addresses decision-maker needs by looking at safety and efficacy, real-world effectiveness and risk, surrogate end points, and long-term outcome—for the right patient—accounting for genetics, comorbidities, and patient preference. The critical success factors for such a learning system going forward will be (1) establishing appropriate methods for research with the EHR as a data source; (2) prioritizing the need for evidence on safety and quality and not just intervention cost; (3) establishing appropriate peer review processes to ensure rigor and timeliness; (4) requiring intensive education and training of health professionals on evidence generation in clinical practice; and (5) using this new information as an adjunct, not a replacement, to RCTs for any purposes, and to ensure agreed upon standards for when such data are sufficient to drive policy and treatment decisions. There are many technical and policy issues, including privacy, that need to be addressed to create this EHR enabled learning framework. We believe a collaborative effort supported by patients, physicians, payers, industry, and regulators can accomplish the goal of a learning healthcare system with an open and transparent process toward developing standards and interoperable capabilities.

ADJUSTING EVIDENCE GENERATION TO THE SCALE OF EFFECTS

Steven M. Teutsch, M.D., M.P.H., and Marc L. Berger, M.D.
Merck & Co., Inc.

With new technologies rapidly introduced fast on the heels of effective older technologies, the demand for high-quality and timely comparative effectiveness studies is exploding. Well-done comparative effectiveness studies tell us which technology is more effective, safer, or for which subpopulation and/or clinical situation a therapy is superior. Clinicians need to understand the incremental benefits and harms of newer treatments compared to standard regimens, particularly with regards to needs of specific patients; and in addition, payers need to know the incremental cost so value can be ascertained. Understanding the magnitude of impact should also guide priorities for quality improvement initiatives.

Systematic evidence reviews of comparative effectiveness are constrained by the limited availability of head-to-head randomized controlled trials of health outcomes for alternative therapies. Such trials are usually costly because they must be large and, for most chronic conditions, long in duration. Indeed, the greatest need for such information is near the time of introduction of a new therapy, before a technology is in widespread use, precisely the time when such information is least likely to be available. Moreover, as challenging as it is to show efficacy of treatments compared to placebos, it is much more difficult and costly to demonstrate differences compared to active comparators and best-available alternatives. Thus, well-conducted head-to-head trials will remain uncommon. In the absence of head-to-head outcomes trials, however, insights may be obtained from trials using surrogate markers, comparisons of placebo controlled trials, or observational studies. The validity and generalizability of these studies for comparative purposes remains a topic of controversy. Observational studies can provide perspective on these issues, although the value of the information gleaned must be balanced against potential threats to validity and uncertainty around estimates of benefit.

While the limitations of different study designs are well known and ways to minimize bias well established, methods for quality assessments and data syntheses need to be refined and standards established to enhance confidence in the information generated. In addition, well-done models can synthesize the information, harness uncertainty to identify critical information gaps, focus attention on core outcomes and surrogates, and provide insights into the relative and absolute differences of therapeutic options. Because of their complexity and potential for bias, we need better processes to reduce the bias and enhance the credibility of models. These include systematic and transparent processes for identifying the key questions to be answered, the options to be evaluated, the structure of models, the parameter estimates, and sensitivity analyses. Mechanisms for validation and accreditation of models would enhance our confidence in their results. Investment in transparent development processes would go a long way to maximizing the value of existing information and identifying critical information needs. All along the way, important stakeholders, including payers and patients, need to participate in deliberative processes to ensure relevance and legitimacy.

For comparative effectiveness studies, there is an additional methodologic issue. Even when available, they typically do not directly provide estimates of absolute benefit or harms applicable to relevant populations. Indeed, most RCTs present results primarily in terms of relative risk reduction. In part this is related to a sense that the relative risk reduction is less variable across a broad range of patients than is the absolute risk reduction. Yet from a clinician's or payer's perspective, what is most important is the absolute change in benefit and harms; accurately estimating this change for specific patient groups is critical to informing bedside choices among alternative therapies. Moreover, estimation of benefits from RCTs may differ substantially from what is achieved for typical patients in real-world practice.

How then should these different sources of information (e.g., randomized clinical trials, effectiveness studies, observational studies, models) be evaluated and what weight should they be given in health policy decisions? We have previously discussed the need to consider the nature of the clinical question to determine the value to be gained from having additional certainty (Teutsch et al. 2005). Djulbegovic et al. (Djulbegovic et al. 2005) have emphasized the "potential for decision regret" to help frame how to deal with uncertainty in different clinical contexts. Some examples may illustrate potential approaches. For prevention, we generally require a high level of confidence that benefits, which generally accrue to a modest proportion of the population, exceed harms, which however uncommon can potentially occur to a large proportion of the population, most of whom will have little or no health benefit from the treatment. The magnitudes of benefits are bounded, of course, by the occurrence of the outcome, the success of identification and treatment of cases when they become clinically apparent, and the effectiveness of treatment. On the other hand, we may accept only small uncertain benefits and the occurrence of real harms for treatment of a fatal condition, such as cancer, for which other therapeutic alternatives have been exhausted.

The magnitude and certainty of net benefit is critical to optimizing the use of healthcare resources. Even for recommended preventive services, the estimated net benefit can vary by orders of magnitude (Maciosek et al. 2006). Understanding which services may provide the greatest benefit can guide providers and health systems to ensure that the greatest attention is paid to those underutilized services with the potential for the greatest health improvement. The same principle applies to diagnostic tests and procedures. Although many technologies may provide some level of benefit, clinical improvement strategies should focus on those technologies that provide the greatest net benefit and should be tailored to the extent possible to the specific subpopulations that have the most to gain.

Currently, there is no general consensus as to what standard—based upon the absolute benefits and harms and the certainty surrounding these estimates—should apply to different clinical recommendations. We have argued that it would be helpful to develop a taxonomy of clinical decision making ex ante to ensure that recommendations are made in a just and equitable manner. Such taxonomy alone would not be sufficient, but combined with procedures that ensure "accountability for reasonableness," it would enhance public trust in such recommendations.

Coverage decisions are perhaps the most critical arbiters of those choices. We need guidance for the information that must be available to warrant positive coverage decisions for the range of medical services. A rational and acceptable process for developing the "rules of the road for coverage decisions" needs to engage all important stakeholders, and a public debate about the trade-offs and consequences is needed to legitimize decisions. It is absolutely plausible that different payers will establish different rules leading to very different coverage decisions at substantially different costs, which will be attractive to different constituencies. However, potential elements in a taxonomy of decisions may include the quality of evidence, the magnitude of effect, the level of uncertainty regarding harms and benefits, the existence or absence of good treatment alternatives, the potential for decision regret, precedent, and acceptability.

We need a marketplace of health technology assessments providing comparative effectiveness information to provide checks and balances of different methods, assumptions, and perspectives. Regardless, a forum needs to be created whereby the methods and results of reports on similar topics are discussed so that methods can be refined and conclusions vetted. In the United States, the Agency for Healthcare Research and Quality has been pivotal to moving the field as far as it has and should continue to play a leadership role. It has spearheaded methods development, fostered the research, and established priorities. It can also capitalize on the extensive experience of groups around the world, such as the Cochrane and Campbell Collaborations, and the National Institute for Health and Clinical Excellence (NICE), among many others. We can also benefit from participation by nontraditional professionals, such as actuaries and operations research scientists, who use different methodologic approaches.

To create a taxonomy of decisions and identify the level of certainty required for each, it will be necessary to convene payers, health professionals, and patients along with methodologic experts. The Institute of Medicine is well-positioned to fulfill this role. More specific guidance can be developed by professional organizations with recognized expertise, such as Society for Medical Decision Making (SMDM), International Society for Pharmacoeconomics and Outcomes Research (ISPOR), and Academy Health, as well as AHRQ-sponsored consortia including the Evidence-based Practice Centers (EPCs), Centers for Education and Research on Therapeutics (CERTs), and the Developing Evidence to Inform Decisions about Effectiveness (DEcIDE) Network. Because of the complexity and need for transparency and legitimacy, the standards have to be the product of a public, deliberative process that includes all important stakeholders including patients, providers, plans, employers, government, and industry. The taxonomy will need to walk a fine line between clarity and overspecification. There is a real risk that when criteria for coverage are too explicit, it may be possible to game the system. This is very apparent with economic evaluations, where having a fixed cutoff for coverage, such as $50,000 per quality-adjusted life year, may lead manufacturers to price products as high as possible while still being below the threshold. Of course, a strict threshold might also work in the other direction where prices might be reduced to ensure cost-effectiveness criteria are met. Whatever the decision criteria, they need to leave room for decision makers to exercise their judgment based on contextual factors such as budget constraints, preferences, and acceptability. Since there is no completely free market for health care, it is important to recognize that decision makers are acting as a proxy for social decision making. Thus, their decisions must be based on criteria recognized as fair and reasonable.

Criteria should not be varied on a decision-by-decision basis for at least two reasons. Fairness requires understanding the "rules of the road" by all stakeholders determined behind a "veil of ignorance" to ensure equity and justice (Rawls 1971) as well as efficiency; this requires that we spend time up front agreeing on the methodology and not delay each decision by revisiting criteria. Thus significant investment in the process must be made up front. Moreover transparency will force disclosure of considerations that heretofore have been only implicit (including preferences, acceptability, and precedent) and not either apparent or explicitly disclosed as critical considerations to the broad range of stakeholders. Other groups are moving ahead with such efforts including America's Health Insurance Plans (AHIP); the specific goal of the AHIP project is to develop explicit guidance on how the certainty of evidence and magnitude of effect should be integrated with the contextual and clinical issues in making coverage decisions. Much as a marketplace of ideas represents a healthy situation for health technology assessments, here too, it will be constructive in the development of a taxonomy acceptable to a broad range of decision makers and stakeholders.

HIPAA AND CLINICAL RESEARCH: PROTECTING PRIVACY

An underlying workshop theme in many discussions of the need for better use of clinical data to assess interventions centers around the effects of privacy regulations, especially HIPAA (see Box 2-1), on current and future efforts to maximize learning from the healthcare system. The potential to collect and combine large quantities of data, including information derived from the point of care, has broad implications for research on clinical effectiveness, as well as on privacy concerns. As we extend our capacity to collect and aggregate data on medical care, researchers are increasingly confronted with limited access to data or burdensome regulatory requirements to conduct research, and privacy regulations are frequently cited as a significant constraint in clinical research.

Concerns cited during the workshop about these HIPAA regulations revealed broad implications for the notion of a learning healthcare system. The prospect of learning as a by-product of everyday care rests on the notion of collecting the data that results from these everyday clinical interactions. Many of the workshop participants cited that HIPAA regulations as limiting on research efforts, and expressed further concern that these limitations would be magnified with efforts to bring together clinical data to generate insights on clinical effectiveness. Throughout this workshop, there was a common concern that protection of privacy is crucial, yet the likely gains for public health need to be taken into account and privacy regulations should be implemented in a manner which is compatible with research. Ensuring that this goal is met will require collaboration between patients and the research community and careful consideration of the concerns of patients and the public at large. In the following piece, Janlori Goldman and Beth Tossell highlight many of the key issues from the patient perspective on privacy issues.

BOX 2-1
HIPPA Privacy Provisions

History of the Privacy Rule: The Health Insurance Portability and Accountability Act (HIPAA) of 1996 (Public Law 104-191) was enacted to improve the portability and continuity of health insurance; combat waste, fraud, and abuse in health insurance and healthcare delivery; promote medical savings accounts; improve access to long-term care services and coverage; and *simplify the administration of health insurance.* The Administrative Simplification "Standards for Privacy of Individually Identifiable Health Information" (the Privacy Rule) arise from this last objective. HIPAA's Administrative Simplification provisions focus on facilitating the electronic exchange of information for financial and administrative functions related to patient care. However, the very advances that make it easier to transmit information also present challenges to preserving the confidentiality of potentially sensitive personal information contained in medical records. Absent further congressional action, the Secretary of Health and Human Services (HHS) was required by the law to develop standards for protecting such information. Within HHS, the Office for Civil Rights (OCR) is responsible for implementing and enforcing the Privacy Rule. The compliance date for most of those affected by the Rule was April 14, 2003.

Provisions of the Privacy Rule: The Privacy Rule addresses the use and disclosure of health information contained in individual health records—"protected health information" (PHI)—by organizations subject to the Privacy Rule—"covered entities." Covered entities include health plans, healthcare clearinghouses, and healthcare providers that transmit health information electronically. All "individually identifiable health information" held or transmitted by a covered entity is protected under the Privacy Rule and considered PHI. This includes data relating to: the individual's past, present, or future physical or mental health or condition; the provision of health care to the individual; or the past, present, or future payment for the provision of health care to the individual. Common items like name, address, birth date, and Social Security Number are included in PHI. "De-identified" health information–information that does not identify an individual or provide the means to do so—is under no disclosure restrictions. The Privacy Rule defines the circumstances under which PHI may be used or disclosed by covered entities. PHI can be used by them in the normal course of providing medical care and the necessary administrative and financial transactions. Most other uses of PHI, including under most circumstances health research, require explicit written authorization by the individual (or personal representative).
SOURCE: Adapted from NIH and OCR guidances accessed August 24, 2003 at http://privacyruleandresearch.nih.gov/pr_02.asp and http://www.hhs.gov/ocr/hipaa.

continued

PROTECTING PRIVACY WHILE LINKING PATIENT RECORDS[3]

Janlori Goldman, J.D., and Beth Tossell
Health Privacy Project

Critical medical information is often nearly impossible to access both in emergencies and during routine medical encounters, leading to lost time, increased expenses, adverse outcomes and medical errors. Imagine the following scenarios:

- You are rushed to the emergency room, unable to give the paramedics your medical history.
- Your young child gets sick on a school field trip, and you are not there to tell the doctor that your child has a life-threatening allergy to penicillin.
- As you are being wheeled into major surgery, your surgeon realizes she must first look at an MRI taken two weeks earlier at another hospital.

If health information were easily available electronically, many of the nightmare scenarios above could be prevented.

But, to many, the potential benefits of a linked health information system are matched in significance by the potential drawbacks. The ability to enhance medical care coexists with the possibility of undermining the

---

[3]Text reprinted from *iHealthBeat*, February 2004, with permission from the California HealthCare Foundation, 2007.

privacy and security of people's most sensitive information. In fact, privacy fears have been a substantial barrier to the development of a national health information network. A 1999 survey by the California HealthCare Foundation showed that even when people understood the huge health advantages that could result from linking their health records, a majority believed that the risks—of lost privacy and discrimination—outweighed the benefits.

The issue does not split along partisan lines; prominent politicians from both parties have taken positions both for and against electronically linking medical records. During speeches to Congress and the public in 1993, Former President Bill Clinton touted a prototype "health security card" that would allow Americans to carry summaries of their medical records in their wallets. In response, Former Senate Minority Leader Bob Dole decried the health plan as "a compromise of privacy none of us can accept." And yet, in his State of the Union address last month, President Bush advocated "computerizing health records [in order to] avoid dangerous medical mistakes, reduce costs, and improve care."

History of Medical Record Linkage

But since the HIPAA privacy rule went into effect last April, the issue of unique health identifiers has resurfaced in the political debate. In November, the Institute of Medicine issued a report urging legislators to revisit the question of how to link patient data across organizations. "Being able to link a patient's health care data from one department location or site to another unambiguously is important for maintaining the integrity of patient data and delivering safe care," the report concluded. In fact, the Markle Foundation's Information Technologies for Better Health program recently announced that the second phase of its Connecting for Health initiative will be aimed at recommending policy and technical options for accurately and securely linking patient records. Decision makers in the health arena are once again grappling with the questions of whether and how to develop a national system of linking health information.

Is It Linkage? Or Is It a Unique Health Identifier?

The initial debate over linking medical records foundered over concern that any identifier created for health care purposes would become as ubiquitous and vulnerable as the Social Security number. At a hearing of the National Committee on Vital and Health Statistics in 1998, one speaker argued that "any identifier issued for use in health care will become a single national identifier . . . used for every purpose under the sun including driver's licenses, voter registration, welfare, employment and tax."

Using a health care identifier for non-health purposes would make people's information more vulnerable to abuse and misuse because the identifier would act as a key that could unlock many databases of sensitive information. To break this impasse, a more expansive approach is needed, focusing on the overarching goal of securely and reliably linking medical information. An identifier is one way to facilitate linkage, but not necessarily the only one. A 1998 NCVHS (National Committee on Vital and Health Statistics) white paper identified a number of possible approaches to linkage, some of which did not involve unique identifiers. At this stage, we should consider as many options as possible. It is simplistic to suggest that creating linkages is impossible simply because some initial proposals were faulty.

Linkage Will Improve Health Care

A reliable, confidential and secure means of linking medical records is necessary to provide the highest quality health care. In this era of health care fragmentation, most people see many different providers, in many different locations, throughout their lives. To get a full picture of each patient, a provider must request medical records from other providers or the patient, a burdensome process that rarely produces a thorough and accurate patient history, and sometimes produces disastrous errors. According to the Institute of Medicine, more than 500,000 people annually are injured due to avoidable adverse drug events in the United States. Linking medical records is, literally, a matter of life and death.

The question, then, is not whether we need to link medical records but what method of linking records will best facilitate health care while also protecting privacy and ensuring security. The time is long overdue for politicians, technical specialists, and members of the health care industry to find a workable solution.

Privacy Must Be Built in from the Outset

If privacy and security are not built in at the outset, linkage will make medical information more vulnerable to misuse, both within health care and for purposes unrelated to care. Even when most records are kept in paper files in individual doctors' offices, privacy violations occur. People have lost jobs and suffered stigma and embarrassment when details about their medical treatment were made public. Putting health information in electronic form, and creating the technical capacity to merge it with the push of a button, only magnifies the risk. Recently, computers containing the medical records of more 500,000 retired and current military personnel were stolen from a Department of Defense contractor. If those computers had been linked to an external network, the thieves might have been able to break into the records without even entering the office. We must therefore make sure that any system we implement is as secure as possible.

Similar Obstacles Have Been Overcome in Other Areas

The fields of law enforcement and banking have succeeded in linking personal information across sectors, companies and locations. Like health care, these fields are decentralized, with many points of entry for data and many organizations with proprietary and jurisdictional differences. Yet the urgent need to link information has motivated them to implement feasible and relatively secure systems. Law enforcement, for example, uses the Interstate Identification Index, which includes names and personal identification information for most people who have been arrested or indicted for a serious criminal offense anywhere in the country. In the banking industry, automated teller machines use a common operating platform that allows information to pass between multiple banks, giving people instant access to their money, anytime, almost anywhere in the world with an ATM card and a PIN.

Although the health care field is particularly diverse, complex, and disjointed, these examples show that, with dedication and creativity, it is possible to surmount both technical and privacy barriers to linking large quantities of sensitive information. A caveat—no information system, regardless of the safeguards built in—can be 100 percent secure. But appropriate levels of protection coupled with tough remedies and enforcement measures for breaches can strike a fair balance.

First Principles

In resolving the conjoined dilemmas of linking personal health information and maintaining confidentiality, the Health Privacy Project urges an adherence to the following first principles:

- Any system of linkage or identification must be secure, limiting disclosures from within and preventing unauthorized outside access.
- An effective system of remedies and penalties must be implemented and enforced. Misuse of the identifier, as well as misuse of the information to which it links, must be penalized.
- Any system of linkage or identifiers must be unique to health care.
- Patients must have electronic access to their own records.
- A mechanism for correcting—or supplementing—the record must be in place.
- Patients must have the ability to opt out of the system.

- Consideration should be given to making only core encounter data (e.g., blood type and drug allergies) accessible in emergencies and developing the capacity for a more complete record to be available with patient consent in other circumstances, such as to another provider.

With these privacy protections built in at the outset, a system of linking medical records may ultimately gain the public's approval.

REFERENCES

Abraham, E, P-F Laterre, R Garg, H Levy, D Talwar, B Trzaskoma, B Francois, J Guy, M Bruckmann, A Rea-Neto, R Rossaint, D Perrotin, A Sablotzki, N Arkins, B Utterback, W Macias, and the Administration of Drotrecogin Alfa in Early Stage Severe Sepsis Study, G. 2005. Drotrecogin alfa (activated) for adults with severe sepsis and a low risk of death. *New England Journal of Medicine* 353(13):1332-1341.

Bhatt, D, M Roe, E Peterson, Y Li, A Chen, R Harrington, A Greenbaum, P Berger, C Cannon, D Cohen, C Gibson, J Saucedo, N Kleiman, J Hochman, W Boden, R Brindis, W Peacock, S Smith Jr., C Pollack Jr., W Gibler, and E Ohman. 2004. Utilization of early invasive management strategies for high-risk patients with non-ST-segment elevation acute coronary syndromes: results from the CRUSADE Quality Improvement Initiative. *Journal of the American Medical Association* 292(17):2096-2104.

Bhatt, D, K Fox, W Hacke, P Berger, H Black, W Boden, P Cacoub, E Cohen, M Creager, J Easton, M Flather, S Haffner, C Hamm, G Hankey, S Johnston, K-H Mak, J-L Mas, G Montalescot, T Pearson, P Steg, S Steinhubl, M Weber, D Brennan, L Fabry-Ribaudo, J Booth, E Topol, for the CHARISMA Investigators. 2006. Clopidogrel and aspirin versus aspirin alone for the prevention of atherothrombotic events. *New England Journal of Medicine* 354(16):1706-1717.

Binanay, C, R Califf, V Hasselblad, C O'Connor, M Shah, G Sopko, L Stevenson, G Francis, C Leier, and L Miller. 2005. Evaluation study of congestive heart failure and pulmonary artery catheterization effectiveness: the ESCAPE trial. *Journal of the American Medical Association* 294(13):1625-1633.

Califf, R. 2006a. Fondaparinux in ST-segment elevation myocardial infarction: the drug, the strategy, the environment, or all of the above? *Journal of the American Medical Association* 295(13):1579-1580.

———. 2006b. Benefit assessment of therapeutic products: the Centers for Education and Research on Therapeutics. *Pharmacoepidemiology and Drug Safety.*

Califf, R, Y Tomabechi, K Lee, H Phillips, D Pryor, F Harrell Jr., P Harris, P Peter, V Behar, Y Kong, and R Rosati. 1983. Outcome in one-vessel coronary artery disease. *Circulation* 67(2):283-290.

Califf, R, R Harrington, L Madre, E Peterson, D Roth, and K Schulman. In press. Curbing the cardiovascular disease epidemic: aligning industry, government, payers, and academics. *Health Affairs.*

CDC Diabetes Cost-Effectiveness Group. 2002. Cost-effectiveness of intensive glycemic control, intensified hypertension control, and serum cholesterol level reduction for type 2 diabetes. *Journal of the American Medical Association* 287(19):2542-2551.

Chiasson, J, R Gomis, M Hanefeld, R Josse, A Karasik, and M Laakso. 1998. The STOP-NIDDM Trial: an international study on the efficacy of an alpha-glucosidase inhibitor to prevent type 2 diabetes in a population with impaired glucose tolerance: rationale, design, and preliminary screening data. Study to Prevent Non-Insulin-Dependent Diabetes Mellitus. *Diabetes Care* 21(10):1720-1725.

Colhoun, H, D Betteridge, P Durrington, G Hitman, H Neil, S Livingstone, M Thomason, M Mackness, V Charlton-Menys, and J Fuller. 2004. Primary prevention of cardiovascular disease with atorvastatin in type 2 diabetes in the Collaborative Atorvastatin Diabetes Study (CARDS): multicentre randomised placebo-controlled trial. *Lancet* 364(9435):685-696.

Connors, A, Jr., T Speroff, N Dawson, C Thomas, F Harrell Jr., D Wagner, N Desbiens, L Goldman, A Wu, R Califf, W Fulkerson Jr., H Vidaillet, S Broste, P Bellamy, J Lynn, and W Knaus. 1996. The effectiveness of right heart catheterization in the initial care of critically ill patients. SUPPORT Investigators. *Journal of the American Medical Association* 276(11):889-897.

Cowley, G, and M Hager. 1996 (September 30). Are catheters safe? *Newsweek*: 71.

Djulbegovic, B, A Frohlich, and C Bennett. 2005. Acting on imperfect evidence: how much regret are we ready to accept? *Journal of Clinical Oncology* 23(28):6822-6825.

Eddy, D, and L Schlessinger. 2003a. Archimedes: a trial-validated model of diabetes. *Diabetes Care* 26(11):3093-3101.

———. 2003b. Validation of the archimedes diabetes model. *Diabetes Care* 26(11): 3102-3110.

Eddy, D, L Schlessinger, and R Kahn. 2005. Clinical outcomes and cost-effectiveness of strategies for managing people at high risk for diabetes. *Annals of Internal Medicine* 143(4):251-264.

FDA (Food and Drug Administration). 1999. *Summary of Safety and Effectiveness: INTER FIX Intervertebral Body Fusion Device*. Available from www.fda.gov/cdrh/pdf/p970015b.pdf. (accessed April 4, 2007).

———. 2002. *Summary of Safety and Effectiveness Data: InFUSE Bone Graft / LT-CAGE Lumbar Tapered Fusion Device by Medtronic*. Available from www.fda.gov/cdrh/pdf/p000058b.pdf. (accessed April 4, 2007).

———. 2004 (March). *Challenge and Opportunity on the Critical Path to New Medical Products*.

———. 2006. *Public Meeting for the Use of Bayesian Statistics in Medical Device Clinical Trials*. Available from http://www.fda.gov/cdrh/meetings/072706-bayesian.html. (accessed April 4, 2007).

Ferguson, T, Jr., L Coombs, and E Peterson. 2002. Preoperative beta-blocker use and mortality and morbidity following CABG surgery in North America. *Journal of the American Medical Association* 287(17):2221-2227.

Fiaccadori, E, U Maggiore, M Lombardi, S Leonardi, C Rotelli, and A Borghetti. 2000. Predicting patient outcome from acute renal failure comparing three general severity of illness scoring systems. *Kidney International* 58(1):283-292.

Flaker, G, J Warnica, F Sacks, L Moye, B Davis, J Rouleau, R Webel, M Pfeffer, and E Braunwald. 1999. Pravastatin prevents clinical events in revascularized patients with average cholesterol concentrations. Cholesterol and Recurrent Events CARE Investigators. *Journal of the American College of Cardiology* 34(1):106-112.

Gerstein, H, S Yusuf, J Bosch, J Pogue, P Sheridan, N Dinccag, M Hanefeld, B Hoogwerf, M Laakso, V Mohan, J Shaw, B Zinman, and R Holman. 2006. Effect of rosiglitazone on the frequency of diabetes in patients with impaired glucose tolerance or impaired fasting glucose: a randomised controlled trial. *Lancet* 368(9541):1096-1105.

Greenfield, S, R Kravitz, N Duan, and S Kaplan. Unpublished. Heterogeneity of treatment effects: implications for guidelines, payment and quality assessment.

Harrington, R, and R Califf. 2006. Late ischemic events after clopidogrel cessation following drug-eluting stenting: should we be worried? *Journal of the American College of Cardiology* 48(12):2584-2591.

Hayward, R, D Kent, S Vijan, and T Hofer. 2005. Reporting clinical trial results to inform providers, payers, and consumers. *Health Affairs* 24(6):1571-1581.

———. 2006. Multivariable risk prediction can greatly enhance the statistical power of clinical trial subgroup analysis. *BMC Medical Research Methodology* 6:18.

Hennessy, S, W Bilker, L Zhou, A Weber, C Brensinger, Y Wang, and B Strom. 2003. Retrospective drug utilization review, prescribing errors, and clinical outcomes. *Journal of the American Medical Association* 290(11):1494-1499.

IOM (Institute of Medicine). 2000. *Interpreting the Volume-Outcome Relationship in the Context of Health Care Quality: Workshop Summary.* Washington, DC: National Academy Press.

———. 2006. *Effect of the HIPAA Privacy Rule on Health Research: Proceedings of a Workshop Presented to the National Cancer Policy Forum.* Washington, DC: The National Academies Press.

Kaplan, S, and S Normand. 2006 (December). Conceptual and analytic issues in creating composite measure of ambulatory care performance. In *Final Report to NQF.*

Kent, D. 2007. In press. Analyzing the results of clinical trials to expose individual patients' risks might help doctors make better treatment decisions. *American Scientist* 95(1).

Kent, D, R Hayward, J Griffith, S Vijan, J Beshansky, R Califf, and H Selker. 2002. An independently derived and validated predictive model for selecting patients with myocardial infarction who are likely to benefit from tissue plasminogen activator compared with streptokinase. *American Journal of Medicine* 113(2):104-111.

Knowler, W, E Barrett-Connor, S Fowler, R Hamman, J Lachin, E Walker, and D Nathan. 2002. Reduction in the incidence of type 2 diabetes with lifestyle intervention or metformin. *New England Journal of Medicine* 346(6):393-403.

Kravitz, R, N Duan, and J Braslow. 2004. Evidence-based medicine, heterogeneity of treatment effects, and the trouble with averages. *The Milbank Quarterly* 82(4):661-687.

Lagakos, S. 2006. The challenge of subgroup analyses—reporting without distorting. *New England Journal of Medicine* 354(16):1667-1669.

LaRosa, J, S Grundy, D Waters, C Shear, P Barter, J Fruchart, A Gotto, H Greten, J Kastelein, J Shepherd, and N Wenger. 2005. Intensive lipid lowering with atorvastatin in patients with stable coronary disease. *New England Journal of Medicine* 352(14):1425-1435.

Lipscomb, B, G Ma, and D Berry. 2005. Bayesian predictions of final outcomes: regulatory approval of a spinal implant. *Clinical Trials* 2(4):325-333; discussion 334-339, 364-378.

Litwin, M, S Greenfield, E Elkin, D Lubeck, J Broering, and S Kaplan. In press. *Total Illness Burden Index Predicts Mortality.*

Maciosek, M, N Edwards, N, Coffield, A, Flottemesch, T, Nelson, W, Goodman, M, and Solberg, L. 2006. Priorities among effective clinical preventive services: methods. *American Journal of Preventive Medicine* 31(1):90-96.

Mamdani, M, K Sykora, P Li, S Normand, D Streiner, P Austin, P Rochon, and G Anderson. 2005. Reader's guide to critical appraisal of cohort studies: 2. Assessing potential for confounding. *British Medical Journal* 330(7497):960-962.

March, J, C Kratochvil, G Clarke, W Beardslee, A Derivan, G Emslie, E Green, J Heiligenstein, S Hinshaw, K Hoagwood, P Jensen, P Lavori, H Leonard, J McNulty, M Michaels, A Mossholder, T Osher, T Petti, E Prentice, B Vitiello, and K Wells. 2004. AACAP 2002 research forum: placebo and alternatives to placebo in randomized controlled trials in pediatric psychopharmacology. *Journal of the American Academy of Child and Adolescent Psychiatry* 43(8):1046-1056.

McGlynn, E, S Asch, J Adams, J Keesey, J Hicks, A DeCristofaro, and E Kerr. 2003. The quality of health care delivered to adults in the United States. *New England Journal of Medicine* 348(26):2635-2645.

Mehta, R, C Montoye, M Gallogly, P Baker, A Blount, J Faul, C Roychoudhury, S Borzak, S Fox, M Franklin, M Freundl, E Kline-Rogers, T LaLonde, M Orza, R Parrish, M Satwicz, M Smith, P Sobotka, S Winston, A Riba, and K Eagle. 2002. Improving quality of care for acute myocardial infarction: the Guidelines Applied in Practice (GAP) Initiative. *Journal of the American Medical Association* 287(10):1269-1276.

Muthen, B, and K Shedden. 1999. Finite mixture modeling with mixture outcomes using the EM algorithm. *Biometrics* 55(2):463-469.

National Health and Nutrition Evaluation Survey, 1998-2002. Available from http://www.cdc. gov/nchs/hnanes.htm. (accessed April 4, 2007).

Normand, S, K Sykora, P Li, M Mamdani, P Rochon, and G Anderson. 2005. Readers guide to critical appraisal of cohort studies: 3. Analytical strategies to reduce confounding. *British Medical Journal* 330(7498):1021-1023.

Pedersen, T, O Faergeman, J Kastelein, A Olsson, M Tikkanen, I Holme, M Larsen, F Bendiksen, C Lindahl, M Szarek, and J Tsai. 2005. High-dose atorvastatin vs usual-dose simvastatin for secondary prevention after myocardial infarction: the IDEAL study: A randomized controlled trial. *Journal of the American Medical Association* 294(19):2437-2445.

Pfisterer, M, H Brunner-La Rocca, P Buser, P Rickenbacher, P Hunziker, C Mueller, R Jeger, F Bader, S Oss-wald, and C Kaiser, for the BASKET-LATE Investigators. In press. Late clinical events after clopidogrel discontinuation may limit the benefit of drug-eluting stents: an observational study of drug-eluting versus bare-metal stents. *Journal of the American College of Cardiology.*

Pocock, S, V McCormack, F Gueyffier, F Boutitie, R Fagard, and J Boissel. 2001. A score for predicting risk of death from cardiovascular disease in adults with raised blood pressure, based on individual patient data from randomised controlled trials. *British Medical Journal* 323(7304):75-81.

Prevention of cardiovascular events and death with pravastatin in patients with coronary heart disease and a broad range of initial cholesterol levels. The Long-Term Intervention with Pravastatin in Ischaemic Disease (LIPID) Study Group. 1998. *New England Journal of Medicine* 339(19):1349-1357.

Randomised trial of cholesterol lowering in 4444 patients with coronary heart disease: the Scandinavian Simvastatin Survival Study (4S). 1994. *Lancet* 344(8934):1383-1389.

Rawls, J. 1971. *A Theory of Justice.* Boston, MA: Harvard University Press.

Rochon, P, J Gurwitz, K Sykora, M Mamdani, D Streiner, S Garfinkel, S Normand, and GM Anderson. 2005. Reader's guide to critical appraisal of cohort studies: 1. Role and design. *British Medical Journal* 330(7496):895-897.

Rothwell, P, and C Warlow. 1999. Prediction of benefit from carotid endarterectomy in individual patients: A risk-modelling study. European Carotid Surgery Trialists' Collaborative Group. *Lancet* 353(9170):2105-2110.

Ryan, J, E Peterson, A Chen, M Roe, E Ohman, C Cannon, P Berger, J Saucedo, E DeLong, S Normand, C Pollack Jr., and D Cohen. 2005. Optimal timing of intervention in non-ST-segment elevation acute coronary syndromes: insights from the CRUSADE (Can rapid risk stratification of unstable angina patients suppress adverse outcomes with early implementation of the ACC/AHA guidelines) Registry. *Circulation* 112(20):3049-3057.

Schlessinger, L, and D Eddy. 2002. Archimedes: a new model for simulating health care systems—the mathematical formulation. *Journal of Biomedical Informatics* 35(1):37-50.

Schneeweiss, S, M Maclure, B Carleton, R Glynn, and J Avorn. 2004. Clinical and economic consequences of a reimbursement restriction of nebulised respiratory therapy in adults: direct comparison of randomised and observational evaluations. *British Medical Journal* 328(7439):560.

Selker, H, J Griffith, J Beshansky, C Schmid, R Califf, R D'Agostino, M Laks, K Lee, C Maynard, R Selvester, G Wagner, and W Weaver. 1997. Patient-specific predictions of outcomes in myocardial infarction for real-time emergency use: a thrombolytic predictive instrument. *Annals of Internal Medicine* 127(7):538-556.

Shah, M, V Hasselblad, L Stevenson, C Binanay, C O'Connor, G Sopko, and R Califf. 2005. Impact of the pulmonary artery catheter in critically ill patients: meta-analysis of randomized clinical trials. *Journal of the American Medical Association* 294(13):1664-1670.

Shepherd, J, S Cobbe, I Ford, C Isles, A Lorimer, P MacFarlane, J McKillop, and C Packard. 1995. Prevention of coronary heart disease with pravastatin in men with hypercholesterolemia. West of Scotland Coronary Prevention Study Group. *New England Journal of Medicine* 333(20):1301-1307.

Shepherd, J, G Blauw, M Murphy, E Bollen, B Buckley, S Cobbe, I Ford, A Gaw, M Hyland, J Jukema, A Kamper, P Macfarlane, A Meinders, J Norrie, C Packard, I Perry, D Stott, B Sweeney, C Twomey, and R Westendorp. 2002. Pravastatin in elderly individuals at risk of vascular disease (PROSPER): a randomised controlled trial. *Lancet* 360(9346):1623-1630.

Singh, A, L Szczech, K Tang, H Barnhart, S Sapp, M Wolfson, and D Reddan. 2006. Correction of anemia with epoetin alfa in chronic kidney disease. *New England Journal of Medicine* 355(20):2085-2098.

Slotman, G. 2000. Prospectively validated prediction of organ failure and hypotension in patients with septic shock: the Systemic Mediator Associated Response Test (SMART). *Shock* 14(2):101-106.

Snitker, S, R Watanabe, I Ani, A Xiang, A Marroquin, C Ochoa, J Goico, A Shuldiner, and T Buchanan. 2004. Changes in insulin sensitivity in response to troglitazone do not differ between subjects with and without the common, functional Pro12Ala peroxisome proliferator-activated receptor-gamma2 gene variant: Results from the Troglitazone in Prevention of Diabetes (TRIPOD) study. *Diabetes Care* 27(6):1365-1368.

Stier, D, S Greenfield, D Lubeck, K Dukes, S Flanders, J Henning, J Weir, and S Kaplan. 1999. Quantifying comorbidity in a disease-specific cohort: adaptation of the total illness burden index to prostate cancer. *Urology* 54(3):424-429.

Teno, J, F Harrell Jr., W Knaus, R Phillips, A Wu, A Connors Jr., N Wenger, D Wagner, A Galanos, N Desbiens, and J Lynn. 2000. Prediction of survival for older hospitalized patients: the HELP survival model. Hospitalized Elderly Longitudinal Project. *Journal of the American Geriatrics Society* 48(5 Suppl.):S16-S24.

Teutsch, S, and M Berger. 2005. Evidence synthesis and evidence-based decision making: related but distinct processes. *Medical Decision Making* 25(5):487-489.

Teutsch, S, M Berger, and M Weinstein. 2005. Comparative effectiveness: asking the right question. Choosing the right method. *Health Affairs* 24:128-132.

Tunis, S, D Stryer, and C Clancy. 2003. Practical clinical trials: Increasing the value of clinical research for decision making in clinical and health policy. *Journal of the American Medical Association* 290(12):1624-1632.

Tuomilehto, J, J Lindstrom, J Eriksson, T Valle, H Hamalainen, P Ilanne-Parikka, S Keinanen-Kiukaanniemi, M Laakso, A Louheranta, M Rastas, V Salminen, and M Uusitupa. 2001. Prevention of type 2 diabetes mellitus by changes in lifestyle among subjects with impaired glucose tolerance. *New England Journal of Medicine* 344(18):1343-1350.

Vijan, S, T Hofer, and R Hayward. 1997. Estimated benefits of glycemic control in microvascular complications in type 2 diabetes. *Annals of Internal Medicine* 127(9):788-795.

Vincent, J, D Angus, A Artigas, A Kalil, B Basson, H Jamal, G Johnson 3rd, and G Bernard. 2003. Effects of drotrecogin alfa (activated) on organ dysfunction in the PROWESS trial. *Critical Care Medicine* 31(3):834-840.

Welke, K, T Ferguson Jr., L Coombs, R Dokholyan, C Murray, M Schrader, and E Peterson. 2004. Validity of the society of thoracic surgeons national adult cardiac surgery database. *Annals of Thoracic Surgery* 77(4):1137-1139.

Zimmerman, J, E Draper, L Wright, C Alzola, and W Knaus. 1998. Evaluation of acute physiology and chronic health evaluation III predictions of hospital mortality in an independent database. *Critical Care Medicine* 26(8):1317-1326.

3

Narrowing the Research-Practice Divide—Systems Considerations

OVERVIEW

Bridging the inference gap, as described in this chapter, is the daily leap physicians must make to piece existing evidence around individual patients in the clinical setting. Capturing and utilizing data generated in the course of care offers the opportunity to bring research and practice into closer alignment and propagate a cycle of learning that can enhance both the rigor and the relevance of evidence. Papers in this chapter illustrate process and analytic changes needed to narrow the research-practice divide and allow healthcare delivery to play a more fundamental role in the generation of evidence on clinical effectiveness.

In this chapter, Brent James outlines the system-wide reorientation that occurred at Intermountain Healthcare as it implemented a system to manage care at the care delivery level. Improved performance and patient care were fostered by a system designed to collect data to track inputs and outcomes and provide feedback on performance—elements that also created a useful research tool that has led to incremental improvements in quality along with discovery and large advancements in care at the practice level. The experience at Intermountain identifies some of the organizational and cultural changes needed, but a key was the utilization of electronic health records (EHRs) and support systems. Walter F. Stewart expands on the immense potential of the EHR as a tool to narrow the inference gap—the gap between what is known at the point of care and what evidence is needed to make a clinical decision. In his paper, he focuses on the potential for EHRs to increase real-time access to knowledge and facilitate the creation of evidence that is more directly relevant to everyday clinical decisions. Stewart views the EHR as a transforming technology and suggests several ways in which appropriate design and utilization of this tool and surrounding support systems can allow researchers to tap into and learn from the heterogeneity of patients, treatment effects, and the clinical environment to accelerate the generation and application of evidence in a learning healthcare system.

Perhaps one of the most substantial considerations will be how these quicker, practice-based opportunities to generate evidence might affect evidentiary standards. Steven Pearson's paper outlines how the current process of assessing bodies of evidence to inform the coverage decision process might not be able to meet future needs, and the potential utility of a means to consider factors such as clinical circumstance in the process. He discusses possible unintended consequences of approaches such as Coverage with Evidence Development (CED) and suggests concepts and processes associated with coverage decisions in need of development and better definition. Finally, Robert Galvin discusses the employer's dilemma of how to get true innovations in healthcare technology to populations of benefit as quickly as possible but guard against the harms that could arise from inadequate evaluation. He suggests that a "cycle of unaccountability" has hampered efforts to balance the need to foster innovation while controlling costs, and discusses some of the issues facing technology developers in the current system and a recent initiative by General Electric (GE), UnitedHealthcare, and InSightec to apply the CED approach to a promising treatment for uterine fibroids. Although this initiative has potential to substantially expand the capacity for evidence generation while accelerating access and innovation, challenges to be overcome include those related to methodology, making the case to employers to participate, and confronting the culture of distrust between payers and innovators.

FEEDBACK LOOPS TO EXPEDITE STUDY TIMELINESS AND RELEVANCE

Brent James, M.D., M.Stat.
Intermountain Healthcare

Quality improvement was introduced to health care in the late 1980s. Intermountain Healthcare, one of the first groups to attempt clinical improvement using these new tools, had several early successes (Classen et al. 1992; James 1989 [2005, republished as a "classics" article]). While those experiences showed that Deming's process management methods could work within healthcare delivery, they highlighted a major challenge: the results did not, on their own, spread. Success in one location did not lead to widespread adoption, even among Intermountain's own facilities.

Three core elements have been identified for a comprehensive quality-based strategy (Juran 1989): (1) Quality control provides core data flow and management infrastructure, allowing ongoing process management. It creates a context for (2) quality improvement—the ability to systematically identify then improve prioritized targets. (3) Quality design encompasses a set of structured tools to identify, then iteratively create new processes and products.

Since the quality movement's inception, most care delivery organizations have focused exclusively on improvement. None have built a comprehensive quality control framework. Quality control provides the organizational infrastructure necessary to rapidly deploy new research findings across care delivery locations. The same infrastructure makes it possible to generate reliable new clinical knowledge from care delivery experience. In 1996, Intermountain undertook to build clinical quality control across its 22 hospitals, 100-plus outpatient clinics, employed and affiliated physician groups (1,250 core physicians, among more than 3,000 total associated physicians), and a health insurance plan (which funds about 25 percent of Intermountain's total care delivery). Intermountain's quality control plan contained 4 major elements: (1) key process analysis; (2) an outcomes tracking system that measured and reported accurate, timely, medical, cost, and patient satisfaction results; (3) an organizational structure to use outcomes data to hold practitioners accountable, and to enable measured progress on shared clinical goals; and (4) aligned incentives, to harvest some portion of resulting cost savings back to the care delivery organization (while in many instances better quality can demonstrably reduce care delivery costs, current payment mechanisms direct most such savings to health payers).

The Intermountain strategy depended heavily upon a new "shared baselines" approach to care delivery, that evolved during early quality improvement projects as a mechanism to functionally implement evidence-based medicine (James 2002): All health professionals associated with a particular clinical work process come together on a team (physicians, nurses, pharmacists, therapists, technicians, administrators, etc.). They build an evidence-based best practice guideline, fully understanding that it will not perfectly fit any patient in a real care delivery setting. They blend the guideline into clinical workflow, using standing order sets, clinical worksheets, and other tools. Upon implementation, health professionals adapt their shared common approach to the needs of each individual patient. Across more than 30 implemented clinical shared baselines, Intermountain's physicians and nurses typically (95 percent confidence interval) modify about 5 to 15 percent of the shared baseline to meet the specific needs of a particular patient. That makes it "easy to do it right" (James 2001), while facilitating the role of clinical expertise. It also is much more efficient. Expert clinicians can focus on a subset of critical issues because the remainder of the care process is reliable. The organization can staff, train, supply, and organize physical space to a single defined process. Shared baselines also provide a structure for electronic data systems, greatly enhancing the effectiveness of automated clinical information. Arguably, shared baselines are the key to successful implementation of electronic medical record systems.

Key Process Analysis

The Institute of Medicine's prescription for reform of U.S. health care noted that an effective system should be organized around its most common elements (IOM 2001). Each year for 4 years, Intermountain attempted to identify high priority clinical conditions for coordinated action, through expert consensus among senior clinical and administrative leaders generated through formal nominal group technique. In practice, consensus methods never overcame advocacy. Administrative and clinical leaders, despite a superficially successful consensus process, still focused primarily on their own departmental or personal priorities. We therefore moved from expert consensus to objective measurement. That involved first, identifying front line work processes. This complex task was aided by conceptually subdividing Intermountain's operations into 4 large classes: (1) work processes centered around clinical conditions; (2) clinical work processes that are not condition-specific (clinical support services, e.g., processes located within pharmacy, pathology, anesthesiology/procedure rooms, nursing units, intensive care units, patient safety); (3) processes associated with patient satisfaction; and (4) administrative support processes. Within each category, we attempted to identify all major work processes that produced value-added results.

These work processes were then prioritized. To illustrate, within clinical conditions we first measured the number of patients affected. Second, clinical risk to the patient was estimated. We used intensity of care as a surrogate for clinical risk, and assessed intensity of care by measuring true cost per case. This produced results that had high face validity with clinicians, while also working well with administrative leadership. Third, basestate variability within a particular clinical work process was measured by calculating the coefficient of variation, based on intensity of care (cost per case). Fourth, using Batalden and Nelson's concept of clinical microsystems specialty groups that routinely worked together on the basis of shared patients were identified along with the clinical processes through which they managed those patients (Batalden and Splaine 2002; Nelson et al. 2002). This was a key element for organizational structure. Finally, we applied two important criteria for which we could not find metrics: we used expert judgment to identify underserved subpopulations, and to balance our rollout across all elements of the Intermountain care delivery system.

Among more than 1,000 inpatient and outpatient condition-based clinical work processes, 104 accounted for almost 95 percent of all of Intermountain's clinical care delivery. Rather than the traditional 80/20 rule (the Pareto principle), we saw a 90/10 rule: Clinical care concentrated massively, on a relative handful of high priority clinical processes (the IOM's Quality Chasm report got it right!). Those processes were addressed in priority order, to achieve the most good for the most patients, while freeing resources to enable traditional, one by one care delivery plans for uncommon clinical conditions.

Outcomes Tracking

Prior to 1996, Intermountain had tried to start clinical management twice. The effort failed each time. Each failure lost $5 million to $10 million in sunk costs, and cashiered a senior vice president for medical affairs. When asked to make a third attempt, we first performed a careful autopsy on the first two attempts. Each time Intermountain had found clinicians willing to step up and lead. Then, each time, Intermountain's planners uncritically assumed that the new clinical leaders could use the same administrative, cost-based data to manage clinical processes, as had traditionally been used to manage hospital departments and generate insurance claims. On careful examination, the administrative data contained gaping holes relative to clinical care delivery. They were organized for facilities management, not patient management.

One of the National Quality Forum's (NQF) first activities, upon its creation, was to call together a group of experts (its Strategic Framework Board—SFB) to produce a formal, evidence-based method to identify valid measurement sets for clinical care (James 2003). The SFB found that outcomes tracking systems work best when designed around and integrated into front-line care delivery. Berwick et al. noted that such integrated data systems can "roll up" into accountability reports for practice groups, clinics, hospitals, regions, care delivery systems, states, and the nation. The opposite is not true. Data systems designed top down for national reporting usually cannot generate the information flow necessary for front-line process management and improvement (Berwick et al. 2003). Such top-down systems often compete for limited front-line resources, damaging care delivery at the patient interface (Lawrence and Mickalide 1987).

Intermountain adopted the NQF's data system design method. It starts with an evidence-based best practice guideline, laid out for care delivery—a shared baseline. It uses that template to identify and then test a comprehensive set of medical, cost, and satisfaction outcomes reports, optimized for clinical process management and improvement. The report set leads to a list of data elements and coding manuals, which generate data marts within an electronic data warehouse (patient registries), and decision support structure for use within electronic medical record systems.

The production of new clinical outcomes tracking data represented a significant investment for Intermountain. Clinical work processes were attacked in priority order, as determined by key process analysis. Initial progress was very fast. For example, in 1997 outcomes tracking systems were completed for the two biggest clinical processes within the Intermountain system. Pregnancy, labor, and delivery represents 11 percent of Intermountain's total clinical volume. Ischemic heart disease adds another 10 percent. At the end of the year, Intermountain had a detailed clinical dashboard in place for 21 percent of Intermountain's total care delivery. Those data were designed for front-line process management, then rolled up into region- and system-level accountability reports. Today, outcomes data cover almost 80 percent of Intermountain's inpatient and outpatient clinical care. They are immediately available through internal websites, with data lag times under one month in all cases, and a few days in most cases.

Organizational Structure

About two-thirds of Intermountain's core physician associates are community-based, independent practitioners. That required an organizational structure that heavily emphasized shared professional values, backed up by aligned financial incentives (in fact, early successes relied on shared professional values alone; financial incentives came quite late in the process, and were always modest in size). The microsystems (Batalden and Splaine 2002) subpart of the key process analysis provided the core organizational structure. Families of related processes, called Clinical Programs, identified care teams that routinely worked together, even though they often spanned traditional subspecialty boundaries. Intermountain hired part-time physician leaders (¼ full time equivalent) for each Clinical Program in each of its 3 major regions (networks of outpatient practices and small community hospitals, organized around large tertiary hospital centers). Physician leaders are required to be in active practice within their Clinical Program; to have the respect of their professional peers; and to complete formal training in clinical quality improvement methods through Intermountain's internal clinical QI training programs (the Advanced Training Program in Clinical Practice Improvement). Recognizing that the bulk of process management efforts rely upon clinical staff, Intermountain also hired full-time "clinical operations administrators." Most of the staff support leaders are experienced nurse administrators. The resulting leadership dyad—a physician leader with a nursing/support staff leader—meet each month with each of the local clinical teams that work within their Clinical Program. They present and review patient outcomes results for each team, compared to their peers and national benchmarks. They particularly focus on clinical improvement goals, to track progress, identify barriers, and discuss possible solutions. Within each region, all of the Clinical Program dyads meet monthly with their administrative counterparts (regional hospital administration, finance, information technology, insurance partners, nursing, and quality management). They review current clinical results, track progress on goals, and assign resources to overcome implementation barriers at a local level.

In addition to their regional activities, all leaders within a particular Clinical Program from across the entire Intermountain system meet together monthly as a central Guidance Council. One of the 3 regional physician leaders is funded for an additional part-time role (¼ time) to oversee and coordinate the system-wide effort. Each system-level Clinical Program also has a separate, full-time clinical operations administrator. Finally, each Guidance Council is assigned at least one full-time statistician, and at least one full-time data manager, to help coordinate clinical outcomes data flow, produce outcomes tracking reports, and to perform special analyses. Intermountain coordinates a large part of existing staff support functions, such as medical informatics (electronic medical records), electronic data warehouse, finance, and purchasing, to support the clinical management effort.

By definition, each Guidance Council oversees a set of condition-based clinical work processes, as identified and prioritized during the key process analysis step. Each key clinical process is managed by a Development Team which reports to the Guidance Council. Development Teams meet each month. The majority of Development Team members are drawn from front-line physicians and clinical staff, geographically balanced across the Intermountain system, who have immediate hands-experience with the clinical care under discussion (technically, "fundamental knowledge"). Development Team members carry the team's activities—analysis and management system results—back to their front-line colleagues, to seek their input and help with implementation and operations. Each Development Team also has a designated physician leader, and Knowledge Experts drawn from each region. Knowledge Experts are usually specialists associated with the Team's particular care process. For example, the Primary Care Clinical Program includes a Diabetes Mellitus Development Team (among others). Most team members are front-line primary care physicians and nurses who see diabetes patients in their practices every day. The Knowledge Experts are diabetologists, drawn from each region.

A new Development Team begins its work by generating a Care Process Model (CPM) for their assigned key clinical process. Intermountain's central Clinical Program staff provides a great deal of coordinated support for this effort. A Care Process Model contains 5 sequential elements:

1. The Knowledge Experts generate an evidence-based best practice guideline for the condition under study, with appropriate links to the published literature. They share their work with the body of the Development Team, who in turn share it with their front-line colleagues, asking "What would you change?" As the "shared baseline" practice guideline stabilizes over time,

2. The full Development Team converts the practice guideline into clinical workflow documents, suitable for use in direct patient care. This step is often the most difficult of the CPM development process. Good clinical flow can enhance clinical productivity, rather than adding burden to front-line practitioners. The aim is to make evidence-based best care the lowest energy default option, with data collection integrated into clinical workflow.

The core of most chronic disease CPMs is a treatment cascade. Treatment cascades start with disease detection and diagnosis. The first (and most important) "treatment" is intensive patient education, to make the patient the primary disease manager. The cascade then steps sequentially through increasing levels of treatment. A font-line clinical team moves down the cascade until they achieve adequate control of the patient's condition, while modifying the cascade's "shared baseline" based upon individual patient needs. The last step in most cascades is referral to a specialist.

3. The team next applies the NQF SFB outcomes tracking system development tools, to produce a balanced dashboard of medical, cost, and satisfaction outcomes. This effort involves the electronic data warehouse team, to design clinical registries that bring together complementary data flows with appropriate pre-processing.

4. The Development Team works with Intermountain's medical informatics groups, to blend clinical workflow tools and data system needs into automated patient care data systems.

5. Central support staff help the Development Team build web-based educational materials for both care delivery professionals, and the patients they serve.

A finished CPM is formally deployed into clinical practice by the governing Guidance Council, through its regional physician/nurse leader dyads. At that point, the Development Team's role changes. The Team continues to meet monthly to review and update the CPM. The Team's Knowledge Experts have funded time to track new research developments. The Team also reviews care variations as clinicians adapt the shared baseline. It closely follows major clinical outcomes, and receives and clears improvement ideas that arise among Intermountain's front-line practitioners and leadership.

Drawing on this structure, Intermountain's CPMs tend to change quite frequently. Knowledge Experts have an additional responsibility of sharing new findings and changes with their front-line colleagues. They conduct regular continuing education sessions, targeted both at practicing physicians and their staffs, for their assigned CPM. Education sessions cover the full spectrum of the coordinated CPM: They review current best practice (the core evidence-based guideline); relate it to clinical workflow; show delivery teams how to track patient results through the outcomes data system; tie the CPM to decision support tools built into the electronic medical record; and link it to a full set of educational materials, for patients and for care delivery professionals.

Chronic disease Knowledge Experts also run the specialty clinics that support front-line care delivery teams. Continuing education sessions usually coordinate the logistics of that support. The Knowledge Experts also coordinate specialty-based nurse care managers and patient trainers.

An Illustrative CPM in Action: Diabetes Mellitus

Through its health plan and outpatient clinics, Intermountain supports almost 20,000 patients diagnosed with diabetes mellitus. Among about 800 primary care physicians who manage diabetics, approximately one-third are employed within the Intermountain Medical Group, while the remainder are community-based independent physicians. All physicians and their care delivery teams—regardless of employment status—interact regularly with the Primary Care Clinical Program medical directors and clinical operations administrators. They have access to regular diabetes continuing education sessions. Three endocrinologists (one in each region) act as Knowledge Experts on the Diabetes Development Team. In addition to conducting diabetes training, the Knowledge Experts coordinate specialty nursing care management (diabetic educators), and supply most specialty services.

Each quarter, Intermountain sends a packet of reports to every clinical team managing diabetic patients. The reports are generated from the Diabetes Data Mart (a patient registry) within Intermountain's electronic data warehouse. The packet includes, first, a Diabetes Action List. It summarizes every diabetic patient in the team's practice, listing testing rates and level controls (standard NCQA HEDIS measures: HbA1c, LDL, blood pressure, urinary protein, dilated retinal exams, pedal sensory exams; Intermountain was an NCQA Applied Research Center that helped generate the HEDIS diabetes measures, using the front-line focused NQF outcomes tracking design techniques outlined above). The report flags any care defect, as reflected either in test frequency or level controls. Front-line teams review lists, then either schedule flagged patients for office visits, or assign them to general care management nurses located within the local clinic. While

Intermountain pushes Diabetes Action Lists out every quarter, front-line teams can generate them on demand. Most teams do so every month.

In addition to Action Lists, front-line teams can access patient-specific Patient Worksheets through Intermountain's web-based Results Review system. Most practices integrate Worksheets into their workflow during chart preparation. The Worksheet contains patient demographics, a list of all active medications, and a review of pertinent history and laboratory focused around chronic conditions. For diabetic patients, it will include test dates and values for the last seven HbA1c, LDLs, blood pressures, urinary proteins, dilated retinal examinations, and pedal sensory examinations. A final section of the Worksheet applies all pertinent treatment cascades, listing recommendations for currently due immunizations, disease screening, and appropriate testing. It will flag out-of-control levels, with next-step treatment recommendations (technically, this section of the Worksheet is a passive form of computerized physician order entry).

The standard quarterly report packet also contains sections comparing each clinical team's performance to their risk-adjusted peers. A third report tracks progress on quality improvement goals, and links them to financial incentives. Finally, a separate summary report goes to the team's Clinical Program medical director. In meeting with the front-line teams, the Clinical Program leadership dyad often share methods used by other practices to improve patient outcome performance, with specific practice flow recommendations.

Intermountain managed more than 20,000 diabetic patients by March, 2006 and Figures 3-1 and 3-2 show system-level performance on representative diabetes outcomes measures, as pulled real-time from the Intermountain outcomes tracking system. Primary care physicians supply almost 90 percent of all diabetes care in the system.

As the last step on a treatment cascade, Intermountain's Diabetes Knowledge Experts tend to concentrate the most difficult patients in their specialty practices. As a result, they typically have worse outcomes than their primary care colleagues.

Using Routine Care Delivery to Generate Reliable Clinical Knowledge

Evidence-based best practice faces a massive evidence gap. The healing professions currently have reliable evidence (Level I, II, or III—randomized trials, robust observational designs, or expert consensus opinion using formal methods (Lawrence and Mickalide 1987) to identify best, patient-specific, practice for less than 20 percent of care delivery choices (Ferguson 1991; Lappe et al. 2004; Williamson 1979). Bridging that gap will strain the capacity of any conceivable research system.

Intermountain designed its Clinical Programs to optimize care delivery

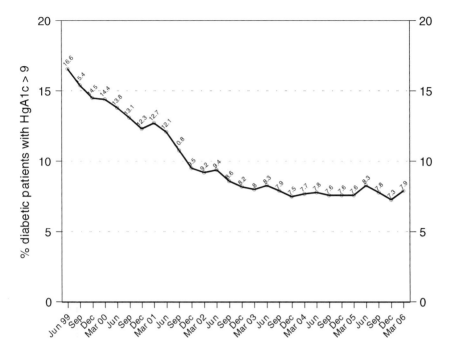

FIGURE 3-1 Blood sugar control with Clinical Program management over time, for all diabetic patients managed within the entire Intermountain system National guidelines recommend that all diabetic patients be managed to hemoglobin A1c levels < 9 percent; ideally, patients should be managed to levels < 7 percent.

performance. The resulting organizational and information structures make it possible to generate robust data regarding treatment effects, as a by-product of demonstrated best care. CPMs embed data systems that directly link outcome results to care delivery decisions. They deploy organized care delivery processes. Intermountain's Clinical Programs might be thought of as effectiveness research, built system-wide into front-line care delivery. At a minimum, CPMs routinely generate Level II-3 information (robust, prospective observational time series) for all key clinical care delivery processes. In such a setting, all care changes get tested. For example, any new treatment, recently released in the published medical literature; any new drug; a new organizational structure for an ICU; a new nurse staffing policy implemented within a hospital can generate robust information to assess its effectiveness in a real care delivery setting.

At need, Development Teams move up the evidence chain as a part of routine care delivery operations. For example, the Intermountain Car-

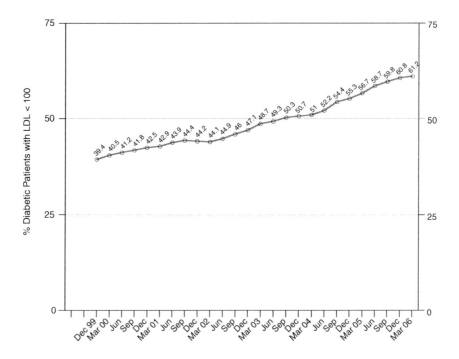

FIGURE 3-2 Lipid (low density lipoprotein/LDL) control with Clinical Program management over time, for all diabetic patients managed within the entire Intermountain system. National guidelines recommend that all diabetic patients should be managed to LDL levels < 100 mg/dL.

diovascular Guidance Council developed robust observational evidence regarding discharge medications for patients hospitalized with ischemic heart disease or atrial fibrillation (Level II-2 evidence) (Lappe et al. 2004). The Mental Health Integration Development Team used the Intermountain outcomes tracking system to conduct a prospective non-randomized controlled trial (Level II-1 evidence) to assess best practice for the detection and management of depression in primary care clinics (Reiss-Brennan 2006; Reiss-Brennan et al. 2006a; Reiss-Brennan et al. 2006b). The Lower Respiratory Infection Development Team ran a quasi-experiment that used existing prospective data flows to assess roll-out of their community-acquired pneumonia (CAP) CPM (Level II-1 evidence) (Dean et al. 2006a; Dean et al. 2001). That led to a randomized controlled trial to identify best antibiotic choices for outpatient management of CAP (Level 1 evidence) (Dean et al. 2006b). With embedded data systems and an existing "shared baseline" care protocol that spanned the Intermountain system, it took less than 3 months to complete the trial. The largest associated expenses were IRB oversight and data analysis—costs that Intermountain underwrote, based on a clear need to quickly generate then apply appropriate evidence to real patient care.

While Intermountain demonstrates the concept of embedded effectiveness research, many other integrated care delivery networks are rapidly deploying similar methods. Embedded effectiveness research is an engine that can make evidence-based care delivery the norm, rather than the exception. It holds massive potential to deliver "best care" to patients, while generating evidence to find the next step in "best care."

ELECTRONIC HEALTH RECORDS AND EVIDENCE-BASED PRACTICE

Walter F. Stewart, Ph.D., M.P.H., and Nirav R. Shah, M.D., M.P.H.
Geisinger Health System

Every day, clinicians engage in a decision process on behalf of patients that requires a leap beyond available evidence. This process, which we characterize as "bridging the inferential gap" (Stewart et al. 2007 [in press]), uses varying degrees of judgment, either because available evidence is not used or because the right evidence does not exist. This gap has widened as the population has aged, with the rapid growth in treatment needs and options, and as the creation of knowledge continues to accelerate. Increasing use of the EHR in practice will help to narrow this gap by substantially increasing real-time access to knowledge (Haynes 1998) and by facilitating creation of evidence that is more directly relevant to everyday clinical decisions (Haynes et al. 1995).

The Twentieth-Century Revolution in Creation of Evidence

In the early twentieth century, medical knowledge creation emerged as a new enterprise with the propagation of an integrated model of medical education, clinical care, and "bench to bedside" research (Flexner 2002; Vandenbroucke 1987) In the United States, this model evolved with the rapid growth in foundation and federal funding, and later with substantial growth in industry funding (Charlton and Andras 2005; Graham and Diamond 2004). Today, this enterprise has exceeded expectations in the breadth and depth of evidence created, but has fallen short in the relevance of evidence to everyday clinical care needs.

Over the last 50 years, rigorous scientific methods have developed as part of this enterprise, in response to challenges with the interpretation of evidence. While observational and experimental methods developed in parallel, the randomized controlled clinical trial became the dominant method for creating clinical evidence, emerging as the "gold standard" in response to demand for a rigorous and reliable approach to answering questions (Meldrum 2000). The application of the RCT naturally evolved in response to regulatory demands for greater accuracy in the interpretation of evidence of treatment benefit and minimizing risk of harm to volunteers. As a consequence, RCTs have tended toward very focused interventions in highly select populations (Black 1996). Often, the questions answered do not fully address more specific questions that arise in clinical practice. Moreover, restricting enrollment to the healthiest subgroup of patients (i.e., with minimal comorbidities) limits the generalizability of the evidence derived. Patients seen in clinical practice tend to be considerably more diverse and more clinically complex than patients enrolled in clinical trials. This gap between existing evidence and the needs of clinical practice does not mean that we should change how RCTs are done. It is not sensible to use the RCT as a routine method to answer practice-specific questions. The resources required to answer a meaningful number of practice-based questions would be too substantial. The time required would often be too long for answers to be relevant.

Accepting that the RCT should continue to be used primarily as a testing and regulatory tool does not resolve the dilemma of the need for an effective means of creating more relevant evidence. We currently do not have the means to create evidence that is rigorous and timely, and answers the myriad of questions common to everyday practice. As a bridging strategy, we have resorted to consensus decisions among clinical experts, replacing evidence with guidance (Greenblatt 1980). Finally, systematic observational studies in general population- or practice-based samples are often cited as a means to address the generalizability limits of evidence from RCTs (Horwitz et al. 1990). Confounding by indication is an important concern with interpretation of evidence from such studies, but this is not the most significant challenge (Salas et al. 1999). Again, the same issues regarding resource limitations and access to timely evidence apply. Most practice-based questions of clinical interest cannot be answered by funding systematic prospective observational studies.

Knowledge Access

While the methods to generate knowledge over the past century have advanced at a remarkable pace and knowledge creation itself is accelerating, the methods to access such knowledge for clinical care have not evolved. Direct education of clinicians continues to be the dominant model for bringing knowledge to practice. This is largely because there are no practical alternatives. While the modes by which knowledge is conveyed (e.g., CDs, Internet) have diversified, all such modes still rely on individual education, a method that was useful when knowledge was relatively limited. Today, however, individual continuing medical education (CME) can be characterized as a hit-or-miss approach to gaining knowledge. There is so little time, yet so much to know. There are also numerous other factors essential to bringing knowledge to practice that individual education does not address. These other factors, downstream from gaining knowledge, probably contribute to variation in quality of care. Specifically, clinicians vary substantially, not just in what they have learned, but in the accuracy of what is retained, in real-time retrieval of what is retained when needed, in the details of what they know or review about the patient during an encounter, in the interpretation of patient data given the retained knowledge that is retrieved during the encounter, and in how this whole process translates into a care decision. Even if incentives (e.g., pay for performance) were logically designed to motivate the best clinical behavior, the options for reducing variation in practice are limited given the numerous other factors that influence the ultimate clinical decision. In the paper-based world of most clinical practices, clinicians will always be constrained by a "pony-express" model of bringing knowledge to practice. That is, with very limited time, clinicians must choose a few things to learn from time to time and hope that they use what they learn effectively when needed.

Just as consensus decision making is used to bridge the knowledge gap, efforts to codify knowledge over the past decade are an important step toward increasing access to knowledge. However, this is only one of the many steps noted above that is relevant to translating knowledge to practice-based decision making. The EHR opens opportunities for a paradigm shift in how knowledge is used in practice-based clinical decisions.

The EHR and New Directions

There are several areas in which the EHR represents the potential for a fundamental shift in research emphasis—in particular, the linkage of research to development, the most common paradigm for research worldwide; the opening of opportunities to explore new models for creating evidence; and the evolving role of decision support in bringing knowledge directly to practice.

Research and Development In the private for-profit sector, the dominant motivation for research is to create value, through its intimate link to the development of better products and services. "Better" generally means that more value is attained because the product or service cost is reduced (e.g., research and development [R&D], which results in a lower cost of production), the product is made more capable at the same or a lower cost, or quality is improved (e.g., more durable, fewer errors) at the same or at lower cost. This R&D paradigm, core to competition among market rivals in creating ongoing value to customers, does exist in certain healthcare sectors (e.g., pharmaceutical and device manufacturers) but does not exist, for the most part, in the U.S. healthcare system, where, notably, value-based competition also does not exist (Porter and Teisber 2006).

The dominant research model in academic institutions is different. Research funding is largely motivated by the mission to create knowledge, recognizing the inherent social value of such an enterprise.[1] The policies and practices in this sector are largely created by academic officials and faculty in collaboration with government or foundation officials. This is in essence a closed system that seeks to fulfill its mission of creating knowledge. It is not a system primarily designed to influence or bring value, as defined above, to health care. Academic research institutions are not representative of where most health care is provided in the United States. Private practice physicians, group practices, community hospitals, and health systems deliver the vast majority of care in the United States. Even if there was a desire to shift some funding toward an R&D focus, the link between academic institutions and the dominant systems of care in the United States may not be substantial enough for research to be directed in a manner that creates value. In contrast, new healthcare strategies and models of care are increasingly tested by the Centers for Medicare and Medicaid Services (CMS), where large-scale demonstration projects are funded to identify new ways of creating value in health care. However, these macro-level initiatives are designed primarily to influence policy, not to create new models of care and, as such, lack a quality of other federally funded research that offers insight on how outcomes are actually obtained.

Even though the pursuit of knowledge is the dominant motivation for research in the academic model, discoveries sometimes result in the creation of new services and products. However, the development process is motivated by a diversity of factors (e.g., investigators' desire to translate their research into concrete end points, unexpected market opportunities that coincide with the timing of research discoveries) that are not causally or specifically directed to development and the need to create value. This process is qualitatively different from what occurs in R&D, where, as we have noted, the intention of research is to create value.

Despite the challenges, adoption of an R&D model for healthcare delivery is not practical, given the constraints of a paper-based world. Moreover, there are numerous structural problems (e.g., lack of alignment between

---

[1]The National Institutes of Health is the steward of medical and behavioral research for the nation. Its mission is science in pursuit of fundamental knowledge about the nature and behavior of living systems and the application of that knowledge to extend healthy life and reduce the burdens of illness and disability.

interests of payers and providers, paying for performance and outcomes versus paying for care) in the U.S. healthcare system that make it very difficult to create value in the traditional sense (Porter and Teisber 2006), even if R&D evolved to how it is in other markets. R&D is, however, sensible in a digital healthcare world and is one of several factors required to achieve a broader solution of providing high-quality care at a lower cost.

Why is the EHR important in this context? Paper-based healthcare settings are fundamentally constrained not only in what is possible, but also in what one imagines is possible. It is somewhat analogous to imagining what could be done in advancing the use of the horse and buggy to go faster, to explore new dimensions of transportation (e.g., as a form of entertainment with the integration of media from radio, CDs, and video with travel), to make use of decision support (e.g., a Global Positioning System [GPS] to provide directions, to find restaurants), and so forth. These new factors were not worth considering until a new technology emerged. The paper-based world is inherently constrained in this manner. Namely, it is almost not worth considering the expansive development and adoption of clinical data standards, expansive use of human independent interactions (e.g., algorithmic ordering of routine preventive health interventions), real-time monitoring of data, detailed feedback on patient management performance, sophisticated means of clinical decision support, and timely creation of evidence, to mention a few. Moreover, a paper-based world is truly limited in the ability to take a solution tested in one clinical setting and export and scale the discovered solution to many other settings.

The EHR is a transforming technology. It is unlikely that the EHR in itself will create substantial value in health care. Rather, we believe it will create unique opportunities to seamlessly link research to development, to ensure that the exporting and scalability problem is solved as part of the research endeavor, and to intentionally create value in health care. Bringing knowledge to practice will be an important part of this enterprise. Figure 3-3 presents a familiar characterization of how EHR-based R&D can influence health care. Efficiency and quality of care can be improved through the integration of new workflows and sophisticated decision support that move more and more tasks to the patient and nonphysician and nonclinical staff. Clinician management should increasingly be reserved for situations where the decisions to be made are less certain and where threats (e.g., adverse events) are possible. The notion behind such a model is to continuously explore new ways in which structure can be added to the care delivery process such that those with less formal training, including patients, assume more responsibility for care.

EHR-based practices also offer the promise of aligning interests around the business value of data and information. As sophisticated models of care (e.g., integration of workflow, evaluation of data, decision support) evolve,

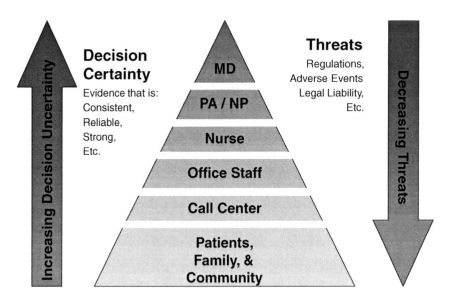

FIGURE 3-3 Who should be responsible for what?

the value of accurate and complete data will increase. This is especially likely to be true if market-sensible expectations (e.g., pay for performance or outcomes) emerge as a dominant force for payment. In this context, data standards and data quality represent business assets to practicing clinicians (i.e., facilitate the ability to deliver higher-quality care at a lower cost), opening the most important path alignment. Moreover, those who pay for care will view data as an essential ingredient to providing high-quality and efficient care.

Discovering What Works in Reality and Beyond

Creating medical evidence is a costly and time-consuming enterprise, with the result that it is not possible to conduct studies to address most questions relevant to health care, and the time required to generate the evidence limits its relevance. Consider, however, three related stages of research relevant to developing new models for creation of evidence: (1) development of new methods designed to extract valid evidence from analysis of retrospective longitudinal patient data; (2) translation of these methods into protocols that can rapidly evaluate patient data in real time as a component of sophisticated clinical decision support; and (3) rapid protocols designed to conduct clinical trials as a routine part of care delivery in the face of multiple treatment options for which there is inadequate evidence to decide what is most sensible (i.e., clinical equipoise).

Valid methods are needed to extract evidence from retrospective analysis of EHR data. For example, one such method may include research on how longitudinal EHR data can be used to replicate the results of prior randomized clinical trials. Such an evaluation might include imposing the same patient inclusion and exclusion criteria, duration of "observation," and other design features used in pivotal trials. Other techniques (e.g., use of propensity scores, interaction terms with treatment used) may have to be used to adjust for underlying differences between clinic patients and trial participants and for confounding by indication and other factors (Seeger et al. 2005). This represents one scenario for how methods may be developed and validated as a first step toward extracting evidence from EHR data. Establishing such a foundation opens opportunities to explore other questions relevant to the generalizability gap between RCT evidence and questions that arise in practice. What would have happened in the trial if, for example, patients who were sicker or older, or patients who had more diverse comorbidities, had been enrolled? What are the profiles of patients who might best (or least) benefit from the treatment? What are the treatment effects on other outcomes not measured in the original trial? Such "virtual" trials could extend the evidence from efficacy studies to those more relevant to clinical practice.

Ultimately, such methods can be used to serve two purposes: to create evidence more relevant to practice and to translate the methods into protocols that rapidly evaluate data to provide real-time decision support. Consider the needs of a patient with comorbid atrial fibrillation, diabetes, and hypertension. If each disease were considered in isolation, thiazides might be prescribed for hypertension, angiotensin receptor blocker for diabetes, and a beta-blocker for atrial fibrillation. Yet in considering the whole patient, clinicians necessarily have to make nuanced decisions (i.e., to optimize the relative benefits of taking numerous medications, simplifying the treatment regimen, reducing cost to the patient, minimizing drug-drug interactions and adverse events, etc.) that are unlikely to ever be based on expert guidelines. A logical extension of the methodological work described above is to apply such methods to the rapid processing of longitudinal, population-based EHR data to facilitate clinical decision making given a patient's profile and preferences.

The above methods could be valuable in both providing decision support and identifying when a decision is completely uncertain. Decision uncertainty has been and will continue to be ever-present. There are no absolute means of closing the loop so that every decision is made with certainty. New questions will continue to arise at an increasingly faster pace, and these questions will always change and evolve. Meaningful advances will emerge by making questions more explicit sooner and by providing answers proximal to when the questions arise. An everyday solution will be required to meet the perpetual growth in demand for new knowledge in medicine (Stewart et al. 2007 [in press]). One such solution may be to use the power of the EHR and new decision methods described above to identify conditions where clinical equipoise between two or more options has occurred. Embedding protocols that randomize the decision under this condition provides a means to conduct RCTs that fundamentally fill the inferential gap.

It is especially important to underscore that to be useful, functional, exportable, and scalable, solutions need to be developed that serve one critical purpose: to create value. Without this ultimate intention, physicians will be reluctant to adopt new methods. Offering improvements to quality as an incentive to adopt new ways of practicing medicine is simply not enough to change behavior. The notion of sophisticated clinical decision support (CDS) will embody many such solutions, as long as these solutions also solve the workflow challenges for such processes. A new term may have to be created to avoid confusion and to distinguish the evolution of CDS from its rudimentary roots and from what exists today (e.g., poorly timed binary alerts, drug interaction checking, simple default orders derived from practice guidelines, access to electronic textbooks and literature). The future of CDS is in developing real-time processes that directly influence clinical care decisions at exactly the right time (i.e., sensing when it is appropriate to present decision options). EHR platforms alone are unlikely to have the capability of managing such processes. They are designed for a different purpose. Rather, these processes are likely to involve sophisticated "machines" that are external to the EHR, but interact with the EHR. "Sophisticated" from today's vantage point means reducing variation in the numerous steps we have previously described that influence a clinical decision, evaluating patient data (i.e., clinical and preferences) in relation to codified evidence-based rules, evaluating data on other patients in this context, presenting concrete support (i.e., not advice but an actionable decision that can be modified), and ensuring that the whole process increases overall productivity and efficiency of care.

We are at a seminal point in the history of medical care, as important as the changes that took place at the turn of the last century and that today have created the demand for new solutions to address the problems created by a century of success. We believe that new opportunities are emerging that will change how evidence is created, accessed, and ultimately used in the care of patients. By leveraging the EHR, we see that providers and others who care for patients will be able move beyond dependence on "old media" forms of knowledge creation to practice real-time, patient-centered care driven by the creation of value. Such a system will not only close the gap in practice between what we know works and what we do, but also allow new means of data creation in situations of clinical equipoise.

STANDARDS OF EVIDENCE

Steven Pearson, M.D.
America's Health Insurance Plans

It is easy to forget that not too long ago, evidence-based medicine often meant if there is no good evidence for harm, the physician was allowed to proceed with the treatment. Now, however, it is clear that we are in a new era in which evidence-based medicine is being used to address an increasing number of clinical questions, and answering these questions requires that some standard for evidence exists that is "beyond a reasonable doubt." Evidence can be applied to make different types of decisions regarding the use of new and existing technologies in health care, including decisions regarding appropriate study designs and safeguards for new treatments, clinical decisions for the treatment of individual patients, and population-level decisions regarding insurance coverage. Coverage decisions are particularly sensitive to a narrowing of the research-practice divide, and this discussion focuses on how evidence standards currently operate in coverage decisions for both diagnostic and therapeutic technologies. Quicker, practice-based research opportunities inherent to a learning healthcare system may affect evidence standards in an unanticipated manner.

In general, following approval, technologies are assessed on how they measure up to various criteria or evidentiary hurdles. Possible hurdles for new technologies include considerations of efficacy, effectiveness versus placebo, comparative effectiveness, and perhaps even cost-effectiveness. As an example, the Technology Evaluation Center (TEC), established by Blue Cross Blue Shield Association (BCBSA) evaluates the scientific evidence for technologies to determine, among other things, whether the technology provides substantial benefits to important health outcomes, or whether the new technology is safer or more beneficial than existing technologies. To answer these questions, technology assessment organizations gather, examine, and synthesize bodies of evidence to determine the strength of evidence.

Strength of evidence, as a concept, is very complicated and not an easy construct to communicate to the population at large. The general concept is that individual studies are assessed within the context of a standing hierarchy of evidence, and issues that often get less visibility include the trade-offs between benefit versus risk. However in considering the strength of evidence, we usually talk about the net health benefit for a patient, and this can often depend on the magnitude and certainty of what we know about both the risks and the benefits. The United States Preventive Task

Force (USPTF) was uniquely visible in advancing the idea of considering not just the quality of individual evidence, but how the strength of evidence can be characterized as it applies to an entire body of evidence—whether this relates to consistencies across different studies or the completeness of the conceptual chain. These concepts have been very important in advancing how groups use evidence in making decisions.

This idea of the *strength* of evidence, however, is still different from a *standard* of evidence. For a standard of evidence, we must be able to give the evidence to a decision-making body, which must be able to do something with it. As an example of how difficult this can be, TEC has five criteria, and careful examination of the criteria indicates that much is left unresolved that might have important implications for coverage decisions. TEC criteria number three, "the technology must improve the net health outcome," might vary depending on the nature of the intervention or circumstance of application. Moreover, TEC only evaluates select technologies and their technology assessments only inform decision-making bodies. When an evaluation goes to a decision-making group, charged with deciding whether something is medically necessary, it is often difficult to know when evidence will be sufficient to make a decision. In part this is because it is difficult to set a uniform standard of evidence. Specifying, for instance, a requirement such as three RCTs with some very specific outcomes clearly would not allow the flexibility needed to deal with the variety of issues and types of data that confront such decision-making bodies.

Although we have made much progress in advancing our thinking about how to understand the strength of a body of evidence, advancing our understanding of how to make a decision based on the strength of evidence is another issue. There are many factors that could modulate a coverage decision, including existence of alternate treatments, severity of disease, and cost. How we might account for these factors and what formal structure might be needed to integrate such "contextual considerations" are concepts that are just now beginning to evolve.

Part of the problem with evidence-based coverage decisions is the fact that evidence itself is lacking. Many of the people that sit on these decision-making bodies will agree that the majority of the time, the evidence is just not adequate for the decisions they need to make. Part of the difficulty is the lack of appropriate studies, but for procedures and devices the lack of evidence is related to the fluid nature of technology development and our evidence base. For example, devices are often rapidly upgraded and improved, and the procedures and practitioner competency with those procedures evolve over time. Evidence developed shortly after a product is developed is thus a snapshot in time, and it is difficult to know what such current evidence means for the effectiveness of the product over the next several years. Likewise, traditional evidence hierarchies are framed around therapeutics and fit poorly for diagnostics. Many new diagnostics represent tests of higher accuracy or may be an addition to an existing diagnostic process. In the latter case, evidence will need to address not just for whom these tests are effective but when in the workup they should be used. There are other types of emerging technologies that pose new challenges to our existing evidentiary approach, such as genetic tests for disease counseling, pharmacogenomic assays, and prognostic studies. Collectively, these technologies pose several questions for our current approach to standards of evidence. As our understanding of heterogeneity of treatment effects expands, how might new modes of diagnosis change therapeutic decision making? As we move to a system that will increasingly utilize interventions that evolve rapidly, how do we establish standards of evidence that are meaningful for current clinical practice? As we begin to utilize data generated at the point of care to develop needed evidence, how might the standards of evidence for their evaluation change?

On top of all these uncertainties and challenges, our current approach to evidentiary assessment and technology appraisal is not well defined beyond taking systematized analyses of existing evidence, giving them to a group, and asking it to decide. As a field, there are many discussions about heterogeneity, meta-analyses, propensity scores, and so forth, but there is very little knowledge about how this information is or should be used by these decision-making bodies and what the process should be.

Consider an alternative approach to standards of evidence and decision making as we move toward a learning healthcare system: think of a dial that can move along a spectrum of evidence—including evidence that is persuasive, promising, or preliminary. There are additional circumstances that can also influence decision making such as the severity of disease and whether this intervention might be considered a patient's last chance. In this case does it mean that we only need preliminary evidence of net health benefit for us to go forward with a coverage decision? What if there are many treatment alternatives? Should the bar for evidence rise? These are the types of issues we need to consider. Decision makers in private health plans have to wrestle with this problem constantly while trying to establish a consistent and transparent approach to evidence.

So what happens to the evidence bar when we move toward a learning healthcare system? Coverage with evidence development has been discussed in an earlier chapter as a movement toward what might be envisioned to be a learning healthcare system. In the case of CED, consider what might happen to the evidence bar in addressing the many important questions. If we are trying to foster promising innovation, will we drop the evidence bar for coverage? What do we mean by "promising"? Do we mean that a technology is safe and effective within certain populations, but now we are considering an expansion of its use? Is it "promising" because we know it is safe, but are not so sure that it is effective? Or is it effective, but we don't know whether the effectiveness is durable over the long term? Are these questions all the same visions of "promising" evidence?

Is CED a new hurdle? Does it lower the one behind it? Does it introduce the opportunity to bring new hurdles such as comparative and cost-effectiveness that we have not had before? Ultimately CED may be used to support studies whose results will enhance the strength of evidence to meet existing standards, certainly part of the vision of CED—but might it also lead to a shift to a lower initial standard of evidence for coverage decisions? As we know when CED policy became known to industry, many groups approached CMS with not "promising" but perhaps even "poor" evidence, asking for coverage in return for the establishment of a registry from which we will all "learn." Resolving these issues is an active area of policy discussion—with individuals at CMS and elsewhere still very early on the learning curve—and is vital to improving approaches as we develop and advance our vision of a learning healthcare system.

IMPLICATIONS FOR ACCELERATING INNOVATION

Robert Galvin, M.D.
General Electric

Technological innovations have substantially improved our nation's health, but they also account for the largest percentage of the cost increases that continue to strain the U.S. healthcare system (Newhouse 1993). The process to decide whether to approve and then provide insurance coverage for these innovations has represented a "push-pull" between healthcare managers—representing healthcare insurers and public payers, trying to control cost increases—and manufacturers, including pharmaceutical companies, biotech startups, and others, looking for return on their investment and a predictable way to allocate new research resources. Employers, providers, and consumers also figure into the process, and the sum of all these stakeholders and their self-interests has, unfortunately, led to a cycle of "unaccountability" and a system that everyone agrees doesn't work well (Figure 3-4). Over the past several years, a single-minded concentration on the rising costs of health care has gradually been evolving into a focus on the "value" of care delivered. In the context of assessing new technologies, evaluation has begun to shift to determining what outcomes are produced from the additional expense for a new innovation. A notable example of this approach is Cutler's (Cutler et al. 2006) examination of cardiac innovations. In weighing technology costs and outcomes, he concluded that several years of additional life were the payback for the additional expense of these new interventions and at a cost that has been considered accept-

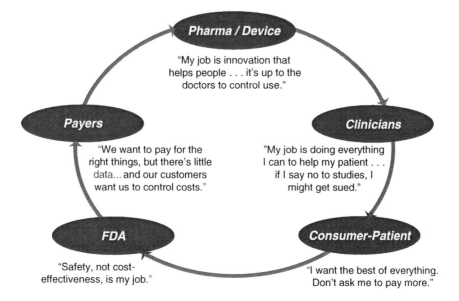

FIGURE 3-4 The cycle of unaccountability.

able in our health system. However for employers and other payers, who look at value a little differently (i.e., what is the best quality achievable at the most controlled cost?), the situation is complex. While applauding innovations that add value—similar to those examined by Cutler—they remain acutely aware of the innovations that either didn't add much incremental value or offered some improvement for specific circumstances but ended up increasing costs at an unacceptable rate due to overuse. A good example of the latter is the case of COX-2 inhibitors for joint inflammation. This modification of nonsteroidal anti-inflammatory drugs (NSAIDs) represented a significant advance for the 3-5 percent of the population who have serious gastric side effects from first-generation NSAIDs; however, within two years of their release, more than 50 percent GE's population on NSAIDs were using COX-2s, an overuse of technology that has cost GE tens of millions of dollars in unnecessary cost. The employers' dilemma is how to get breakthrough innovations to populations as fast as possible, but used by just those who will truly benefit, and not overpay for innovations whose costs exceed their benefits.

How Coverage Decisions Work Today

Although a lot of recent attention has focused on Food and Drug Administration (FDA) approval, employers are impacted most directly by decisions about coverage and reimbursement. Although approval and coverage are linked, it is often not appreciated that they are distinctly different processes. FDA approval does not necessarily equate to insurance coverage. Payers, most often CMS and health insurance companies, make coverage decisions. CMS makes national coverage decisions in a minority of cases and otherwise delegates decision making to its regional carriers, largely Blue Cross insurance plans. Final coverage decisions vary among these Blue Cross plans and other commercial health insurers, but in general, a common process is followed.

The method developed by the TEC, sponsored by the Blue Cross Blue Shield Association and composed of a committee of industry experts, is typical. The TEC decides what new services to review and then gathers all available literature and evaluates the evidence against five criteria (BlueCross BlueShield Association 2007). There is a clear bias toward large, randomized, controlled trials. If the evidence is deemed insufficient to meet the TEC criteria, a new product will be designated "experimental." This has significant implications for technology developers, as payers, following their policy of reimbursing only for "medically necessary" services, uniformly do not pay for something considered experimental.

This process has many positives, particularly the insistence on double blinding and randomization, which minimizes "false positives" (i.e., interventions that appear to work but turn out not to). Certain innovations have significant potential morbidity and/or very high cost (e.g., some pharmaceuticals or autologous bone marrow transplants for breast cancer), and having a high bar for coverage protects patients and payers. However, the process also has several negatives. It is a slow process working in the fast-moving world of innovation, and new services that greatly help patients can be unavailable for years after the FDA has approved them. Large, randomized controlled trials are often not available or feasible, and take a significant amount of time to complete Also, RCTs are almost exclusively performed in academic medical centers, and results achieved in this setting frequently cannot be extrapolated to the world of community-based medical care, where the majority of patients receive their care. The process overall is better at not paying for unproven innovations that it is at providing access to and encouraging promising new breakthroughs.

The coverage history for digital mammography provides an example of these trade-offs. Digitizing images of the breast leads to improvements in sensitivity and specificity in the diagnosis of breast cancer, which most radiologists and oncologists believe translates into improved treatment of the disease. Although the FDA approved this innovation in 2000, it was deemed "experimental" in a 2002 TEC report due to insufficient evidence. Four years elapsed before a subsequent TEC review recommended coverage, and very soon after, all payers reimbursed the studies. In an interesting twist, CMS approved reimbursement in 2001 but at the same rate as film-based mammography, a position that engendered controversy among radiologists and manufacturers. While the goal of not paying for an unproven service was met, the intervening four years between approval and coverage did not lead to improvement in this "promising" technology but rather marked the time needed to develop and execute additional clinical studies. The current process therefore falls short in addressing one part of the employer dilemma, speeding access of valuable new innovations to their populations.

What is particularly interesting in the context of today's discussion is that the process described is the *only* accepted process. Recognizing that innovation needed to occur in technology assessment and coverage determination, CMS developed a new process called CED—Coverage with Evidence Development (Tunis and Pearson 2006). This process takes promising technologies that have not accumulated sufficient patient experience and instead of calling them "experimental" and leaving it to the manufacturer to gather more evidence, combines payment of the service in a selected population with evidence development. Evidence development can proceed through submission of data to a registry or through practical clinical trials, and the end point is a definitive decision on coverage. This novel approach addresses three issues simultaneously: by covering the service, those patients most in need have access; by developing information on a large population, future tailoring of coverage to just those subpopulations who truly benefit can mitigate overuse; and by paying for the service, the manufacturer collects revenue immediately and gets a more definitive answer on coverage sooner—a potential mechanism for accelerating innovation.

To date, CMS has applied CED to several interventions. The guidelines were recently updated with added specification on process and selection for CED. However, given the pace of innovations, it is not reasonable to think that CMS can apply this approach in sufficient volume to meet current needs. Because one-half of healthcare expenditures come from the private sector in the form of employer-based health benefits, it makes sense for employers to play a role in finding a solution to this cycle of unaccountability. On this basis, GE, in its role as purchaser, has launched a pilot project to apply CED in the private sector.

Private Sector CED

General Electric is working with UnitedHealthcare, a health insurer, and InSightec, an Israel-based manufacturer of healthcare equipment, to apply the CED approach to a new, promising treatment for uterine fibroids. The treatment in question is magnetic resonance (MR) based focused ultrasound (MRgFUS), in which ultrasound beams directed by magnetic resonance imaging are focused at and destroy the fibroids (Fennessy and Tempany 2005). The condition is treated today by either surgery (hysterectomy or myomyectomy) or uterine artery embolization. The promise of the new treatment is that it is completely noninvasive and greatly decreases the time away from work that accompanies surgery.

The intervention has received FDA pre-market approval on the basis of treatment in approximately 500 women (FDA 2004), but both CMS and TEC deemed the studies not large enough to warrant coverage and the service has been labeled "experimental" (TEC Assessment Program October 2005). As a result, no major insurer currently pays for the treatment. Both CMS and TEC advised InSightec to expand its studies to include more subjects and measure whether there was recurrence of fibroids. InSightec is a small company that has been having trouble organizing further research, due to both the expense and the fact that the doctors who generally treat fibroids, gynecologists, have been uninterested in referring treatment to radiologists. The company predicts that it will likely be three to five years before TEC will perform another review.

All stakeholders involved in this project are interested in finding a noninvasive treatment for these fibroids. Women would certainly benefit from a treatment with less morbidity and a shorter recovery time. There are also economic benefits for the three principals in the CED project: GE hopes to pay less for treatment and have employees out of work for a shorter time; UnitedHealthcare would pay less for treatment as well, plus it would have the opportunity to design a study that would help target future coverage to specific subpopulations where the benefit is greatest; and InSightec would have the opportunity to develop important evidence about treatment effectiveness while receiving a return on its initial investment in the product.

The parties agreed to move forward and patterned their project on the Medicare CED model, with clearly identified roles. General Electric is the project sponsor and facilitator, with responsibility for agenda setting, meeting planning, and driving toward issue resolution. As a self-insured purchaser, GE will pay for the procedure for its own employees. UnitedHealthcare has several tasks: (1) market the treatment option to its members; (2) establish codes and payment rates and contract with providers performing the service; (3) extend coverage to its insured members and its own employees in addition to its self-funded members; and (4) co-develop the research protocol with InSightec, including data collection protocols and parameters around study end-points and future coverage decisions. Finally, as the manufacturer, InSightec is co-developing the research protocol, paying for the data collection and analysis (including patient surveys), and soliciting providers to participate in the project.

Progress to Date and Major Challenges

The initiative has progressed more slowly than originally planned, but data collection is set to begin before the end of 2006. The number and intensity of challenges has exceeded the expectations of the principals, and addressing them has frankly required more time and resources than anyone had predicted. However, the three companies recognize the importance of creating alternative models to the current state of coverage determination, and their commitment to a positive outcome is, if anything, stronger than it was at the outset of the project. There are challenges.

Study Design and Decision End Points

From a technical perspective this area has presented some very tough challenges. There is little information or experience about how to use data collected from nonrandomized studies in coverage decisions. The RCT has so dominated the decision making in public and private sectors that little is known about the risks or benefits of using case controls or registry data. What level of certainty is required to approve coverage? If a treatment is covered and turns out to be less beneficial than thought, should this be viewed as a faulty coverage process that resulted in wasted money or a "reasonable investment" that didn't pay off? Who is the "customer" in the coverage determination process: the payers, the innovators, or the patients? If it is patients, how should their voice be integrated in the process?

Another set of issues has to do with fitting the coverage decision approach to the new technology in question. It is likely that some innovations should be subject to the current TEC-like approach while others would benefit from a CED-type model. On what criteria should this decision be made and who should be the decision maker?

Engaging Employers

Private sector expenditures, whether through fully insured or self-funded lines of business, ultimately derive from employers (and their workers). Although employers have talked about value rather than cost containment over the past five years, it remains to be seen how many of them will be willing to participate in CED. Traditionally employers have watched "detailing" by pharmaceutical sales people and direct-to-consumer advertising lead to costly overuse and they may be reluctant to pay even more for technologies that would otherwise not be covered. The project is just reaching the stage in which employers are being approached to participate, so it is too early to tell how they will react. Their participation may, in part, be based on how CED is framed. If the benefit to employees is clearly described and there is a business case to offer them (e.g., that controlled accumulation of evidence could better tailor and limit future use of the innovation), then uptake may be satisfactory. However, employers' willingness to participate in the CED approach is critical.

Culture of Distrust

The third, and most surprising, challenge is addressing the degree of distrust between payers and innovators. Numerous difficult issues arise in developing a CED program (e.g., pricing, study end points, binding or nonbinding coverage decisions), and as in any negotiation, interpersonal relationships can be major factors in finding a compromise. Partly from simply not knowing each other, partly from suspiciousness about each other's motives, the lack of trust has slowed the project. Manufacturers believe that payers want to delay coverage to enhance insurance margins, and payers believe that manufacturers want to speed coverage to have a positive impact on their own profit statements. Both sides have evidence to support their views, but both sides are far more committed to patient welfare than they realize. If CED or other innovations in coverage determinations are going to expand, partnership and trust are key. The system would benefit by having more opportunities for these stakeholders to meet and develop positive personal and institutional relationships.

The current processes to determine coverage for innovations are more effective at avoiding paying for new service that may turn out not to be beneficial than they are at getting new treatments to patients quickly or helping develop needed evidence. These processes protect patients from new procedures that may lead to morbidity and are consistent with the "first, do no harm" approach of clinical medicine. However, this approach also slows access to new treatments that could reduce morbidity and improve survival and inadvertently makes investing in new innovations more difficult. With a rapidly growing pipeline of innovations from the device, biotechnology, and imaging industries, there is growing interest in developing additional models of evidence development and coverage determination. Three companies began an initiative in early 2006 to adopt a promising approach called Coverage with Evidence Development, pioneered by CMS, to the private sector. The initiative has made steady progress but it has also faced significant challenges, primarily the lack of experience in pricing, study design, and negotiating study end points in a non-RCT context. A major and unexpected issue is the lack of trust between payers and manufacturers. With the stakes for patients, payers, and innovators growing rapidly, pursuing new approaches to evidence development and coverage determination and addressing the resulting challenges should be a high priority for healthcare leaders.

REFERENCES

Batalden, P, and M Splaine. 2002. What will it take to lead the continual improvement and innovation of health care in the twenty-first century? *Quality Management in Health Care* 11(1):45-54.

Berwick, D, B James, and M Coye. 2003. Connections between quality measurement and improvement. *Medical Care* 41(1 Suppl.):130-138.

Black, N. 1996. Why we need observational studies to evaluate the effectiveness of health care. *British Medical Journal* 312(7040):1215-1218.

BlueCross BlueShield Association. 2007. *Technology Evaluation Center* [accessed 2006]. Available from www.bcbs.com/tec/teccriteria.html.

Charlton, B, and P Andras. 2005. Medical research funding may have over-expanded and be due for collapse. *QJM: An International Journal of Medicine* 98(1):53-55.

Classen, D, R Evans, S Pestotnik, S Horn, R Menlove, and J Burke. 1992. The timing of prophylactic administration of antibiotics and the risk of surgical-wound infection. *New England Journal of Medicine* 326(5):281-286.

Cutler, D, A Rosen, and S Vijan. 2006. The value of medical spending in the United States, 1960-2000. *New England Journal of Medicine* 355(9):920-927.

Dean, N, M Silver, K Bateman, B James, C Hadlock, and D Hale. 2001. Decreased mortality after implementation of a treatment guideline for community-acquired pneumonia. *American Journal of Medicine* 110(6):451-457.

Dean, N, K Bateman, S Donnelly, M Silver, G Snow, and D Hale. 2006a. Improved clinical outcomes with utilization of a community-acquired pneumonia guideline. *Chest* 130(3):794-799.

Dean, N, P Sperry, M Wikler, M Suchyta, and C Hadlock. 2006b. Comparing gatifloxacin and clarithromycin in pneumonia symptom resolution and process of care. *Antimicrobial Agents and Chemotherapy* 50(4):1164-1169.

FDA (Food and Drug Administration). 2004 (October 22). *Pre-Market Approval Letter: Ex-Ablate 2000 System*, [accessed November 30 2006]. Available from http://www.fda.gov/cdrh/pdf4/P040003.html.

Fennessy, F, and C Tempany. 2005. MRI-guided focused ultrasound surgery of uterine leiomyomas. *Academic Radiology* 12(9):1158-1166.

Ferguson, J. 1991. Forward: research on the delivery of medical care using hospital firms. Proceedings of a workshop. April 30 and May 1, 1990, Bethesda, MD. *Medical Care* 29(7 Suppl.):JS1-JS2.

Flexner, A. 2002. Medical education in the United States and Canada. From the Carnegie Foundation for the Advancement of Teaching, Bulletin Number Four, 1910. *Bull World Health Organ* 80(7):594-602.

Graham, H, and N Diamond. 2004. *The Rise of American Research Universities: Elites and Challengers in the Postwar Era*. Baltimore, MD: Johns Hopkins University Press.

Greenblatt, S. 1980. Limits of knowledge and knowledge of limits: an essay on clinical judgment. *Journal of Medical Philosophy* 5(1):22-29.

Haynes, R. 1998. Using informatics principles and tools to harness research evidence for patient care: evidence-based informatics. *Medinfo* 9(1 Suppl.):33-36.

Haynes, R, R Hayward, and J Lomas. 1995. Bridges between health care research evidence and clinical practice. *Journal of the American Medical Informatics Association* 2(6):342-350.

Horwitz, R, C Viscoli, J Clemens, and R Sadock. 1990. Developing improved observational methods for evaluating therapeutic effectiveness. *American Journal of Medicine* 89(5):630-638.

IOM (Institute of Medicine). 2001. *Crossing the Quality Chasm: A New Health System for the 21st Century.* Washington, DC: National Academy Press.

James, B. 1989 (2005, republished as a "classics" article). *Quality Management for Health Care Delivery* (monograph). Chicago, IL: Hospital Research and Educational Trust (American Hospital Association).

———. 2001. Making it easy to do it right. *New England Journal of Medicine* 345(13): 991-993.

———. 2002. Quality improvement opportunities in health care. Making it easy to do it right. *Journal of Managed Care Pharmacy* 8(5):394-399.

———. 2003. Information system concepts for quality measurement. *Medical Care* 41(1 Suppl.):171-179.

Juran, J. 1989. *Juran on Leadership for Quality: An Executive Handbook.* New York: The Free Press.

Lappe, J, J Muhlestein, D Lappe, R Badger, T Bair, R Brockman, T French, L Hofmann, B Horne, S Kralick-Goldberg, N Nicponski, J Orton, R Pearson, D Renlund, H Rimmasch, C Roberts, and J Anderson. 2004. Improvements in 1-year cardiovascular clinical outcomes associated with a hospital-based discharge medication program. *Annals of Internal Medicine* 141(6):446-453.

Lawrence, R, and A Mickalide. 1987. Preventive services in clinical practice: designing the periodic health examination. *Journal of the American Medical Association* 257(16): 2205-2207.

Meldrum, M. 2000. A brief history of the randomized controlled trial. From oranges and lemons to the gold standard. *Hematology/Oncology Clinics of North America* 14(4):745-760, vii.

Nelson, E, P Batalden, T Huber, J Mohr, M Godfrey, L Headrick, and J Wasson. 2002. Microsystems in health care: Part 1. Learning from high-performing front-line clinical units. *Joint Commission Journal on Quality Improvement* 28(9):472-493.

Newhouse, J. 1993. An iconoclastic view of health cost containment. *Health Affairs* 12(suppl.): 152-171.

Porter, M, and E Teisber. 2006. *Redefining Health Care: Creating Value-Based Competition on Results.* 1 ed. Cambridge, MA: Harvard Business School Press.

Reiss-Brennan, B. 2006. Can mental health integration in a primary care setting improve quality and lower costs? A case study. *Journal of Managed Care Pharmacy* 12(2 Suppl.):14-20.

Reiss-Brennan, B, P Briot, W Cannon, and B James. 2006a. Mental health integration: rethinking practitioner roles in the treatment of depression: the specialist, primary care physicians, and the practice nurse. *Ethnicity and Disease* 16(2 Suppl.):3, 37-43.

Reiss-Brennan, B, P Briot, G Daumit, and D Ford. 2006b. Evaluation of "depression in primary care" innovations. *Administration and Policy in Mental Health* 33(1):86-91.

Salas, M, A Hofman, and B Stricker. 1999. Confounding by indication: an example of variation in the use of epidemiologic terminology. *American Journal of Epidemiology* 149(11):981-983.

Seeger, J, P Williams, and A Walker. 2005. An application of propensity score matching using claims data. *Pharmacoepidemiology and Drug Safety* 14(7):465-476.

Stewart, W, N Shah, M Selna, R Paulus, and J Walker. 2007 (In press). Bridging the inferential gap: the electronic health record and clinical evidence. *Health Affairs (Web Edition).*

TEC Assessment Program. October 2005. *Magnetic Resonance-Guided Focused Ultrasound Therapy for Symptomatic Uterine Fibroids.* Vol. 20, No. 10.

Tunis, S, and S Pearson. 2006. Coverage options for promising technologies: medicare's "coverage with evidence development." *Health Affairs* 25(5):1218-1230.

Vandenbroucke, J. 1987. A short note on the history of the randomized controlled trial. *Journal of Chronic Disease* 40(10):985-987.

Williamson, J, P Goldschmidt, and I Jillson. 1979. Medical Practice Information Demonstration Project: Final Report. Office of the Assistant Secretary of Health, Department of Health Education and Welfare, Contract #282-77-0068GS. Baltimore, MD: Policy Research, Inc.

4

New Approaches—
Learning Systems in Progress

OVERVIEW

Incorporation of data generation, analysis, and application into health-care delivery can be a major force in the acceleration of our understanding of what constitutes "best care." Many existing efforts to use technology and create research networks to implement evidence-based medicine have produced scattered examples of successful learning systems. This chapter includes papers on the experiences of the Veterans Administration (VA) and the practice-based research networks (PBRNs) that demonstrate the power of this approach as well as papers outlining the steps needed to knit together these existing systems and expand these efforts nationwide toward the creation of a learning healthcare system. Highlighted in particular are key elements—including leadership, collaboration, and a research-oriented culture—that underlie successful approaches and their continued importance as we take these efforts to scale.

In the first paper, Joel Kupersmith discusses the use of the EHR to further evidence-based practice and research at the VA. Using diabetes mellitus as an example, he outlines how VistA (Veterans Health Information Systems and Technology Architecture) improves care by providing patient and clinician access to clinical and patient-specific information as well as a platform from which to perform research. The clinical data within electronic health records (EHRs) are structured such that data can be aggregated from within VA or with other systems such as Medicare to provide a rich source of longitudinal data for health services research (VA Diabetes Epidemiology Cohort [DEpiC]). PBRNs are groups of ambulatory practices, often partnered with hospitals, academic health centers, insurers, and others to perform research and improve the quality of primary care. These networks constitute an important portion of the clinical research enterprise by providing insight from research at the "coalface" of clinical care. Robert L. Phillips suggests that many lessons could be learned about essential elements in building learning communities—particularly the organization and resources necessary—as well as how to establish such networks between many unique practice environments. The electronic component of the Primary Care Research Network PBRN has the potential to extend the capacity of existing PBRNs by providing an electronic connection that would enable the performance of randomized controlled trials (RCTs) and many other types of research in primary care practices throughout the United States.

While the work of the VA and PBRNs demonstrates immense potential for the integration of research and practice within our existing, fragmented, healthcare system, the papers that follow look at how we might bring their success to a national scale. George Isham of HealthPartners lays out a plan to develop a national architecture for a learning healthcare system and discusses some recent activities by the AQA (formerly the Ambulatory Care Quality Alliance) to promote needed systems cooperation and use of data to bring research and practice closer together. In particular, AQA is focused on developing a common set of standardized measures for quality improvement and a strategy for their implementation; a unified approach to the aggregation and sharing of data; and common principles to improve public reporting. Citing a critical need for rapid advance in the evidence base for clinical care, Lynn Etheredge makes the case for the potential to create a rapidly learning healthcare system if we build wisely on existing resources and infrastructure. In particular he focused on the potential for creating virtual research networks and the improved use of EHR data. Through the creation of national standards, the many EHR research registries and databases from the public and private sectors could become compatible. When coupled with the anticipated expansion of databases and registry development these resources could be harnessed to provide insights from data that span populations, health conditions, and technologies. Leadership and stable funding are needed along with a shift in how we think about access to data. Etheredge advances the idea of the "economics of the commons" as one to consider for data access in which researchers would give up exclusive access to some data but benefit from access to a continually expanding database of clinical research data.

IMPLEMENTATION OF EVIDENCE-BASED PRACTICE IN THE VA[1]

Joel Kupersmith, M.D.
Veterans Administration

As the largest integrated delivery system in the United States, the Veterans Health Administration serves 5.3 million patients annually across nearly 1,400 sites of care. Although its patients are older, sicker, and poorer than the general U.S. population, VA's performance now surpasses other health systems on standardized quality measures (Asch et al. 2004; Kerr et al. 2004; Jha et al. 2003). These advances are in part related to VA's leadership in the development and use of the electronic health record, which has fostered veteran-centered care, continued improvement, and research. Human and system characteristics have been essential to the transformation of VA care.

Adding computers to a care delivery system unprepared to leverage the advantages of health information can create inefficiency and other negative outcomes (Himmelstein and Woolhandler 2005). In contrast, during the period of time in which VA deployed its EHR, the number of veterans seen increased from less than 3 million to nearly 5 million, while costs per patient and full-time employees per patient both decreased (Evans et al. 2006; Perlin et al. 2004). To understand how this could be possible, it is important to highlight historical and organizational factors that were important to the adoption of VA's EHR.

VA health care is the product of decades of innovation. In 1930, Congress consolidated programs for American veterans under VA. Facing more than 1 million returning troops following World War II, VA partnered with the nation's medical schools, gaining access to faculty and trainees and adding research and education to its statutory missions. That bold move created an environment uniquely suited to rapid learning. At present, VA has affiliations with 107 medical schools and trains almost 90,000 physicians and associated health professionals annually.

The VA was originally based on inpatient care, and administrative and legal factors created inefficiency and inappropriate utilization. By the 1980s, the public image of the VA was poor. In 1995, facing scrutiny from Congress, VA reorganized into 22 integrated care networks. Incentives were created for providing care in the most appropriate setting, and legislation established universal access to primary care.

---

[1]This paper is adapted from an article copyrighted and published by Project HOPE/*Health Affairs* as Kupersmith et al., "Advancing Evidence Based Care in Diabetes Through Health Information Technology: Lessons from the Veterans Health Administration, *Health Affairs*, 26(2),w156-w168, 2007. The published article is archived and available online at www. healthaffairs.org.

These changes resulted in a reduction of 40,000 inpatient beds and an increase of 650 community-based care sites. Evidence-based practice guidelines and quality measures were adopted and safeguards were put in place for vulnerable groups such as the mentally ill and those needing chronic care while VA's performance management system held senior managers accountable for evidence-based quality measures. All of these changes created a strong case for robust information systems and spurred dramatic improvements in quality (Jha et al. 2003; Perlin et al. 2004).

VistA: VA's Electronic Health Record

Because VA was both a payer and a provider of care, its information system was developed to support patient care and its quality with clinical information, rather than merely capture charges and facilitate billing. In the early 1980s, VA created the Decentralized Hospital Computer Program (DHCP), one of the first EHRs to support multiple sites and healthcare settings. DHCP developers worked incrementally with a network of VA academic clinicians across the country, writing and testing code locally and transmitting successful products electronically to other sites where they could be further refined. Over time, the group had created a hospital information system prototype employing common tools for key clinical activities. The system was launched nationally in 1982, and by 1985, DHCP was operational throughout VA.

DHCP evolved to become the system now known as VistA, a suite of more than 100 applications supporting clinical, financial, and administrative functions. Access to VistA was made possible through a graphical user interface known as the Computerized Patient Record System (CPRS). With VistA-CPRS, providers can securely access patient information at the point of care and, through a single interface, update a patient's medical history, place orders, and review test results and drug prescriptions. Because VistA also stores medical images such as X-rays and photographs directly in the patient record, clinicians have access to all the information needed for diagnosis and treatment. As of December 2005, VistA systems contained 779 million clinical documents, more than 1.5 billion orders, and 425 million images. More than 577,000 new clinical documents, 900,000 orders, and 600,000 images are added *each workday*—a wealth of information for the clinician, researcher, or healthcare administrator.

Clinicians were engaged at the onset of the change process. This meant working incrementally to ensure usability and integration of the EHR with clinical processes. Both local and national supports were created (e.g., local "superusers" were designated to champion the project), and a national "Veterans Electronic Health University" facilitated collaboration among local, regional, and national sponsors of EHR rollout. National performance measures, as well as the gradual withdrawal of paper records, made use of the EHR an inescapable reality. With reductions in time wasted searching for missing paper records and other benefits, over time, staff came to view VistA-CPRS as an indispensable tool for good clinical care (Brown et al. 2003).

VistA-CPRS allows clinicians to access and generate clinical information about their individual patients, but additional steps are needed to yield insights into population health. Structured clinical data in the EHR can be aggregated within specialized databases, providing a rich source of data for VA administrators and health services researchers (Figure 4-1). Additionally, unstructured text data, such as clinician notes, can be reviewed and abstracted electronically from a central location. This is of particular benefit to researchers—VA multisite clinical trials and observational studies are facilitated by immediate 100 percent chart availability. Furthermore, VA has invested in an External Peer Review Program (EPRP), in which an independent external contractor audits the electronic text records to assess clinical performance using evidence-based performance criteria. Finally, data derived

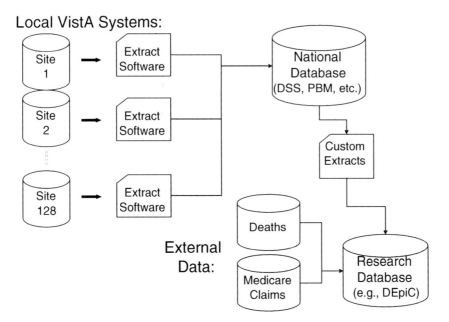

FIGURE 4-1 The sources and flow of the data most often used by VA researchers for national studies. Most data originate from the VistA system but VA data can also be linked with external data sources such as Medicare claims data and the National Death Index.

from the EHR can be supplemented by information from other sources such as Medicare utilization data or data from surveys of veterans.

Leveraging the EHR: Diabetes Care in VA

Much of the work that follows has been supported by VA's Office of Research and Development through its Health Services Research and Development and Quality Enhancement Research Initiative (QUERI) programs (Krein 2002). Diabetes care in the VA illustrates advantages of a national EHR supported by an intramural research program. Veterans with diabetes comprise about a quarter of those served, and the VA was an early leader in using the EHR for a national diabetes registry containing clinical elements as well as administrative data. While VA's EHR made a diabetes registry possible, operationalizing data transfer and transforming it into useful information did not come automatically or easily. In the early 1990s, VA began extracting clinical data from each local VA database into a central data repository. By the year 2000, the VA diabetes registry contained data for nearly 600,000 patients receiving care in the VA, including medications, test results, blood pressure values, and vaccinations. This information has subsequently been merged with Medicare claims data to create the DEpiC (Miller et al. 2004).

Of diabetic veterans, 73 percent are eligible for Medicare and 59 percent of dual eligibles use both systems. Adding Medicare administrative data results in less than 1 percent loss to followup, and while it is not as rich as the clinical information in VA's EHR, its addition fills gaps in follow-up, complication rates, and resource utilization (Miller, D. Personal communication, March 10, 2006.) Combined VA and Medicare data also reveal a prevalence of diabetes among veterans exceeding 25 percent. The impact of the diabetic population on health expenditures is considerable, including total inpatient expenditures (VA plus Medicare) of $3.05 billion ($5,400 per capita) in fiscal year 1999 (Pogach and Miller 2006).

The rich clinical information made possible through the EHR yields other insights. For example, VA has identified a high rate of comorbid mental illness (24.5 percent) among patients with diabetes and is using that information to understand the extent to which newer psychotropic drugs, which promote weight gain, as well as mental illness itself, contribute to poor outcomes (Frayne et al. 2005). The influence of gender and race or ethnicity can also be more fully explored using EHR data (Safford et al. 2003).

Delineating and tracking diabetic complications are also facilitated by the EHR, for example, the progression of diabetic kidney disease. Using clinical data from the EHR allows identification of early chronic kidney disease in a third of veterans with diabetes, less than half of whom have renal impairment indicated in the record (Kern et al. 2006). VA is able to use the EHR to identify patients at high risk for amputation and is distributing that information to clinicians in order to better coordinate their care (Robbins, J. 2006. Personal communication, February 17, 2006).

EHR-Enabled Approaches to Monitoring Quality and Outcomes

Traditional quality report cards may provide incentives to health providers to disenroll the sickest patients (Hofer et al. 1999). VA's EHR provides a unique opportunity to construct less "gameable" quality measures that assess how well care is managed for the same individual over time for diseases such as diabetes where metrics of process quality, intermediate outcomes, and complications (vision loss, amputation, renal disease) are well defined.

Using the VA diabetes registry, longitudinal changes within individual patients can be tracked. In Figure 4-2, case-mix-adjusted glycosylated hemoglobin values among veterans with diabetes decreased by –0.314 percent (range –1.90 to 1.03, $p < .0001$) over two years, indicating improved glycemic control over time, rather than simply the enrollment of healthier veterans (Thompson et al. 2005). These findings provide a convincing demonstration of effective diabetic care.

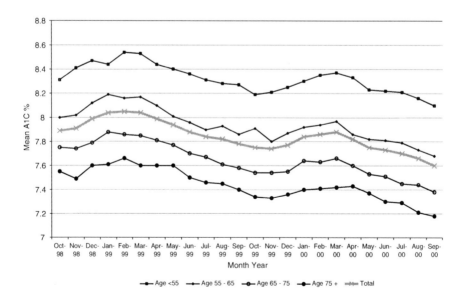

FIGURE 4-2 Trends in mean hemoglobin A1c levels.

Longitudinal data have other important uses. For example, knowledge of prior diagnoses and procedures can distinguish new complications from preexisting conditions. This was shown to be the case for estimates of amputation rates among veterans with diabetes, which were 27 percent lower once prior diagnoses and procedures were considered. Thus longitudinal data better reflect the effectiveness of the management of care and can help health systems avoid being unfairly penalized for adverse selection (Tseng et al. 2005). Longitudinal data from the EHR are also important for evaluating the safety and effectiveness of treatments, which are critical insights for national formulary decisions.

Advancing Evidence-Based Care

Figure 4-3 shows the trends in VA's national performance scorecard for diabetes care based on EHR data. In addition to internal benchmarking, this approach has compared VA performance to commercial managed care (Kerr et al. 2004; Sawin et al. 2004). While these performance data are currently obtained by abstracting the electronic chart, the completion of a national Health Data Repository with aggregated relational data will eventually support automatic queries about quality and outcomes ranging from the individual patient to the entire VA population (see below).

The richness of EHR data allows VA to refine its performance measures.

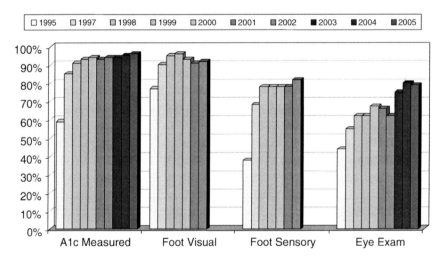

FIGURE 4-3 Improvement in VA diabetes care (based on results from the VA External Peer Review Program).

VA investigators were able to demonstrate that annual retinal screening was inefficient for low-risk patients and inadequate for those with established retinopathy (Hayward et al. 2005). As a consequence, VA modified its performance metrics and is developing an approach to risk-stratified screening that will be implemented nationally.

The greatest advantage of the EHR in the VA is its ability to improve performance by influencing the behavior of patients, clinicians, and the system itself. For instance, VA's diabetes registry has been used to construct performance profiles for administrators, clinical managers, and clinicians. These profiles included comparisons between facilities and identified the proportion of veterans with substantial elevations of glycosylated hemoglobin, cholesterol, and blood pressure. Patient lists also facilitated follow-up with high-risk individuals. Additionally, the EHR allowed consideration of the actions taken by clinicians to intensify therapy in response to elevated levels (e.g., starting or increasing a cholesterol medication when the low-density lipid cholesterol is elevated). This approach credits clinicians for providing optimal treatment and also informs them about what action might be required to improve care (Kerr et al. 2003).

Data from the EHR and diabetes registry also demonstrated the critical importance of defining the level of accountability in diabetes quality reporting. EHR data show that for most measures in the VA, only a small fraction (≤ 2 percent) of the variance is attributable to *individual* primary care providers (PCPs), and unless panel sizes are very large (200 diabetics or more), PCP profiling will be inaccurate. In contrast, much more variation (12-18 percent) was attributed to overall performance at the site of care, a factor of relevance for the design of approaches to rewarding quality. It also highlights the important influence of organizational and system factors on provider adherence to guidelines (Krein 2002).

The EHR can identify high-risk populations and can facilitate targeted interventions. For instance, poor blood pressure control contributes significantly to cardiovascular complications, the most common cause of death in diabetics. VA investigators are currently working with VA pharmacy leaders to find gaps in medication refills or lack of medication titration and thereby proactively identify patients with inadequate blood pressure control due to poor medication adherence or inadequate medication intensification. Once identified, those patients can be assigned proactive management by clinical pharmacists integrated into primary care teams and trained in behavioral counseling (Choe et al. 2005). Other approaches currently being tested and evaluated using EHR data are group visits, peer counseling, and patient-directed electronic reminders.

VistA-CPRS provides additional tools to improve care at the point of service. For example, PCPs get reminders about essential services (e.g., eye exams, influenza vaccinations) at the time they see the patient, and CPRS functions allow providers and patients to view trends in laboratory values and blood pressure control. Perhaps most importantly, the VA's EHR allows for effective care coordination across providers in order to communicate patients' needs, goals, and clinical status as well as to avoid duplication of services.

Care Coordination and Telehealth for Diabetes

In-home monitoring devices now can collect and transmit vital data for high-risk patients from the home to a care coordinator who can make early interventions that might prevent the need for institutional intervention (Huddleston and Cobb 2004). Such a coordinated approach is possible only with an EHR. Based on promising pilot data as well as needs projections, VA has implemented a national program of Care Coordination through Home Telehealth (CCHT) (Chumbler et al. 2005).

Information technology also supports cost-effective access to specialized services. VA recently piloted the use of digital retinal imaging to screen for diabetic retinopathy and demonstrated it could be a cost-effective alternative to ophthalmoscopy for detecting proliferative retinopathy (Conlin et al. 2006). Diabetic retinopathy is not only a preventable complication but also a biomarker for other end-organ damage (e.g., kidney damage). In October 2005, VA began implementing a national program of teleretinal imaging to be available on VistA-CPRS for use by clinicians and researchers. In the future, computerized pictorial analysis and new tools for mining text data across millions of patient records have the potential to transform the clinical and research enterprise by identifying biomarkers of chronic illness progression.

Limits of the EHR in VA

Although VA has one of the most sophisticated EHRs in use today, VistA is not a single system, but rather a set of 128 interlinked systems, each with its own database (i.e., a decentralized system with central control). This limits its ability to make queries against all of a patient's known data. In addition, lack of standardization for laboratory values such as glycosylated hemoglobin and other data elements creates challenges for aggregating available data for administrative and research needs. The VA diabetes registry, while a product of the EHR, took years of effort to ensure data integrity.

A national data standardization project is currently under way to ensure that data elements are compliant with emerging health data standards and data management practices. Extracting data from free-text data fields, a challenge for all electronic records, will be addressed by defining moderately structured data elements for public health surveillance, population health, clinical guidelines compliance, and performance monitoring. Mapping of legitimate local variations to standard representations will allow easier creation of longitudinal registries for a variety of conditions.

The care of diabetes is complex and demanding, and delivering all indicated services may require more time than is typically available in a follow-up visit (Parchman, Romero, and Pugh 2006). Studies of the impact of the EHR on workflow and efficiency in VA and other settings have shown conflicting results (Overhage et al. 2001). While it is unlikely that the EHR saves time during the office encounter, downstream benefits such as better care coordination, reduction of duplicative and administrative tasks, and new models of care (e.g., group visits) translate into a "business case" when the reimbursement structure favors population management.

Creating Patient-Centered, Community-Based Care: My HealtheVet

VA's quality transformation since 1996 involved shifting from inpatient to integrated care. The next phase will involve empowering patients to be more actively engaged and moving care from the clinic to the community and home. Again, health information technology has been designed to support the new delivery system.

My HealtheVet (MHV) is a nationwide initiative intended to improve the overall health of veterans and support greater communication between VA patients and their providers. Through the MHV web portal, veterans can securely view and manage their personal health records online, as well as access health information and electronic services. Veterans can request copies of key portions of their VA health records and store them in a personal "eVAult," along with self-entered health information and assessments, and can share this information with their healthcare providers and others inside and outside VA. The full functionality of MHV will help patients plan and coordinate their own care through online access to care plans, appointments, laboratory values, and reminders for preventive care (U.S. Department of Veterans Affairs 2006). Research itself can be facilitated by MHV—patients will be able to identify ongoing clinical studies for which they are eligible to enroll, communicate with investigators via encrypted e-mail, have their outcomes tracked through computer-administered "smart surveys," and even provide suggestions for future studies. In addition, the effectiveness of patient-centered care can be evaluated.

The Twenty-first Century EHR

The next phase of VistA-CPRS will feature open-source applications and relational database structures. One benefit of the conversion will be easier access to national stores of clinical data through a unified Health Data Repository (HDR) that will take the place of the current 128 separately located VistA systems. The HDR is under construction and currently contains records from nearly 16 million unique patients, with more than 900 million vital sign recordings and 461 million separate prescriptions.

Additionally, a clinical observations database linked to SNOMED (Systematized Nomenclature of Medicine) terms and semantic relationships will greatly expand the scope of data available for research data-mining activities. Enhanced decision support capabilities will help clinicians provide care according to guidelines and understand situations where it is appropriate to deviate from guidelines. The reengineered EHR will also link orders and interventions to problems, greatly enhancing VA's clinical data-mining capabilities.

To support the delivery of consistent information to all business units, VA is developing a Corporate Data Warehouse (CDW; Figure 4-4), which will include the Health Data Repository as the primary source of clinical data but also encompass other administrative and financial datasets (including Medicare data) to create a unified view of the care of veterans. Among other things, the CDW will supplement the capabilities of VistA by provid-

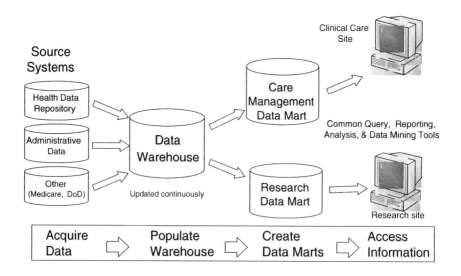

FIGURE 4-4 VA Corporate Data Warehouse architecture.

ing an integrated analytical system to monitor, analyze, and disseminate performance measures. This will greatly enhance population-based health services research by offering standardized data across all the subjects it contains, tools for rapidly performing hypothesis testing, and ease of data acquisition. Unlike VA's current diabetes registry, which has been labor-intensive to create and maintain, future registries based on the CDW will be easier to construct and update. The CDW will eventually facilitate personalized medicine by allowing the linkage of genomic information collected from veterans to longitudinal outcome information.

These changes will introduce a greater degree of central control than was present during the early days of VA's EHR, but clinicians and researchers will continue their involvement in developing innovations.

VA has been an innovator in the EHR, developing a clinically rich system "from the ground up" that has become so integrated into the delivery of care and the conduct of research that one cannot imagine a VA health system without it. However, many factors in addition to the EHR contributed to VA's quality transformation, including a culture of academician-clinicians that valued quality, scientific evidence, and accountability (for which EHR became an organizer and facilitator); the presence of embedded researchers who themselves were active clinicians, managers, policy makers, and developers of VistA-CPRS; and a research infrastructure that could be applied to this topic (Greenfield and Kaplan 2004; Perlin 2006). While the data structures themselves are complex and sometimes flawed, they are, because of their user origins, effectively linked to the needs of clinicians and researchers, who in turn incorporate their input into the further evolution of VA's EHR.

The design of the VA system also ensures that overall incentives are aligned to realize the beneficial externalities of EHR. VA benefits, for instance, by being able to eliminate duplicative test ordering when veterans seek care at different facilities (Kleinke 2005). The cost of maintaining the EHR amounts to approximately $80 per patient per year, roughly the amount saved by eliminating one redundant lab test per patient per year (Perlin 2006). It should be noted that VA also benefits greatly by being an interactive, permeable entity in a free market system—VA is an enrollment system, not an entitlement program or a safety-net provider, and thus has incentives for maintaining high satisfaction and perceived value among those it serves.

For patient care management, VA's EHR has developed an infrastructure and system for collecting and organizing information from which a diabetes database (DEpiC) evolved to provide valuable information related to disease prevalence, comorbidities, and costs that are necessary for quality improvement, system-wide planning, and research. Longitudinal within-cohort assessment, made possible by the EHR, is a substantial advance in attaining precise measures of quality that mitigate the effects of adverse patient selection and has the potential to facilitate a variety of clinical care advances.

Home telehealth linked to EHR has made possible novel patient-provider interactions of which the care coordination and teleretinal imaging initiatives are among the earliest prototypes. This approach has the capacity to expand care delivery to many others, and the benefits are not limited to the home-bound—a new generation of Internet-savvy veterans will appreciate 24/7 access for health care the same way they do for instant messaging and shopping. MHV, which is in its launch phase, is part of the future plan to give individuals control over their health and includes many possibilities for research.

One more important initiative enabled by the EHR has a capacity to substantially change the practice of medicine—adding genomic information to the medical record. With its voluminous EHR database, VA has an unprecedented opportunity to identify the genetic correlates of disease and drug response, which may transform medical practice from a process of statistical hunches to one of targeted, personalized care. Because of the vastly larger scale of the healthcare enterprise and the changing needs of veterans, VA's focus now has models in place to shift to issues involving clinical decision support, content standardization, and enhanced interaction between patients, VA providers, and other systems. These capabilities are made possible by VA's EHR, and the VA experience may provide a model for how federal health policies can help the United States create a learning healthcare system.

PRACTICE-BASED RESEARCH NETWORKS

Robert L. Phillips, Jr., M.D., M.S.P.H., The Robert Graham Center
James Mold, M.D., M.P.H., University of Oklahoma
Kevin Peterson, M.D., M.P.H., University of Minnesota

The development of practice-based research networks was a natural response to the disconnect between national biomedical research priorities and intellectual curiosity and questions arising at the "coalface" of clinical care. The physician's office is where the overwhelming majority of people in the United States seek care for illness and undifferentiated symptoms (White et al. 1961). Forty years later, there has been almost no change in this ecology of medicine (Green et al. 2001). The growth in investment in biomedical research over those same four decades has been tremendous, but it has largely ignored the place where nearly a billion visits to a highly trained professional workforce take place. Curiosity is an innately human property, and many of the early PBRNs formed around collections of clinicians who could not find answers in the literature for the questions that arose in their practices, who did not recognize published epidemiologies, and who did not feel that interventions of proven *efficacy* in controlled trials could achieve equivalent *effectiveness* in their practices. PBRNs began to formally appear more than four decades ago to fill the gaps in knowledge identified in primary care and have been called by the IOM "the most promising infrastructure development that [the committee] could find to support better science in primary care" (Green 2000; IOM 1996). PBRNs are proven clinical laboratories critical to closing the gaps between what is known and what we need to know and between what is possible and what we currently do.

More recently, PBRNs have begun to blur the lines between research and quality improvement, forming learning communities that "use both traditional and nontraditional methods to identify, disseminate, and integrate new knowledge to improve primary care processes and patient outcomes" (Mold and Peterson 2005). The interface of discovery, research, and its application—the enterprise of quality improvement—is a logical outcome when the location of discovery is also the location of care delivery. Networks move quality improvement out of the single practice and into a group process so that the processes and outcomes can be compared and studied across clinics and can be generalized more easily.

The successful combination of attributes that creates a learning community within PBRNs has definite characteristics. Six characteristics of a professional learning community have been identified: (1) a shared mission and values, (2) collective inquiry, (3) collaborative teams, (4) an action orientation including experimentation, (5) continuous improvement, and (6) a results orientation (Mold and Peterson 2005). PBRNs demonstrating these characteristics are among the members of the Institute for Healthcare Improvement's Breakthrough Series Collaboratives and recognized by the National Institutes of Health (NIH) Inventory and Evaluation of Clinical Research Networks. The networks in Prescription for Health, a program funded by the Robert Wood Johnson Foundation (RWJF) in collaboration with AHRQ, are innovating to help people change unhealthy behaviors, testing different interventions using common measures that permits pooling data from approximately 100 practices. As other types of clinical networks are developed, they will need similar orientations to realize the benefits of integrating research and practice.

Primary care PBRNs can be instructive to other clinical networks in understanding the resources and organization necessary for successfully integrating research and practice, and for translating external research findings into practice, acting in many ways like any other adaptive, learning entity (Green and Dovey 2001). The Oklahoma Primary Care Research and Resource Network (OKPRN) is a good example of one such learning community. The OKPRN organizes its practices into pods—geographically organized clinic groupings of about eight practices. The pods rely on a central core research and quality improvement (QI) support team that provides grant, analytic, research design, and administration support. Each pod is supported by a Practice Enhancement Assistant (PEA) who acts as a quality improvement coordinator; research assistant; disseminator of ideas between practices; identifier of areas requiring research, development, or education; and facilitator, helping practices apply research findings. This support structure enables the pods and the larger network to do research and integrate findings into practice. The system also promotes the maturation and confidence of clinicians as researchers and leaders of clinical care improvement.

The electronic Primary Care Research Network, ePCRN, is a very different, but likewise instructive PBRN that is testing the capacity of electronic integration to facilitate research and research translation with funding support from the NIH. Beyond the normal PBRN functions, ePCRN's highly integrated electronic backbone facilitates the performance of randomized controlled trials in primary care practices anywhere in the United States and promotes the rapid integration of new research findings into primary care. This electronic backbone can perform many research and QI functions such as routinely identifying patients eligible for ongoing studies, analyzing patient registries to conduct benchmarking of clinical quality measures, or providing prevention reminders at the point of care. Its robust electronic infrastructure is also instructive for what other learning networks might be capable of accomplishing with the right resources.

While the practices that participate in PBRNs are not well integrated into the traditional "road map" of research, they are integral to the healthcare system and have many natural connections to entities on the roadmap that could be used more effectively for research and research translation. Many PBRNs do enable practices to partner with hospitals, academic health centers, insurers, specialty societies, quality improvement organizations (e.g., National Committee for Quality Assurance, National Quality Forum [NQF], Quality Improvement Organizations), community organizations, nonprofits, and federal funding entities to perform studies and improve care in integrated efforts. The clinicians who participate in PBRNs have natural connections to the entities that form the traditional research infrastructure, but these connections lack the resources to support learning communities, to support practice-based research, and to translate research into practice. Even if the practices in a learning healthcare system are not organized into formal PBRNs, they will need to share some of the same characteristics and have some of the same resources to be successful. These include (1) expert clinician scientists who are financially supported to stay in practice while formulating researchable questions and executing studies, (2) modernized institutional review board policies, and (3) stabilized funding that is not tied to a particular study, but rather sustains operations and communication systems across and between research projects. There is some evidence that this is beginning to happen:

- Several institutes have formed or are evaluating clinical trial networks including the National Cancer Institute; the National Heart, Lung, and Blood Institute; and the National Institute of Neurological Disorders and Stroke. There have also been collaborations between the National Cancer Institute and the Agency for Healthcare Research and Quality to fund PBRN studies of cancer screening. However, in most of these cases, networks are composed primarily of physicians participating in research on specific diseases and specialty-based offices, and generally provide subsets of the population seen in primary care.
- The National Institute of Dental and Craniofacial Research recently awarded $75 million for three seven-year grants to form a national PBRN for the evaluation of everyday issues in oral health care.
- In 2006, three PBRN networks were funded as pilot programs under the NIH Roadmap for the National Electronics and Clinical Trials (NECTAR) network: (1) the ePCRN, which potentially includes all primary care clinicians; (2) the Health Maintenance Organization Research Network (HMORN), which includes physician researchers from managed care organizations; and (3) the Regional Health Organization (RHIO) Network, which includes providers caring primarily for the underserved. The early success of these efforts resulted in development of important research resources for primary care that could provide a platform for interconnection and interoperability between several thousand participating primary care clinics currently serving approximately 30 million patients. Unfortunately, just one year into funding, the NIH decided to stop funding these programs in lieu of support for other Roadmap initiatives.
- The Agency for Healthcare Research and Quality (AHRQ) is developing a network of 5 to 10 primary care PBRNs engaged in rapid turnaround research leading to new knowledge and information that contributes to improved primary care practice.

An investment of $30 million or more per year for five years would potentially support 15 to 20 PBRNs selected through a competitive Request for Application (RFA) open to eligible primary care PBRNs and supported by a national center. More than 100 primary care PBRNs currently exist. Virtually all existing PBRNs can be identified through registrations and inventories kept at the IECRN (Inventory and Evaluation of Clinical Research Networks), the AHRQ PBRN Resource Center, and the Federation of Practice-Based Research Networks. If each PBRN recruited and trained 250 to 1,000 community clinicians in human subjects protection and in preparation for clinical trials and translational research, nearly 100 million patients would be served by this cadre of up to 50,000 clinical research associates. The PBRNs would provide regional support for clinicians and be coordinated through the national center. Resources would be available to all NIH institutes and centers for appropriate clinical trials and translational research. In effect, this investment would promote the development of clinical learning communities that care for nearly one-third of all Americans.

The development of a national research infrastructure that provides value and function to the basic scientist and the community clinical investigator is both feasible and practical. This will require the development of new partnerships with academic centers in the discovery of new knowledge and the pursuit of better practice. These partnerships provide the best hope to deliver NIH's achievements in improving health rapidly and effectively for the American people. Through the NIH Roadmap's Clinical Translational Science Awards (CTSA), NIH has begun to develop a home for clinical research. Some of the academic centers receiving this funding, including Duke University, the University of California at San Francisco, and the University of Oregon, are reaching out to their local community clinics or regional clinical research networks, primarily through their community engagement functions. Although the CTSA program will stimulate the development of regionally strong translational centers and some of these centers will provide a pathway for participation of local or regional communities, the promise of transformational change that brings the national primary care community into the clinical research enterprise remains unfulfilled.

The CTSA builds on an academically centered model that presumes new translational resources will be shared with practice-based community investigators over time. Although primary care has made important inroads in some academic centers, many academic centers lack PBRNs and have too few experienced ambulatory care investigators to ensure a bidirectional exchange of information or provide enough sharing of resources to stabilize an ambulatory care research infrastructure.

A learning healthcare system can learn a great deal from PBRNs, particularly for ambulatory care—the bulk of the clinical enterprise, the location most neglected by research and quality improvement efforts, and the setting where most Americans receive medical care. There is a timely opportunity for the NIH, federal agencies, and philanthropic foundations to create an interconnected and interoperable network that assists ambulatory clinicians in integrating discovery into clinical practice. Funding for the initial practice-based research infrastructure would serve an important role for the translation of research into the community and for promoting the integration of the national community of ambulatory care-based investigators into the clinical research enterprise. Such an investment will also support the essential elements of learning communities—a constant state of inquiry and a desire to improve among all clinicians.

NATIONAL QUALITY IMPROVEMENT
PROCESS AND ARCHITECTURE

George Isham, M.D., M.S.
HealthPartners

If consistent improvement in health and care is to be achieved across the entire country, individual learning healthcare organizations will need to be knit together by a national infrastructure in a learning system for the nation. If this is not done, individual examples of progress such as the Veterans Administration, Mayo Clinic, Kaiser Permanente, and HealthPartners will remain exceptions in a disconnected fragmented healthcare system. This paper discusses what is needed to take us beyond these examples and create that learning system for the nation—a National Quality Improvement Process and Architecture (NQIPA). The AQA, previously known as the Ambulatory care Quality Alliance, is an important element enabling the NQIPA.

That the healthcare system is broken has been highlighted by a number of Institute of Medicine (IOM) reports (IOM 1999, 2001), and arguably, it does not really exist as a system. The IOM's recent report on performance measurement (IOM 2005) pointed out that "there are many obstacles to rapid progress to improve the quality of health care but none exceeds the fact that the nation lacks a coherent, goal-oriented, and efficient system to assess and report the performance of the healthcare system."

To illustrate this point, HealthPartners' informatics department put together a map of some of the measurement sets that are relevant to our work as a health organization; see Figure 4-5 (HealthPartners 2006). Each of these standard measurement sets affects one of our activities as a medical group, hospital, health plan, or an organization regulated in Minnesota. Many of these standard sets are similar or measure the same issue or condition slightly differently. As an example, we have been required to measure mammography screening many different ways for different standard measurement sets required by different organizations or standards.

Other obstacles to creating the needed coherent, goal-oriented, and

204

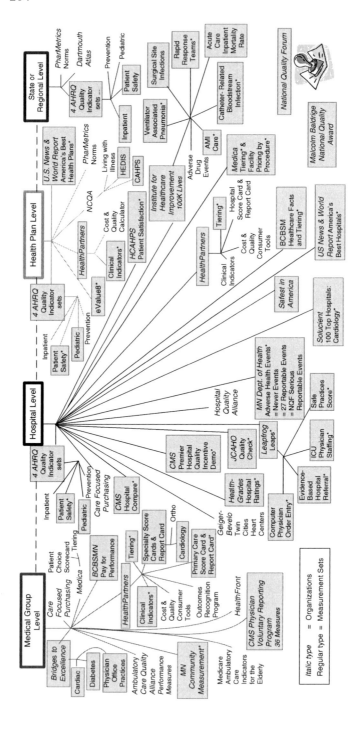

FIGURE 4-5 A map of some of the measurement sets that are relevant to the work of HealthPartners (HealthPartners, Private Analysis 2006) illustrates obstacles presented by the lack of a clear and efficient national system to assess and report the performance of the healthcare system.

efficient system include a lack of clear goals and objectives for improving quality in health care, the lack of leadership focus on improving quality, the lack of a culture of quality and safety in our organizations, the lack of comparative information on what works and what doesn't that is based on scientific evidence, the lack of an environment that creates systematic incentives and supports for improving quality by individual organizations and healthcare professionals, and the lack of the universal availability of an electronic health record system that is interoperable with other EHRs and designed for decision support at the point of care and quality reporting. One of the most critical obstacles is the lack of social mechanisms and institutions on the national and regional levels that enable the collaboration necessary for individual organizations and professionals to work with each other to evaluate and improve the quality of care across the country.

A National Quality Improvement Process and Architecture

To knit together a learning system for the country and create an NQIPA, a national strategy and infrastructure is needed that enables individual healthcare providers and their organizations to know the quality of care they deliver, to have the incentives and tools necessary to improve care, and to provide information critical to individual patients and the public about the quality of care they receive. The work may be described as a seven-step process model for quality improvement (Isham and Amundson October 2002):

1. Establish Focus and Target Goals: Set broad population health goals.
2. Agree on Guidelines: Develop best-practice guidelines with physicians.
3. Devise Standard Measurements: Formulate evaluation standards for each goal.
4. Establish Targets: Set clinical care performance improvement targets.
5. Align Incentives: Reward medical groups for achieving targets.
6. Support Improvement: Assist medical groups in implementation.
7. Evaluate and Report on Progress: Disseminate information on outcome

Some progress has been made at the national and regional levels on some elements of a national support system to ensure health, safety, and quality (IOM 2006). For example, recently there has been significant progress in establishing this support system for quality improvement in Minnesota. In August 2006, the governor of Minnesota signed an executive order directing the state agencies to use incentives in the purchasing of health care that are based on established statewide goals, against the achievement of performance using specific targets and standard quality measures based on evidence-based clinical standards (Office of Governor Tim Pawlenty 2006). This initiative (QCARE) was designed by a work group that used the seven-step model in developing its recommendations.

Institutions in place in Minnesota that enable this model include the Institute for Clinical Systems Improvement, which is a collaborative of Physician Medical Groups and Health Plans that develops and implements evidence-based clinical practice guidelines and provides technical assistance to improve clinical care (Institute for Clinical Systems Improvement 2006). The Institute for Clinical Systems Improvement is an effective way to engage the support of local practicing physicians for evidence-based standards of care. The Institute for Clinical Systems Improvement involves group practices large and small that represent 75 percent of the non-federal physicians practicing in the state.

Minnesota Community Measurement, a second Minnesota collaborative of medical providers, health plans, purchasers, and consumers that collects and publicly reports clinical quality using standard measures grounded in the evidence-based, clinical standards work of the Institute for Clinical Systems Improvement is also a critical component that enables the support system for quality in Minnesota (MN Community Measurement 2006). Incentives for working on improving quality are not only provided by the governor's QCARE program, but also by the private health plans in their pay for performance programs, and by Bridges to Excellence, a national pay for performance program (Bridges to Excellence 2006). All of these use the Institute for Clinical Systems Improvement and Minnesota Community Measurement as the common mechanism for creating incentives founded on evidence-based clinical standards, guidelines, targets, and measures. The individual organizational quality results are publicly reported.

The Minnesota experience can be used in the effort to create a national system to support the improvement of quality of care across the country. NQIPA would be most effective as a federation of regional systems with the ability to engage local providers of care that are knit together by a national system of standards and rules and supported by mechanisms to aggregate data from national and regional sources for two purposes. The first is to report quality improvement progress on a national level for Medicare and other national purchasers. The second is to feed back performance at a regional level to enable local healthcare organizations and providers to be engaged in and part of the process of actually improving the quality of care over time. It is also critical that Medicare, national medical specialty societies, national purchasers, and others with national perspectives and needs be a part of and served well by this system. It is important, therefore, that NQIPA implement national standards and priorities uniformly in each region of the country and be able to aggregate data and information at the multiregional and national levels.

Progress has been made at the national level, although there is much yet to be done. National goals have been suggested (IOM 2003). What is needed next are the top 10 quality issues and problems by specialty to drive the development of evidence-based guidelines, measures, and incentives by specialty, including underuse, overuse, and misuse issues and problems. Many groups produce useful evidence-based recommendations and guidelines, but what is needed now are more evidence-based reviews of acute care, chronic care, and comparative drug effectiveness.

In addition, many organizations use incentives. In 2005, 81 commercial health plans had pay for performance programs, and the Centers for Medicare and Medicaid Services (CMS) was sponsoring six pay for performance demonstrations (Raths 2006). In August 2006, the President signed an executive order promoting quality and efficient health care in federal government-administered or sponsored healthcare programs (The White House 2006). Already mentioned above is the effort by large employers to support incentives through the national Bridges to Excellence Program not only in Minnesota but in many states across the country. Needed now are more healthcare purchasing organizations synchronizing their incentives to standard targets against standard measures that address the most important quality issues across the private and public sectors. There are effective national and regional efforts that engage healthcare organizations and individual physicians in improving the quality of care (Institute for Clinical Systems Improvement 2006; Institute for Healthcare Improvement 2006). Unfortunately, all physician practices and regions of the country are not taking advantage of these healthcare improvement resources. More regional collaboratives are necessary to facilitate improvement in care in all regions of the country. Above all, these individual efforts need to be knit together to form a national strategy and support system—that is, NQIPA.

The AQA Alliance

The AQA Alliance (www.aqaalliance.org) is a broad-based national collaborative of physicians, consumers, purchasers, health insurance plans, and others that has been founded to improve healthcare quality and patient safety through a collaborative process. Key stakeholders agree on a strategy for measuring performance of physicians and medical groups, collecting and aggregating data in the least burdensome way, and reporting meaningful information to consumers, physicians, and stakeholders to inform choices and improve outcomes. The effort's goals are to reach consensus as soon as possible on:

- A set of measures for physician performance that stakeholders can use in private health insurance plan contracts and with government purchasers;
- A multiyear strategy to roll out additional measurement sets and implement measures in the marketplace;
- A model (including framework and governing structure) for aggregating, sharing, and stewarding data; and
- Critical steps needed for reporting useful information to providers, consumers, and purchasers.

Currently there are more than 125 AQA alliance-affiliated organizations including the American College of Physicians, American Academy of Family Physicians, American College of Surgeons, American Association of Retired Persons, Pacific Business Group on Health, America's Health Insurance Plans, and many others. Much progress has been made since the AQA alliance was established in late 2005.

The performance measures workgroup (www.aqaalliance.org/performancewg.htm) has established a framework for selection measures, principles for the use of registries in clinical practice settings, a guide for the selection of measures for medical subspecialty care, principles for efficiency measures along with a starter set of conditions for which cost of care measures should be developed first, and 26 primary care measures as a starter set. In addition, eight cardiology measures, as well as measures for dermatology, rheumatology, clinical endocrinology, radiology, neurology, ophthalmology, surgery, and orthopedic and cardiac surgery, have been approved. The AQA parameters for the selection of measures emphasize that "measures should be reliable, valid and based on sound scientific evidence. Measures should focus on areas which have the greatest impact in making care safe, effective, patient-centered, timely, efficient or equitable. Measures which have been endorsed by the NQF should be used when available. The measure set should include, but not be limited to, measures that are aligned with the IOM's priority areas. Performance measures should be developed, selected and implemented though a transparent process" (AQA Alliance 2006).

The data-sharing and aggregation workgroup (www.aqaalliance.org/datawg.htm) has produced principles for data sharing and aggregation; provided a recommendation for a National Health Data Stewardship Entity (NHDSE) to set standards, rules, and policies for data sharing and aggregation, described desirable characteristics of an NHDSE; developed guidelines and key questions for physician data aggregation projects, and established principles to guide the use of information technology systems that support performance measurement and reporting so as to ensure that electronic health record systems can report these data as part of routine practice. As a consequence of this workgroup's effort, six AQA pilot sites were announced in March 2006. They include the California Cooperative Healthcare Reporting Initiative, Indiana Health Information Exchange, Massachusetts Health Quality Partners, Minnesota Community Measurement, Phoenix Regional Healthcare Value Measurement Imitative, and Wisconsin Collaborative for Healthcare Quality. These pilots are to serve as learning labs to link public and private datasets and assess clinical quality, cost of care, and patient experience. Each of these sites has strong physician leadership, a rich history of collaboration on quality and data initiatives, and the necessary infrastructure and experience to support public and private dataset aggregation. The collaboration across health plans and providers in these six pilot efforts yield a comprehensive view of physician practice. The lessons from the pilot sites can provide valuable input in the establishment of a national framework for measurement, data sharing, and reporting (NQIPA).

The third AQA alliance workgroup is the reporting workgroup (www. aqaalliance/reportingwg.com). It has produced principles for public reporting as well as principles for reporting to clinicians and hospitals, and has had discussions on reporting models and formats.

There are significant opportunities and challenges for the work of the AQA alliance. Among the opportunities are expansion of the measurement sets to address the critical quality issues in all specialties and expansion of the six pilot sites to form a national network of regional data aggregation collaboratives covering all regions of the country. The engagement and support of all medical and surgical specialty groups as well as physicians and their organizations are critical to the success of this work. Determining a business model and funding sources for the expansion of the pilot sites and the operation of the NHDSE are significant challenges. The expansion of the measurement set to address cost of care, access to care, equity, and patient-centered issues represents a major opportunity as well a significant methodological challenge. Determining the best legal structure and positioning between the public and private sectors of the NHDSE will be critical to its success in setting standards and rules for data aggregation for the public and private sectors.

Establishing a common vision for the NQIPA will be important for mobilizing the effort necessary to maximize the value of priority setting, evidence-based medicine, target setting, measurement development, data aggregation, incentives for improved performance, and the public reporting of performance. Getting on with the task of implementing this vision is urgent. Every year that goes by without effective action represents another year of a quality chasm not bridged, of lives lost needlessly, of quality of life diminished unnecessarily.

ENVISIONING A RAPID LEARNING HEALTHCARE SYSTEM

Lynn Etheredge
George Washington University

The United States can develop a rapid learning healthcare system. New research capabilities now emerging—large electronic health record databases, predictive computer models, and rapid learning networks—will make it possible to advance clinical care from the experience of tens of millions of patients each year. With collaborative initiatives in the public and private sectors, a national goal could be for the health system to learn about the best uses of new technologies at the same rate that it produces new technologies. This could be termed a rapid learning health system (Health Affairs 2007).

There is still much to be done to reach that goal. Biomedical researchers and technology firms are expanding knowledge and clinical possibilities much faster than the health system's ability to assess these technologies. Already, there are growing concerns about the evidence base for clinical care, its gaps and biases (Avorn 2004; Kassirer 2005; Abramson 2004; Ioannidis 2005; Deyo and Patrick 2005). Technological change is now the largest factor driving our highest-in-the world health spending, which is now more than $2 trillion per year. With advances in the understanding of the human genome and a doubling of the NIH research budget to more than $28 billion, there may be an even faster stream of new treatment options. Neither government regulation, healthcare markets, consumers, physicians, nor health plans are going to be able to deal with these technology issues, short of rationing, unless there are more rapid advances in the evidence base for clinical care.

The "inference gap" concept, described by Walter Stewart earlier in this volume, incisively captures the knowledge issues that confront public officials, physicians, and patients for the 85 million enrollees in the Medicare and Medicaid programs. As he notes, the clinical trials database is built from randomized clinical trials mostly using younger populations with single diagnoses. The RCT patients are very different from Medicare and Medicaid enrollees who are mostly older patients with multiple diagnoses and treatments, women and children, and individuals with seriously disabling conditions. With Medicare and Medicaid now costing more than $600 billion annually—and projected to cost $3.5 trillion over the next five years— there is a fiscal, as well as a medical, imperative to learn more rapidly about what works in clinical care. As a practical matter, we cannot learn all that we would like to know, as rapidly as we need to know it, through RCTs and need to find powerful and efficient ways to learn rapidly from practice-based evidence.

Large EHR research databases are the key development that makes it possible to create a rapid learning health system. The VA and Kaiser Permanente are the public and private sector leaders; their new research databases each have more than 8 million EHRs. They are likely to add genomic information. New networks with EHR databases—"virtual research organizations"—add even more to these capacities. For instance, HMORN with 14 HMOs has 40 million enrollees and is sponsoring the Cancer Research Network (which has about 10 million patient EHRs) with the National Cancer Institute, as well as the Vaccine Safety Datalink (which has about 6 million patient records) with the Centers for Disease Control and Prevention (CDC). Institutions with EHR databases and genome data include Children's Hospital of Philadelphia, Marshfield, Mayo, and Geisinger. Large research projects that need to access paper health records from multiple sites are now administratively complicated, time-consuming, expensive, and done infrequently. In contrast, studies with computerized EHR databases and new research software will be done from a computer terminal in hours, days, or a few weeks. Thousands of large population studies will be doable quickly and inexpensively.

A fully operational national rapid learning system could include many such databases, sponsors, and networks. It could be organized in many different ways, including by enrolled populations (the VA, Medicare, Medicaid, private health plans); by healthcare professions (specialist registries); by institution (multispecialty clinics and academic health centers); by health condition (disease registries and national clinical studies databases); by technology (drug safety and efficacy studies, coverage with evidence development studies); by geographic area (Framingham study); by age cohort (National Children's Study); or by special population (minorities, genomic studies). With national standards, all EHR research registries and databases could be compatible and multiuse.

The key short-term issues for advancing a rapid learning strategy include leadership and development of learning networks, development of research programs, and funding. As reflected in the spectacularly rapid advances of the Human Genome Project and its sequels, we should be thinking about creating a number of leading-edge networks that cut across traditional organizational boundaries. Among potential new research initiatives, it is notable that large integrated delivery systems, such as Kaiser and VA, have been early leaders and that many parts of NIH could be doing much more to develop ongoing national research networks (see paper by Katz, Chapter 5) and EHR databases. With respect to new databases, the NIH could require reporting of all its publicly funded clinical studies, in EHR-type formats, into national computer-searchable NIH databanks; peer-reviewed journals could require that the datasets of the clinical studies they publish also be available to the scientific community through such NIH databanks (National Cancer Institute 2005). This rapid learning strategy would take advantage of what we economists term the "economics of the commons"; each individual researcher would give up exclusive access to some data, but would benefit, in return, from access to a vast and expanding treasure trove of clinical data from the international research community. With these carefully collected, rich data resources, powerful mathematical modeling approaches will be able to advance systems biology, "virtual" clinical trials, and scientific prediction-based health care much more rapidly. There will also be benefits for research on heterogeneity of treatment responses and the design of "practical clinical trials" to fill evidence gaps (see papers by Tunis, Chapter 1, and by Eddy and Greenfield, Chapter 2). Another important research initiative would be to develop "fast track" learning strategies to evaluate promising new technologies. One model suggested is to establish study designs for new technologies when they are first approved and to review the evidence from patient experience at a specified date (e.g. three years later) to help guide physicians, patients, and future research as these technologies diffuse into wider use (Avorn 2004).

To implement a national learning strategy, the Department of Health and Human Services (HHS) health agencies and the VA could be designers and funders of key public or private initiatives. HHS first-year initiatives could include expanding on the National Cancer Institute's (NCI's) Cancer Research Network with NIH networks for heart disease and diabetes; starting national computer searchable databases for NIH, the Food and Drug Administration (FDA), and other clinical studies; a broad expansion of AHRQ's research to address Medicare Rx, Medicaid, national health spending, socioeconomic and racial disparities, effectiveness, and quality issues; expanding CDC's Vaccine Safety Datalink network and FDA's post-market surveillance into a national FDA-CDC program for evaluation of drug safety and efficacy, including pharmacogenomics; starting national EHR research programs for Medicaid's special needs populations; and initiating a national "fast track" learning system for evaluating promising new technologies. A first-year budget of $50 million for these initiatives takes into account that research capabilities are still capacity limited by EHR database and research tool development. Within five years, a national rapid learning strategy could be taken to scale with about $300 million a year.

To move forward, a national learning strategy also needs vision and consensus. The IOM is already having a key catalytic role through this workshop and publication of these papers. This paper identifies many opportunities for the public and private sectors to collaborate in building a learning healthcare system.

REFERENCES

Abramson, J. 2004. *Overdosed America*. New York: HarperCollins.

Asch, S, E McGlynn, M Hogan, R Hayward, P Shekelle, L Rubenstein, J Keesey, J Adams, and E Kerr. 2004. Comparison of quality of care for patients in the Veterans Health Administration and patients in a national sample. *Annals of Internal Medicine* 141(12):938-945.

AQA Alliance. 2006 (April) *AQA Parameters for Selecting Measures for Physician Performance*. Available from http://www.aqaalliance.org/files/AQAParametersforSelectingAmbulatoryCare.doc. (accessed April 4, 2007).

Avorn, J. 2004. *Powerful Medicines*. New York: Alfred A. Knopf.

Bridges to Excellence. 2006. *Bridges to Excellence Overview*. Available from http://www.bridgestoexcellence.org/bte/about_us/home.htm. (accessed November 30, 2006).

Brown, S, M Lincoln, P Groen, and R Kolodner. 2003. Vista-U.S. Department of Veterans Affairs national-scale HIS. *International Journal of Medical Informatics* 69(2-3):135-156.

Choe, H, S Mitrovich, D Dubay, R Hayward, S Krein, and S Vijan. 2005. Proactive case management of high-risk patients with Type 2 diabetes mellitus by a clinical pharmacist: a randomized controlled trial. *American Journal of Managed Care* 11(4):253-260.

Chumbler, N, B Neugaard, R Kobb, P Ryan, H Qin, and Y Joo. 2005. Evaluation of a care coordination/home-telehealth program for veterans with diabetes: health services utilization and health-related quality of life. *Evaluation and the Health Professions* 28(4):464-478.

Conlin, P, B Fisch, J Orcutt, B Hetrick, and A Darkins. 2006. Framework for a national teleretinal imaging program to screen for diabetic retinopathy in Veterans Health Administration patients. *Journal of Rehabilitation Research and Development* 43(6):741-748.

Deyo, R, and D Patrick. 2005. *Hope or Hype*. New York: American Management Association/AMACOM Books.

Evans, D, W Nichol, and J Perlin. 2006. Effect of the implementation of an enterprise-wide electronic health record on productivity in the Veterans Health Administration. *Health Economics, Policy, and Law* 1(2):163-169.

Frayne, S, J Halanych, D Miller, F Wang, H Lin, L Pogach, E Sharkansky, T Keane, K Skinner, C Rosen, and D Berlowitz. 2005. Disparities in diabetes care: impact of mental illness. *Archives of Internal Medicine* 165(22):2631-2638.

Green, L. 2000. Putting practice into research: a 20-year perspective. *Family Medicine* 32(6):396-397.

Green, L, and S Dovey. 2001. Practice based primary care research networks. They work and are ready for full development and support. *British Medical Journal* 322(7286):567-568.

Green, L, G Fryer Jr., B Yawn, D Lanier, and S Dovey. 2001. The ecology of medical care revisited. *New England Journal of Medicine* 344(26):2021-2025.

Greenfield, S, and S Kaplan. 2004. Creating a culture of quality: the remarkable transformation of the department of Veterans Affairs Health Care System. *Annals of Internal Medicine* 141(4):316-318.

Hayward, R, C Cowan Jr., V Giri, M Lawrence, and F Makki. 2005. Causes of preventable visual loss in type 2 diabetes mellitus: an evaluation of suboptimally timed retinal photocoagulation. *Journal of General Internal Medicine* 20(5):467-469.

Health Affairs. 2007. A rapid learning health system. *Health Affairs* (collection of articles, special web edition) 26(2):w107-w118.

Himmelstein, D, and S Woolhandler. 2005. Hope and hype: predicting the impact of electronic medical records. *Health Affairs* 24(5):1121-1123.

Hofer, T, R Hayward, S Greenfield, E Wagner, S Kaplan, and W Manning. 1999. The unreliability of individual physician "report cards" for assessing the costs and quality of care of a chronic disease. *Journal of the American Medical Association* 281(22):2098-2105.

Huddleston, M, and R Cobb. 2004. Emerging technology for at-risk chronically ill veterans. *Journal of Healthcare Quality* 26(6):12-15, 24.

Institute for Clinical Systems Improvement. 2006. Available from http://www.icsi.org/about/index.asp. (accessed November 30, 2006).

Institute for Healthcare Improvement. 2006. Available from http://www.ihi.org/ihi. (accessed December 3, 2006).

IOM (Institute of Medicine). 1996. *Primary Care: America's Health in a New Era*. Washington, DC: National Academy Press.

——. 1999. *To Err Is Human: Building a Safer Health System*. Washington, DC: National Academy Press.

——. 2001. *Crossing the Quality Chasm: A New Health System for the 21st Century*. Washington, DC: National Academy Press.

——. 2003. *Priority Areas for National Action: Transforming Health Care Quality*. Washington, DC: The National Academies Press.

——. 2005. *Performance Measurement: Accelerating Improvement*. Washington, DC: The National Academies Press.

——. 2006. *The Richard and Hilda Rosenthal Lectures 2005: The Next Steps Toward Higher Quality Health Care*. Washington, DC: The National Academies Press.

Ioannidis, J. 2005. Contradicted and initially stronger effects in highly cited clinical research. *Journal of the American Medical Association* 294(2):218-228.

Isham, G, and G Amundson. 2002 (October). A seven step process model for quality improvement. *Group Practice Journal* 40.

Jha, A, J Perlin, K Kizer, and R Dudley. 2003. Effect of the transformation of the Veterans Affairs Health Care System on the quality of care. *New England Journal of Medicine* 348(22):2218-2227.

Kassirer, J. 2005. *On The Take*. New York: Oxford University Press.

Kern, E, M Maney, D Miller, C Tseng, A Tiwari, M Rajan, D Aron, and L Pogach. 2006. Failure of ICD-9-CM codes to identify patients with comorbid chronic kidney disease in diabetes. *Health Services Research* 41(2):564-580.

Kerr, E, D Smith, M Hogan, T Hofer, S Krein, M Bermann, and R Hayward. 2003. Building a better quality measure: are some patients with "poor quality" actually getting good care? *Medical Care* 41(10):1173-1182.

Kerr, E, R Gerzoff, S Krein, J Selby, J Piette, J Curb, W Herman, D Marrero, K Narayan, M Safford, T Thompson, and C Mangione. 2004. Diabetes care quality in the Veterans Affairs Health Care System and commercial managed care: the TRIAD study. *Annals of Internal Medicine* 141(4):272-281.

Kleinke, J. 2005. Dot-gov: market failure and the creation of a national health information technology system. *Health Affairs* 24(5):1246-1262.

Krein, S. 2002. Whom should we profile? Examining diabetes care practice variation among primary care providers, provider groups, and health care facilities. *Health Services Research* 35(5):1160-1180.

Miller, D, M Safford, and L Pogach. 2004. Who has diabetes? Best estimates of diabetes prevalence in the Department of Veterans Affairs based on computerized patient data. *Diabetes Care* 27(Suppl.):2, B10-B21.

MN Community Measurement. 2006. *Our Community Approach*. Available from http://mnhealthcare.org/~wwd.cfm. (accessed November 30, 2006).

Mold, J, and K Peterson. 2005. Primary care practice-based research networks: working at the interface between research and quality improvement. *Annals of Family Medicine* 3(Suppl.):1, S12-S20.

National Cancer Institute. 2005 (June). *Restructuring the National Cancer Clinical Trials Enterprise*. Available from http://integratedtrials.nci.nih.gov/ict/. (accessed May 24, 2006).

Office of Governor Tim Pawlenty. 2006 (July 31). *Governor Pawlenty Introduces Health Care Inititative to Improve Quality and Save Costs.* Available from http://www.governor.state. mn.us/mediacenter/pressreleases/PROD007733.html. (accessed November 30, 2006.

Overhage, J, S Perkins, W Tierney, and C McDonald. 2001. Controlled trial of direct physician order entry: effects on physicians' time utilization in ambulatory primary care internal medicine practices. *Journal of the American Medical Informatics Association* 8(4):361-371.

Parchman, M, R Romero, and J Pugh. 2006. Encounters by patients with Type 2 diabetes—complex and demanding: an observational study. *Annals of Family Medicine* 4(1):40-45.

Perlin, J. 2006. Transformation of the U.S. Veterans Health Administration. *Health Economics, Policy, and Law* 1(2):99-105.

Perlin, J, R Kolodner, and R Roswell. 2004. The Veterans Health Administration: quality, value, accountability, and information as transforming strategies for patient-centered care. *American Journal of Managed Care* 10(11.2):828-836.

Pogach, L, and D Miller. 2006. *Merged VHA-Medicare Databases: A Tool to Evaluate Outcomes and Expenditures of Chronic Diseases.* Poster Session, VHA Health Services Research and Development Conference, February 26, 2006.

Raths, D. 2006 (February). *9 Tech Trends: Pay for Performance.* Healthcare Informatics Online. Available from http://healthcare-informatics.com/issues/2006/02/48. (accessed December 2, 2006).

Safford, M, L Eaton, G Hawley, M Brimacombe, M Rajan, H Li, and L Pogach. 2003. Disparities in use of lipid-lowering medications among people with Type 2 diabetes mellitus. *Archives of Internal Medicine* 163(8):922-928.

Sawin, C, D Walder, D Bross, and L Pogach. 2004. Diabetes process and outcome measures in the Department of Veterans Affairs. *Diabetes Care* 27(Suppl.):2, B90-B94.

Thompson, W, H Wang, M Xie, J Kolassa, M Rajan, C Tseng, S Crystal, Q Zhang, Y Vardi, L Pogach, and M Safford. 2005. Assessing quality of diabetes care by measuring longitudinal changes in hemoglobin A1c in the Veterans Health Administration. *Health Services Research* 40(6.1):1818-1835.

Tseng, C, M Rajan, D Miller, G Hawley, S Crystal, M Xie, A Tiwari, M Safford, and L Pogach. 2005. Use of administrative data to risk adjust amputation rates in a national cohort of Medicare-enrolled veterans with diabetes. *Medical Care* 43(1):88-92.

U.S. Department of Veterans Affairs. 2006. *My HealtheVet.* Available from http://www.my-health.va.gov. (accessed August 21, 2006).

White, K, T Williams, and B Greenberg. 1961. The ecology of medical care. *New England Journal of Medicine* 265:885-892.

White House. 2006 (August 22). *Executive Order: Promoting Quality and Efficient Health Care in Federal Government Administered or Sponsored Health Care Programs.* Available from http://www.whitehouse.gov/news/releases/2006/08/20060822-2.html. (accessed April 4, 2007)

5

Developing the Test Bed—
Linking Integrated Service Delivery Systems

OVERVIEW

Many extensive research networks have been established to conduct clinical, basic, and health services research and to facilitate communication between the different efforts. The scale of these networks ranges from local, uptake-driven efforts to wide-ranging efforts to connect vast quantities of clinical and research information. This chapter explores how various integrated service delivery systems might be better linked to expand our nation's capacity for structured, real-time learning—in effect, developing a test bed to improve development and application of evidence in healthcare decision making.

In the first paper, Steven I. Katz outlines the efforts of the National Institutes of Health (NIH) Roadmap for Medical Research to accelerate biomedical research on a basic level as well as accelerate translational research by connecting existing research networks and maintaining necessary infrastructure for more efficient conduct of clinical research through the National Electronics and Clinical Trials Research network (NECTAR). Cynthia Palmer then discusses efforts of the Agency for Healthcare Research and Quality (AHRQ) to build on the experience of the Integrated Delivery Systems Research Network and establish a vehicle for translation of research into practice by linking healthcare systems with health services researchers. Through rapid cycle, applied research, AHRQ's Accelerating Change and Transformation in Organizations and Networks initiative has begun to establish a network that fosters demand-driven research and the uptake of innovative approaches to care.

Eric B. Larson discusses the Health Maintenance Organization (HMO) Research Network as a potential model for a national test bed. Many ongoing activities of these 15 linked integrated delivery systems illustrate the potential for these networks to facilitate needed two-way learning between research and healthcare systems. Finally, Michael Mustille presents the history and progress of the Council for Accountable Physician Practices (CAPP) to demonstrate how this network of multispecialty medical groups has accelerated the redesign of physician practice—improving the uptake of evidence-based approaches to care, the translation of research to practice, and the outcomes and efficiency of care.

NIH AND REENGINEERING CLINICAL RESEARCH

Stephen I. Katz, M.D., Ph.D.
National Institutes of Health

The NIH Roadmap for Medical Research was developed to increase synergy across NIH and accelerate the pace of discoveries and their translation. It was launched in order to identify major opportunities and gaps in biomedical research that the agency as a whole needed to address to have the greatest impact on the progress of medical research. Roadmap dollars represent 0.8 percent of the total NIH budget and are planned to reach $500 million by 2008. The Roadmap project is meant to address the questions that no one of the 27 different institutes or centers could address on its own but that we could address collectively. This is not a single initiative, but more than 345 individual awards were given, in FY 2005: 40 percent for basic, 40 percent for translational, and 20 percent for high-risk research.

The NIH Roadmap Strategy was to build on the paradigm of bringing basic science and discovery to clinical practice. Roadmap initiatives are grouped under three main headings: New Pathways to Discovery, Research Teams of the Future, and Reengineering the Clinical Research Enterprise. These are all initiatives that are meant to facilitate bench-to-bedside translation of research. New Pathways to Discovery addresses the fundamental issues that need to be overcome to accelerate research at the basic level. Most notable here are the molecular libraries and imaging advances that will enable high-throughput screening of molecular pathways that have been identified as of interest. Research Teams of the Future embodies the commitment of NIH to an interdisciplinary research approach and the promotion of high-risk research through Pioneer Awards.

About one-third of the Roadmap awards are in the area of Reengineering the Clinical Research Enterprise. These initiatives include the Clinical and Translational Science Awards (CTSAs) and a number of projects that are investigating the integration of clinical research networks. We have heard repeatedly that the clinical research enterprise is broken. Some of the responsibility for fixing this enterprise falls to NIH, and this paper considers some of the major issues and focuses in particular on the work of some of our translational initiatives on clinical research informatics and integrated research networks.

One of the central challenges to clinical research lies in the regulatory requirements that govern it. Human subjects protection is one issue, but across the board, whether it is HMOs, pharmaceutical research, or the biotech industry, there is no harmonization of clinical research regulatory requirements. For example, the requirements related to reporting adverse events are not uniform across NIH and certainly not across agencies. It took 2.5 years to get uniformity across the NIH and the Food and Drug Administration (FDA) just in the reporting of adverse events of gene therapy trials. The work continues to extend this uniformity across all government agencies as well as outside the government to industry.

Enhancing clinical research workforce training has also been identified as a key need, prompting NIH to institute loan repayment programs and encourage more workforce training at earlier levels in medical schools. Also lending support for enhanced workforce training are the CTSAs, which represent the largest of our investments from the NIH Roadmap for Medical Research. This investment addresses the question of how to best respond to the demand created by recent biomedical discoveries for the evolution of clinical science. CTSAs will create homes for clinical research, researchers, and trainees and are meant to lower barriers between disciplines and encourage creative, innovative approaches to solve complex medical mysteries. These awards are designed to encourage change on a number of dimensions, including the development of novel clinical and translational methodologies; pilot collaborative translational and clinical studies; biomedical informatics; design, biostatistics, and ethics; regulatory knowledge and support; participant and clinical interactions resources; community engagement; translational technologies and resources, and education and career development. In the first round of applications, CTSAs have been awarded to 12 academic health centers, with 60 institutions expected to be part of this new consortium by 2012. This is clearly a sea change in terms of what can go on at academic medical centers. Most academic research centers remain structured in the same way they were 50 years ago and the Clinical and Translational Science Awards are meant to catalyze change—breaking silos, breaking barriers, and breaking conventions. If this works the way we hope it should work, it will clearly change the research enterprise.

The Clinical Research Networks project is part of the Reengineering the Clinical Research Enterprise Roadmap aimed at promoting and expanding clinical research networks that can rapidly conduct high-quality clinical studies that address multiple research questions. Specifically, NIH is developing the NECTAR network. While research networks currently exist, this initiative is meant to link those networks so that clinical trials can be conducted more effectively. This is particularly important for the NIH where each institute supports clinical research, but does so independently. As a result, to conduct a clinical study, infrastructure is repeatedly built up and broken down. This continual building up and breaking down of infrastructure is a complete loss of money, not to mention the people and resources needed. This is particularly important, for example, in pediatric research, in which most diseases studied are uncommon and can only be done through linked clinical research networks.

However, there are signs of change. For example, in the area of pediatric rheumatic diseases, the Arthritis Foundation helped to build a network across pediatric rheumatic disease allowing many clinical trials to be done simultaneously, leveraging our resources from one trial to other ongoing and planned trials.

As a first step toward establishing a broader network, an inventory of existing clinical research networks will explore existing informatics and training infrastructures. By identifying characteristics that promote or inhibit successful network interactivity, productivity, and expansion, this inventory will lead to the dissemination of "best practices" that can enhance the efficiency of clinical research networks. Pilot projects will then explore how best to combine and extend clinical networks. The initial NECTAR inventory provided current status of about 250 clinical research networks and evaluated best practices. NECTAR pilot projects have been developed with a broad coverage, including medical disciplines such as cancer, heart, critical care, psychiatry, and transplants; populations and settings (primary care, rural, minority, HMO); ages (pediatric, adult, geriatric); information systems (data standards, informatics, tools, platforms); and geographic locations (U.S. and global).

Collectively, these initiatives—CTSA, NECTAR pilot projects, and the inventory of networks—are complementary programs. CTSA focuses on the academic institutions, and NECTAR focuses on linking organizations together in an electronic research network. CTSA is intended to build the homes for clinical and translational science, emphasizing internal and interinstitutional nationwide interoperable informatics. The NECTAR inventory will also discover best practices for existing clinical network management, helping to define the needed common language and standards. There is strong consensus on the potential to use these linked systems to build a test bed and enhance learning. What is needed is leadership, commitment, passion, and a commitment to funding. Funding in particular will drive the development of needed linkages and infrastructure for a learning healthcare system. Commitment of long-term funding however cannot just be the responsibility of the NIH or the Veterans Administration (VA), but must extend to states as well as to other forms of support.

In this respect, the President's Health Information Technology Strategic Plan has great potential to expand the involvement and improve the efficiency and power of clinical and translational research. To truly transform clinical practice we must interconnect physicians, improve our understanding of population health, and empower patients. Our initiatives will optimize efficiency and productivity of biomedical research, encourage the basic exploration of bioinformatics and computational biology, and accelerate research translation through CTSAs. However developing the needed test bed will require substantial cross-agency and cross-sector work and collaboration.

AHRQ AND THE USE OF
INTEGRATED SERVICE DELIVERY SYSTEMS

Cynthia Palmer, M.Sc.
Agency for Healthcare Research and Quality

Often, health services research findings are not implemented in practice and thus fail to improve the quality of health care that Americans receive. With its program Accelerating Change and Transformation in Organizations and Networks (ACTION), the Agency for Healthcare Research and Quality places the responsibility of investing in the implementation of good ideas, once proven, directly on those who produce, use, and fund such research. ACTION is a five-year implementation model of field-based contract research that fosters public-private collaboration in rapid-cycle, applied studies. With a goal of turning research into practice, 15 ACTION partner organizations and approximately 150 collaborating organizations link many of the nation's largest healthcare systems with its top health services researchers. ACTION provides health services in a wide variety of organizational care settings to at least 100 million Americans. The partnerships span all states and provide access to large numbers of providers, major health plans, hospitals, long-term care facilities, ambulatory care settings, and other care sites. Each partnership includes healthcare systems with large, robust databases, clinical and research expertise, and the authority to implement healthcare interventions. ACTION is the successor to the Integrated Delivery System Research Network (IDSRN), a five-year implementation initiative that was completed in 2005. To maximize the likelihood of uptake of innovation, the ACTION program emphasizes projects that are of interest to the partnerships' own operational leaders as well as the project funders, that are broadly responsive to user needs and operational interests, and that are expected to be generalizable across a number of settings.

Prior to developing the call for proposals for ACTION participants, the IDSRN was evaluated carefully. AHRQ continues to use the findings of that evaluation, and its own perceptions, to help shape and direct the ACTION program. ACTION is meant to help AHRQ achieve its goals by promoting uptake of innovation to change practice, through the capture of information about how people change the way they behave to achieve higher-quality delivery of care. Knowing the right thing to do, even when we have evidence-based practices, is not enough. Getting people to actually do the right thing is the real dilemma. AHRQ recognizes the value of nurturing "receptor sites," or "test beds," where care is actually delivered and is trying to foster user-driven or demand-driven research.

One of the members of AHRQ's current National Advisory Committee developed a model (Balas and Boren 2000), which is quite telling in terms of one of the key issues, suggesting that it takes typically about 17 years after the first study results are published to turn about 14 percent of that research into the benefit of patient care. This sobering concept suggests the need for a shift toward more demand-driven research—in which we bring the producers of work and the users of work together to study how to change practice. In addition, while publications are acknowledged as important, we place a stronger emphasis and focus on other types of products that are in forms that can be more easily disseminated and utilized in other settings.

IDSRN and ACTION represent networks of healthcare delivery-based partnerships in which hospitals, ambulatory care facilities, long-term care facilities, and health plans work in conjunction with health services consultants and researchers through five-year master contracts. Contractors (partners) compete for task orders on a rolling basis with the idea of sustaining networks through five years of studies, keep those partnerships in place so they can grow and develop their infrastructure, and continue to have opportunities to work together over a reasonable period of time. The focus is on rapid-cycle, applied research of interest to AHRQ, the partnerships' own operational leaders, and others. Since AHRQ is a small agency with limited funding to support this endeavor, funding is secured from other organizations to conduct some of the studies. For example, other Department of Health and Human Services (HHS) agencies and some foundations have contributed funds for several studies. In 2005, about two-thirds of ACTION's funding was obtained through interagency agreements or other mechanisms.

The IDSRN and ACTION emphasize demand-driven, practical, applied, rapid-cycle work across a broad range of topics. The 93 task orders issued by the IDSRN between 2000 and 2005 were completed on average in 15 months. Through ACTION, AHRQ will attempt to take implementation and the uptake of innovation to scale. The IDSRN evaluation found evidence in about 60 percent of task orders (projects) of demonstrable uptake of innovation. Most uptake of innovation was local, suggesting that the organizations that conducted the research used the results to improve the quality of care delivery. Part of ACTION's charge is to extend that kind of uptake more broadly, even nationwide where possible.

To help with dissemination, ACTION partnerships include firms with expertise in communication, dissemination, marketing, and other areas to improve both dissemination and uptake of innovation by the partnerships themselves. Dissemination projects are accomplished under contract rather than through grants—funding studies to procure tools, products, and strategies that are felt to be generalizable and sustainable within other delivery systems.

ACTION has several strategic advantages. Collectively, the partnerships serve more than 100 million individuals through a variety of providers working in widely diverse settings of care. ACTION also has broad diversity in payer, geographic, and demographic mix. This is important to AHRQ's goal to focus on priority populations such as children, the elderly, the disabled, minorities, and other underserved individuals. ACTION's partnerships have access to large robust datasets and nationally recognized academic and field-based researchers with expertise in data manipulation methods and emerging organizational and management issues. The partnerships' operational leaders are committed to helping set the network's agenda and using findings of value to their organizations. Perhaps ACTION's most important strategic advantage is speed; the time between the release of a Request for Proposal and an award is approximately 9 to 12 weeks, and the average project is completed in 15 months. Finally, although ACTION is too new to have tested the impact of project findings, the IDSRN had significant impact, with dozens of local to international examples of uptake of tools and strategies developed and tested in IDSRN projects. This occurred in part because, in addition to publications in peer-reviewed and trade journals, AHRQ asks for deliverables such as presentations to the healthcare operational leadership and at live or web-assisted conferences; scalable, scenario-appropriate models; training curricula, workshops, and workshop tools; and "how-to" guides, workbooks, DVDs, and webcasts.

THE HMO RESEARCH NETWORK AS A TEST BED

Eric B. Larson, M.D., M.P.H., M.A.C.P.
Group Health Cooperative's Center for Health Studies
for the HMO Research Network[1]

Learning from experience is something that individuals do continually and automatically. For a country whose health care has been widely

[1]Acknowledgments: Sarah Greene, Paul Fishman, Joe Selby, Andrew Nelson, Rich Platt, James Ralston, Karin Johnson, and Rebecca Hughes.

characterized as costly, inefficient, dangerous, and often falling well short of best practices, learning from experience should serve as a driving force in our efforts to *cross the quality chasm* (IOM 2001). Making this happen, however, remains a tremendous challenge. If we were truly able to improve health care constantly by learning from experience, presumably we would have already solved the problems highlighted in recent Institute of Medicine (IOM) reports on health care and quality (IOM 2007a, 2007b, 2006a, 2006b, 2004a, 2004b, 2004c, 2004d, 2003a, 2003b, 2002). What we need is a setting equipped to conduct observational investigations under normal working conditions. Engineers call this a test bed.

HMORN's Key Features

The HMO Research Network (HMORN) links 15 integrated delivery systems (Figure 5-1). Collectively and individually, these member organizations are examples of learning healthcare systems that can—and *do*—learn through direct experience. Over the past decade, HMORN has collected evidence from both its own research and research in general, translating that evidence into both better and best practices. This paper explores some key questions that a learning organization such as HMORN faces, a few of the lessons learned, and several of the priorities and needs required to foster healthcare systems that are truly devoted to learning.

A learning healthcare system such as HMORN faces five key questions:

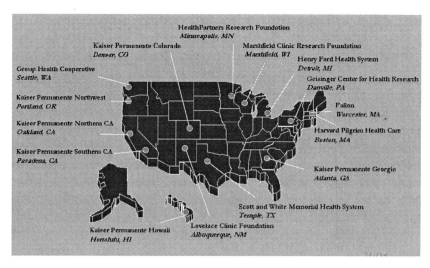

FIGURE 5-1 Sites in the HMO Research Network.

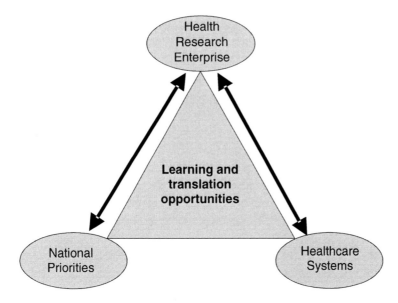

FIGURE 5-2 Reciprocal exchange between research and both healthcare and national priorities.

(1) What is structured real time learning? (2) What are some seminal features of integrated delivery systems? (3) Why are integrated delivery systems well suited to structured real-time learning? (4) Why might linking integrated delivery systems surpass single integrated delivery systems for real-time learning? (5) What is the potential of HMORN, and what are some of the priority areas in which we could accelerate the benefits of such linkages? Answering these questions illuminates the unique features of HMORN and sets the stage for discussing both the network's potential and the priorities for using it as a real-time test bed, or a learning healthcare system.

Structured Real-Time Learning

The HMORN seeks to achieve two-way (bidirectional or reciprocal) learning between health research and both national priorities and healthcare systems (Figure 5-2). This can occur when researchers take advantage of opportunities to respond to important national research issues in a real-world setting—*and* also use insights gained through that setting to advance the nation's research agenda. In this way, a healthcare research enterprise such as HMORN can mediate the exchange of learning and translation between healthcare systems and national priorities. The knowledge exchange between these two spheres, especially when conducted in a way that promotes *implementation* of new knowledge, can greatly accelerate advances in health care through opportunities for translation.

Seminal Features of Integrated Delivery Systems

Integrated delivery systems offer close ties between care delivery, financing, administration, and patients. Ideally, this leads to closer alignment of incentives, especially for ongoing efforts to improve quality. HMORN centers have shared administrative claims and clinical databases. Where researchers enjoy effective relationships with administrators, clinicians, and even health plan members, interest in research projects can be truly shared—and research results are more likely to be translated appropriately. Partnerships with the parent organizations can then lead to research teams that include practicing clinicians and HMORN scientific collaborators.

Another key feature is that institutional review boards (IRBs) oversee all research activities. These IRBs typically include administrators, clinicians, local researchers, and members of the public. The local IRB is a critical control point for all research in an integrated delivery system. Unlike other healthcare research, which enrolls participants from the community, HMORN research typically involves health plan members as participants. Therefore, the HMORN IRBs review research protocols that can have real and perceived influences on the members' relationships with their HMO (Greene and Geiger 2006).

Fit with Structured Real-Time Learning

Healthcare systems can—and in fact do—serve as natural laboratories for applied research questions: thus they have an ongoing role in efforts to optimize health and health care. When these efforts are combined with appropriate measurement strategies designed to answer defined research questions, healthcare systems offer unparalleled learning opportunities. The collective experiences of HMORN members include a wide array of pioneering trials in dozens of clinical and population-based areas, as well as epidemiological, cost-effectiveness, and clinical studies (Raebel et al. 2005; Fishman et al. 2004; Elmore et al. 2005; Geiger et al. 2006; Paasche-Orlow et al. 2006). At this writing, these include research in diabetes prevention, warfarin metabolism, communication around genetic testing, and strategies to increase enrollment in clinical trials. The longest running longitudinal study of aging in the US has operated continuously for over five decades, located in a Seattle HMO (Group Health) (Schaie 1993). That same HMO for the past two decades, now facilitated by real time comprehensive member data, is the setting for ongoing cohort studies of aging and dementia using representative random samples of a very stable population of persons over age 65. (Larson et al. 2006). This partial list illustrates the variety of cutting-edge clinical research opportunities, which include many other types of studies.

Advantage of Linked over Single Integrated Delivery Systems

This is really the question of the moment. The answer hinges on the fact that the larger and broader the scope of the study, the more heterogeneity one can achieve both in patient populations and in approaches to care and quality. Linked integrated delivery systems offer significant advantages over single ones: heterogeneous patient populations—and heterogeneous approaches to care—combined with an enduring commitment to translate research into practice and improve quality. This heterogeneity provides more insights into patient-, provider-, and system-level factors that affect care. The ability to examine these multiple factors has formed the cornerstone of several HMORN projects (Leyden et al. 2005; Taplin et al. 2004; Quinn et al. 2005; Stevens et al. 2005). Multisite studies improve generalizability, especially studies of interventions and evaluations.

The HMORN offers an unparalleled opportunity to study rare disorders in a more natural setting; by contrast, when studies are based only in referral centers, their samples are often highly selective. The scale of the population base (more than 15 million), plus electronic medical records, accurate diagnostic databases, and engaged scientists, should facilitate unique opportunities for studying rare disorders (as well as treatment effects in various subpopulations and common conditions).

A growing number of multisite studies, involving various combinations of HMORN, demonstrate the utility and value of linking integrated delivery systems:

- *The HMO Cancer Research Network (CRN)* has been funded by NCI since 1999 to study the effectiveness of cancer control interventions across the spectrum of cancer from prevention to palliative care (Hornbrook et al. 2005; Wagner et al. 2005). The CRN was recently highlighted as an example of a "best-practice" research consortium at the 2006 National Leadership Forum on clinical research networks (Inventory and Evaluation of Clinical Research Networks 2006).
- *The Vaccine Safety Datalink* is a collaborative project between the National Immunization Program of the Centers for Disease Control and Prevention (CDC) and eight large HMOs (DeStefano 2001). The project began in 1990 with the primary purpose of rigorously evaluating concerns about the safety of vaccines.

- *The Centers for Education and Research on Therapeutics (CERT)* is a national demonstration program funded by AHRQ to conduct research and provide education that advances the optimal use of therapeutics (drugs, medical devices, and biological products) (Platt et al. 2001).
- *The DEcIDE Network (Developing Evidence to Inform Decisions about Effectiveness)* is also funded by AHRQ. A collaborative research and practice-based network program, it helps AHRQ and other federal agencies to implement Section 1013 of the Medicare Modernization Act of 2003.
- *The NIH Roadmap Initiative on Reengineering the Clinical Research Enterprise,* under which HMORN formed the Coordinated Clinical Studies Network (CCSN), is devoted to improving the systems and processes that support our many multisite studies (Greene et al. 2005a).

HMORN, Priority Areas, and Potential

The considerable potential of HMORN is illustrated by the priority areas in which we could accelerate the benefits of such linkages:

Natural experiments in health services research are ongoing: How do benefit changes, new health insurance products, and organization and policy shifts affect outcomes? How do increased prescription copayments affect adherence? When clinicians receive faxed alerts because their patients fail to renew prescriptions, how are outcomes affected? How does the use of "carve-out" disease management systems compare with that of integrated disease management systems that maintain intact primary care relationships? What happens when we provide physicians with performance feedback? What happens when new electronic medical records offer opportunities for more personalized care and real-time evaluation, including asynchronous direct communication with doctors and healthcare teams? How do patient behavior and healthcare utilization change when patients have direct access to specialty care?

Surveillance of the enrollee populations in the network is another general area in which HMORN can meet immediate needs: from biosafety to more focused post-marketing surveillance. The network offers size, data systems, and persons with programming, biostatistical, epidemiologic, and clinical expertise. In therapeutics, the CDC's Vaccine Safety Datalink (eight HMORN plans) is the world's foremost source of vaccine safety data. Ten HMORN health plans make up the largest component of the FDA's population-based drug safety surveillance program. In infectious diseases, five plans have developed methods for early identification and reporting of acute illness clusters that might represent outbreaks of influenza, severe acute respiratory syndrome (SARS), or bioterrorist events. CDC's national BioSense initiative has adopted these methods. Members of HMORN have developed automatic reporting systems for notifiable diseases (including tuberculosis, Lyme disease, hepatitis C, and *Chlamydia*). In one intriguing example, a surveillance case study involved researchers and clinicians, working in real time, to address an urgent public health concern: at Kaiser Permanente Colorado, researchers compared the ability to detect influenza A through syndromic surveillance by providers, sentinel provider diagnosis, and laboratory-confirmed cases. The study concluded that syndromic surveillance can be useful for detecting clusters of respiratory illness in various settings (Ritzwoller et al. 2005).

The HMORN is creating the largest observational test bed for IOM's aims for patient-centered *health information technology* (IOM 2001). Several plans have functioning web-based patient portals, and others are in development. These respond to the IOM care redesign rules that encourage transparency, free flow of information, and patient control. This is an area ripe for discovery and close examination. Web-based patient portals, secure messaging between patients and providers, and the accompanying transformation of the doctor-patient interaction could lead to dramatic changes in cost and quality of care and market dynamics. HMORN is uniquely positioned to study the impact. HMORN plans have conducted randomized trials and quasi-experimental studies of computerized physician order entry (CPOE) systems, including studies of different kinds of alerts and academic detailing to reduce prescribing errors. Additionally, two HMORN randomized controlled trials (RCTs) are testing tailored health behavior change interventions (for fruit and vegetable consumption and smoking cessation) that could eventually be integrated into these portals. Finally, at the levels of both health plans and research centers, we are participating in the dialogue about the structure, function, and standards that would compose a national healthcare infrastructure. Interoperability of healthcare data (allowing data sharing among disparate systems) will influence—and, we hope, enhance—the depth and breadth of research that HMORN could undertake.

The HMORN is extremely well-suited to developing and implementing *clinical trials* based either on individual or on "cluster" randomization (i.e., intact groups of individuals are assigned randomly to receive different interventions). Of particular relevance in HMORN are practical clinical trials (Tunis et al. 2003), marked by heterogeneous populations and practice settings and their ability to study a broad range of clinically meaningful health outcomes. Information systems will routinely include data on all aspects of care useful for screening populations for eligible participants. In stable HMOs, these systems can provide opportunities for automated, less resource intensive, and longer follow-up, providing real-world outcomes over time. A newly funded HMORN study will examine ways to reduce barriers to trial accrual (Somkin et al. 2005), focusing on the effect of patient- and provider-level notification systems that can flag potentially eligible patients for specified cancer clinical trials. In systems that enjoy high levels of trust from patients and healthcare professionals, clinical trials can have high enrollment rates and excellent follow-up rates. The HMORN's NIH Roadmap project has developed infrastructure and tools designed to determine easily how feasible a given clinical trial is in subject availability, budget, more efficient coordination of human subjects review processes, enrollment manuals, data collection processes, adherence to Health Insurance Portability and Accountability Act (HIPAA) rules, and coordinated close-out processes. This project is now working on improving the readability of consent forms and other subject materials and improvements in cluster randomized trial methodologies. These efforts should greatly facilitate the ability to perform clinical trials in HMORN and may lower the costs of launching these trials.

The HMORN has consistently proved its ability to conduct studies designed to *enhance the quality of patient care*. Such studies, which have direct application in delivery systems, run the gamut. Case-control studies of late-stage breast and cervical cancer showed that failure to screen ever, or within the past three years, explained more than half of all cases of delayed diagnoses (Leyden et al. 2005; Taplin et al. 2004). This, in turn, led to systematic redesign of screening outreach programs among HMOs participating in this study. Studies of clinicians' use of the "five As" framework (ask, advise, assist, agree, arrange) to encourage patients to quit smoking resulted in two sites changing their tobacco cessation programs (Solberg et al. 2004). Perhaps the most notable example of an HMO-based effort to improve the quality of patient care was the development of the Chronic Care Model (Greene et al. 2005b). This model, which has been widely adopted throughout HMORN and worldwide, is distinguished by its strong evidence base and comprehensive attention to the many drivers that influence the quality and outcome of the patient-practitioner interaction. Finally, physician-focused interventions have demonstrated how techniques such as computerized physician order entry reminders, "academic detailing," or physician feedback (comparing physicians with their peers) can improve appropriate prescribing in older patients and compliance with guidelines (Simon et al. 2006; Smith et al. 2006).

Improving the HMORN Test Bed

To realize fully an ongoing system of structured real-time learning, several structural innovations are needed. These innovations must facilitate two-way knowledge transfer and the ability to share and apply research lessons that will benefit not only members of HMORN but U.S. health care overall. Today, the leadership of HMORN has developed mechanisms for HMO researchers and clinicians to create and implement new studies. Currently, these mechanisms are somewhat ad hoc but can be memorialized in everyday processes and procedures. Task order funding models allow development of rapid-cycle research proposals and projects. However, the rapid cycle is challenging, both for smaller centers with less infrastructure and for multisite studies. Ideally, these funding mechanisms would include some allowance for infrastructure support and even the resources and time to embed lessons in the delivery system. That support would then cover staff needed for enhanced processes and procedures across the network.

A durable infrastructure in a network-based setting would greatly reduce inefficiencies and speed the cycle of research and translation. One of the key findings of the national study of clinical research networks was the amount of redundancy and reinvention that takes place in collaborative research (Inventory and Evaluation of Clinical Research Networks 2006). By now, there should be ways to simplify and institutionalize many processes that are common to all studies. Through the NIH Roadmap's CCSN, HMORN has begun to develop new approaches to coordinate IRB reviews of multisite studies, which can be among the more time-consuming aspects of collaborative projects. It would be mutually beneficial for NIH, the Office for Human Research Protections (OHRP), and other bodies responsible for harmonizing regulations and developing new guidance for the protection of human subjects to work with groups such as HMORN to ensure that innovations to minimize redundancy and rework (which plague multisite studies today) are feasible and, if so, incorporated into national models for research review.

The HMORN has, at best, informal—and, at worst, inconsistent—systems to collect, disseminate, and translate innovations and best practices among its members and to help meet its mission as a nonproprietary, public interest research group (Greene, Hart, and Wagner 2005b). If the United States continues to rely on private "market forces" to render efficiencies in its healthcare system, an invaluable adjunct would be a mechanism to collect, disseminate, and translate innovations and best practices (especially those funded by public and not-for-profit foundation sources). The HMORN might be ideally suited to take on this important task as a demonstration project. The general inclination of leaders in HMORN is to support the general good, rather than the private good, through their research efforts and results. However, in our current market-driven system, and in the absence of such a demonstration project, researchers are exposed to understandable conflicts in their need to balance proprietary and national interests.

An ongoing challenge that all HMORN centers face is how to involve operational staff, including physicians and other professionals, in research. Experience has shown that when front-line staff participate in design and implementation, such research is more likely to be relevant and "field-ready" for translation. However, it is usually difficult to justify costs for such persons in today's research budgets. Funding agencies should consider including front-line staff as a specification in certain Requests for Applications (RFAs)—particularly those that emphasize translation and dissemination. Learning organizations such as the members of HMORN would likely be able to demonstrate or at least respond to such specifications, because integrated delivery systems typically take an organized approach to determining the applicability of research findings and translating research into practice.

In summary, we believe the HMO Research Network affords the possibility of a structured real-time learning test bed that approaches the ideal. This paper emphasizes that HMORN is uniquely poised to take advantage of opportunities for two-way learning, and we have described several areas in which the Network and its members have conducted—and can further conduct—research that will improve the development and application of evidence to improve healthcare quality and effectiveness. Figure 5-3 illustrates what this might look like. The figure's important features are its reliance on reciprocity and its ability to link real-world care and research to public health goals. If we are to learn from experience about approaches to improving the health of the public, the accumulated experiences of HMORN are a logical place to begin.

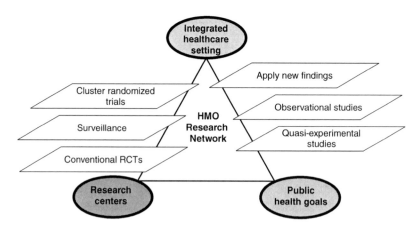

FIGURE 5-3 Idealized intersections among priorities in health care, research, and public health.

COUNCIL OF ACCOUNTABLE PHYSICIAN PRACTICES

Michael A. Mustille, M.D.
The Permanente Federation

The healthcare sector is beset by a constellation of perceived failures. Cost inflation threatens the affordability of care not only for individuals but for businesses, government entities, and ultimately, for the nation as a whole. Quality of care appears mediocre in general and does not seem to be substantially better now than it was 15 years ago (McGlynn et al. 2003). What is known of the science of medicine is too often not accomplished in the practice of medicine. Acquisition, management, and sharing of medical information are inhibited by a combination of anachronistic paper record keeping and scarce, idiosyncratic automated systems that are designed primarily for financial, not clinical, transactions. Underlying these shortcomings is a payment structure too often poorly aligned, and sometimes contradictory, with regard to incentives and priorities that would lead to improvements in care quality and cost.

These failures are complex in origin, and the corrections needed to remedy them will not be simple. However, one element of the solution that offers promise has largely been absent from public debates on health sector problems—namely, care delivery system redesign and, in particular, redesign of physician practice. There are clear examples of physician group practices that have been very successful in delivering high-quality care at reasonable cost despite the general health sector failures outlined above. A recent paper in *Health Services Research* examined multispecialty medical groups (MSMGs) and showed the positive relationship between delivery system organization and Health Plan Employer and Data Information Set (HEDIS) Effectiveness of Care measure scores (Gillies et al. 2006). This cross-sectional, multivariate regression analysis examined the impact of health plan organizational characteristics (i.e., tax status, size, age, type of system used to deliver care) on clinical process and patient satisfaction measures. The analysis of HEDIS scores showed that delivery systems organized around multispecialty staff or group practices outperformed other less integrated delivery models on clinical process measures, while member satisfaction as measured by Consumer Assessment of Health Care Providers and Systems (CAHPS) was no different. These organized delivery systems have succeeded for years, and in many cases for decades, in dealing with issues of cost, quality, and trust. A physician voice from these systems could point to characteristics and features of their groups that would be helpful to those seeking solutions for the complex problems plaguing the healthcare sector.

In 2002, a number of physician leaders from successful MSMGs across the United States gathered to discuss the issue of physician practice redesign and founded a not-for-profit organization called the Council of Accountable Physician Practices. A look at the roster of CAPP members shows that they are located throughout the nation and indicates that MSMGs have been successful in a variety of different geographies and settings:

Austin Regional Clinic, *Texas*
Billings Clinic, *Montana*
Cleveland Clinic, *Ohio*
Dean Health System, *Wisconsin*
Duluth Clinic, *Minnesota*
Everett Clinic, *Washington*
Fallon Clinic, *Massachusetts*
Geisinger Clinic, *Pennsylvania*
Group Health Permanente, *Idaho, Washington*
Harvard Vanguard Medical Associates, *Massachusetts*
HealthCare Partners Medical Group, *Southern California*
HealthPartners, *Minnesota*
Henry Ford Medical Group, *Michigan*
Intermountain Health Care, *Utah*
Jackson Clinic, *Tennessee*
Lahey Clinic, *Massachusetts*
Marshfield Clinic, *Wisconsin*
Mayo Clinic, *Arizona, Florida, Minnesota*
Mayo Health System, *Iowa, Minnesota, Wisconsin*
Nemours, *Delaware, Florida, Maryland, New Jersey, Pennsylvania*
Ochsner Clinic, *Louisiana*
Palo Alto Medical Foundation, *Northern California*
Permanente Federation, *Northern and Southern California, Colorado, District of Columbia, Georgia, Hawaii, Maryland, Ohio, Oregon, Virginia, Washington*
Scott and White, *Texas*
Sharp Rees-Stealy Medical Group, *Southern California*
Virginia Mason Clinic, *Washington*
Wenatchee Valley Medical Center, *Washington*

Since 2002, CAPP has gathered evidence from its members and from the medical literature about the achievements of multispecialty medical groups and is supporting further research to refine the understanding of key success factors. CAPP's array of MSMGs offers an opportunity to study the design elements and characteristics of successful physician practice and can serve as a model for delivery system redesign.

An example serves to illustrate the potential benefits in studying MSMGs. Physicians from Group Health Cooperative of Puget Sound were able to rapidly translate the benefits of groundbreaking heart disease research into improved medical treatment for diabetics, with a great reduction in cardiovascular complications over the expected result. Less than two years after publication of the Heart Protection Study on the use of statins (Gurm and Hoogwerf 2003) and the preceding Heart Outcomes Prevention Evaluation (HOPE) trial on angiotensin-converting enzyme (ACE) inhibitor use in patients with diabetes (Yusuf et al. 2000), Group Health had developed new clinical practice recommendations for medication management in diabetes based on these studies, embedded them into its population care management system, developed educational materials for primary care clinicians and patients, and redesigned important roles and tasks in care teams to ensure their implementation. By comparison, some estimate that it generally takes 17 years to translate evidence-based care practices from the literature into general use in medical practice (Balas and Boren 2000). Knowing the critical elements that enabled this advance in care and having some insight as to how they were put in place would greatly advance physician practice redesign.

CAPP's 35 MSMGs share a common vision as learning organizations dedicated to the improvement of clinical care. Their features include physician leadership and governance; commitment to evidence-based care management processes; well-developed quality improvement systems; team-based care; the use of advanced clinical information technology; and the collection, analysis, and distribution of clinical performance information. These features are congruent with the IOM recommendations on key elements needed to redesign delivery systems. The *Chasm* report (IOM 2004a) envisions a delivery system capable of meeting six challenges: (1) evidence-based care processes; (2) effective use of information technology; (3) knowledge and skills management; (4) development of effective teams; (5) coordination of care across patient conditions, services, and settings over time; and (6) use of performance and outcome measurement for continuous quality improvement and accountability.

Physician governance is a key characteristic of MSMGs. These are physician-led organizations that are guided by ethical and medical principles important to physicians, creating a professional and scientific approach to governance that is deeply rooted in the quality improvement processes of peer review and information sharing, thus cultivating an environment that fosters care improvement. Group responsibility is a clearly articulated commitment. Physicians in MSMGs are responsible not only for the individual and unique patient they are currently treating, but for all of the patients cared for by the practice. Colleagues in group practice have adopted performance management practices to hold one another accountable to provide the best quality of care possible and to contribute to the improvement of the quality of care over time.

MSMG processes and infrastructure characteristics include an evidence-based approach to care. One of the areas of general health sector failure involves the identification and dissemination of successful practices. MSMGs have an organized quality improvement structure that supports identification of important literature contributions to care improvement, analyzes physician and group care practices in light of the science base, can widely disseminate and implement needed changes to care practices based on the evidence, and can monitor physician implementation of the successful practices. Physicians practicing together using a shared medical record, a single organizational structure, and a common payment and incentive system are better able to improve not only the quality of care but also the efficiency of resource use. Because processes and outcomes can systematically be tracked in such a practice, administrative and clinical redundancy and waste are easily recognized and can effectively be eliminated.

Effective knowledge management tools are central to successful learning systems, and in the case of health care, clinical information technology is a critical component. Multispecialty medical groups are at the forefront of using health information technology (HIT) and electronic health records (EHR) to support advanced systems of care. Since MSMGs typically share a common, often automated, medical record, they have access to every part of the patient's experience from ambulatory through hospital to convalescent and end-of-life care. Providing services across the full continuum of care enables them to collect data across this continuum. Such a depth of timely, accurate, clinically relevant information, shared among all providers and available for detailed analysis and reporting, not only supports high-quality, efficient care, but is also a key resource for identifying practice redesign elements.

Common information systems complement team-based care because all team members have access to a shared medical record as they collaborate to manage both illness and health. Collaboration is critical in treating patients with chronic conditions, especially those with multiple, comorbid conditions. The chronic care model (Wagner 1998) provides a clear framework for understanding how shared information is central to success in treating these patients. The team has access to timely and accurate clinical data, and to the extent that information is effectively shared with the patient and the family, all team members are well prepared to collaborate in developing and executing the treatment plan. Shared systems enable the coordination of care within the group and can be used to personalize care through shared decision making such that the patient becomes the focal point of care.

Recently, attention has focused on the availability and sharing of accurate performance information, a process that has come to be called "transparency." Measuring and sharing performance among providers is a critical first step to achieving transparency, and because of shared clinical information systems, the MSMGs are designed to enable consistent individual physician performance monitoring. Transparency among physicians within the group is the central characteristic of MSMG peer review. It provides the opportunity to compare individual physicians against group benchmarks, permits even broader transparency in comparisons outside the group, and ultimately enables reporting to patients, payers, and the general public. This process of acquiring and reporting accurate information on performance supports a consumer's decisions when choosing a physician practice or a treatment team, carrying out treatment plans, and assuming responsibility for self-management, thus finally linking the chain of transparency to informed and effective action to improve health.

Multispecialty medical groups can fill what are currently research gaps between clinical trial research, epidemiological research, and the real-world delivery of care. The multispecialty medical group is a practically oriented healthcare delivery system that translates what is known from research into what is done in practice and, ultimately, what improves the outcomes and efficiency of care. Studying the factors that enhance or impair this process will be illuminating. CAPP, as an example, is currently sponsoring research that examines the impact of the electronic health record on the management of diabetes and explores the correlation between various care management practices supported by the EHR and geographic area variation in medical quality outcomes and resource use. Such studies are generally not possible in non-integrated delivery models where inconsistency in practice and data capture inhibits accurate observation.

The Institute of Medicine can play a critical role in enhancing our ability to learn from the successes of MSMGs. The IOM has already enunciated principles that serve to point the direction to accomplish the task. In 2003, the IOM identified 20 Priority areas for national action. The 20 areas included not only complex chronic conditions, such as diabetes, that greatly benefit from integrated care, but also what the IOM termed "cross-cutting" areas, such as care coordination and self-management or health literacy (IOM 2003c). Coordinated care is at the heart of MSMG systems of care.

Further elaboration came in 2005 with the *Performance Measurement* report that envisioned an organized research agenda, jointly sponsored by federal and private stakeholders (IOM 2006b):

Recommendation 5 (IOM, 2006b): The National Quality Coordination Board should formulate and promptly pursue a research agenda to support the development of a national system for performance measurement and reporting. The board should develop this agenda in collaboration with federal agencies and private-sector stakeholders. The agenda should address the following:

• Development, implementation, and evaluation of new measures to address current gaps in performance measurement.
• Applied research focused on underlying methodological issues, such as risk adjustment, sample size, weighting, and models of shared accountability.
• Design and testing of reporting formats for consumer usability.
• Evaluation of the performance measurement and reporting system.

Several issues critical to improvement of the care delivery system could well be examined in such a research agenda by formulating studies using multispecialty medical groups as the test bed. The IOM should make recommendations in these specific areas:

• Encourage studies using common measurement sets across multiple delivery system models in a way that can compare their impact on coordination of care, clinical quality, patient satisfaction, and efficiency of resource use. Studies must consider both MSMGs and nonintegrated practices by incorporating measures and methods to compare practice-level and group-level performance in addition to individual physician performance. The AQA (Ambulatory Care Quality Alliance) has recently endorsed a set of quality measures that are intended to be applied to all physicians regardless of practice type and will eliminate the gap in performance data from non-group and small-group practices that has hampered such comparisons in the past (Crosson 2005).

• Encourage physician leaders to design and create more integrated care systems. Most physician leaders have historically reacted defensively to the quality and cost challenges we face in the healthcare sector, rather than proactively redesigning the system of care. In contrast, MSMG leaders have generally demonstrated greater innovation and success in meeting these challenges. The IOM should recommend programs, incentives, and legislation that encourage more leaders interested in designing and developing such organizations to come forward.

• Encourage studies to elucidate the most effective method to incentivize physicians to improve quality and efficiency. The impact of rewarding individual physician performance versus physician group performance is likely quite different, and there is little evidence available on how to balance incentives at different levels to achieve the most effective care system and the best care outcomes. Pay-for-performance programs for physicians are proliferating in the healthcare sector and should be designed by using an evidence-based approach.

REFERENCES

Balas, E, and S Boren. 2000. Managing clinical knowledge for healthcare improvements. In *Yearbook of Medical Informatics*, edited by V Schatauer. Stuttgart, Germany: Schattauer Publishing.

Crosson, F. 2005. The delivery system matters. *Health Affairs* 24(6):1543-1548.

DeStefano, F. 2001. The Vaccine Safety Datalink project. *Pharmacoepidemiology and Drug Safety* 10(5):403-406.

Elmore, J, L Reisch, M Barton, W Barlow, S Rolnick, E Harris, L Herrinton, A Geiger, R Beverly, G Hart, O Yu, S Greene, N Weiss, and S Fletcher. 2005. Efficacy of breast cancer screening in the community according to risk level. *Journal of the National Cancer Institute* 97(14):1035-1043.

Fishman, P, M Hornbrook, R Meenan, and M Goodman. 2004. Opportunities and challenges for measuring cost, quality, and clinical effectiveness in health care. *Medical Care Research and Review* 61(3 Suppl.):124S-143S.

Geiger, A, C West, L Nekhlyudov, L Herrinton, I Liu, A Altschuler, S Rolnick, E Harris, S Greene, J Elmore, K Emmons, and S Fletcher. 2006. Contentment with quality of life among breast cancer survivors with and without contralateral prophylactic mastectomy. *Journal of Clinical Oncology* 24(9):1350-1356.

Gillies, R, K Chenok, S Shortell, G Pawlson, and J Wimbush. 2006. The impact of health plan delivery system organization on clinical quality and patient satisfaction. *Health Services Research* 41(4 Pt. 1):1181-1199.

Greene, S, and A Geiger. 2006. A review finds that multicenter studies face substantial challenges but strategies exist to achieve Institutional Review Board approval. *Journal of Clinical Epidemiology* 59(8):784-790.

Greene, S, E Larson, D Boudreau, K Johnson, J Ralston, R Reid, and P Fishman. 2005a. The Coordinated Clinical Studies Network: a multidisciplinary alliance to facilitate research and improve care. *The Permanente Journal* 9(4):33-35.

Greene, S, G Hart, and E Wagner. 2005b. Measuring and improving performance in multicenter research consortia. *Journal of the National Cancer Institute Monographs* (35):26-32.

Gurm, H, and B Hoogwerf. 2003. The Heart Protection Study: high-risk patients benefit from statins, regardless of LDL-C level. *Cleveland Clinic Journal of Medicine* 70(11):991-997.

Hornbrook, M, G Hart, J Ellis, D Bachman, G Ansell, S Greene, E Wagner, R Pardee, M Schmidt, A Geiger, A Butani, T Field, H Fouayzi, I Miroshnik, L Liu, R Diseker, K Wells, R Krajenta, L Lamerato, and C Neslund Dudas. 2005. Building a virtual cancer research organization. *Journal of the National Cancer Institute Monographs* 35:12-25.

IOM (Institute of Medicine). 2001. *Crossing the Quality Chasm: A New Health System for the 21st Century.* Washington, DC: National Academy Press.

———. 2002. *Guidance for the National Healthcare Disparities Report.* Washington, DC: The National Academies Press.

———. 2003a. *Financing Vaccines in the 21st Century: Assuring Access and Availability.* Washington, DC: The National Academies Press.

———. 2003b. *Describing Death in America: What We Need to Know.* Washington, DC: The National Academies Press.

———. 2003c. *Priority Areas for National Action: Transforming Health Care Quality.* Washington, DC: The National Academies Press.

———. 2004a. *1st Annual Crossing the Quality Chasm Summit: A Focus on Communities.* Washington, DC: The National Academies Press.

———. 2004b. *Health Literacy: A Prescription to End Confusion*. Washington, DC: The National Academies Press.

———. 2004c. *Insuring America's Health: Principles and Recommendations*. Washington, DC: The National Academies Press.

———. 2004d. *Quality Through Collaboration: The Future of Rural Health*. Washington, DC: The National Academies Press.

———. 2006a. *Improving the Quality of Health Care for Mental and Substance-Use Conditions: Quality Chasm Series*. Washington, DC: The National Academies Press.

———. 2006b. *Performance Measurement, Accelerating Improvement*. Washington, DC: The National Academies Press.

———. 2007a. *Hospital-Based Emergency Care: At the Breaking Point*. Washington, DC: The National Academies Press.

———. 2007b. *Preventing Medication Errors: Quality Chasm Series*. Washington, DC: The National Academies Press.

Inventory and Evaluation of Clinical Research Networks. 2006 (July 28). *IECRN Best Practices Study Profile of Networks*. Available from http://www.clinicalresearchnetworks. org/documents/BPNetworkProfiles.pdf. (accessed November 26, 2006).

Larson, E, L Wang, J Bowen, W McCormick, L Teri, P Crane, and W Kukull. 2006. Exercise is associated with reduced risk for incident dementia among persons 65 years of age and older. *Annals of Internal Medicine* 144(2):73-81.

Leyden, W, M Manos, A Geiger, S Weinmann, J Mouchawar, K Bischoff, M Yood, J Gilbert, and S Taplin. 2005. Cervical cancer in women with comprehensive health care access: attributable factors in the screening process. *Journal of the National Cancer Institute* 97(9):675-683.

McGlynn, E, S Asch, J Adams, J Keesey, J Hicks, A DeCristofaro, and E Kerr. 2003. The quality of health care delivered to adults in the United States. *New England Journal of Medicine* 348(26):2635-2645.

Paasche-Orlow, M, D Schillinger, S Greene, and E Wagner. 2006. How health care systems can begin to address the challenge of limited literacy. *Journal of General Internal Medicine* 21(8):884-887.

Platt, R, R Davis, J Finkelstein, A Go, J Gurwitz, D Roblin, S Soumerai, D Ross-Degnan, S Andrade, M Goodman, B Martinson, M Raebel, D Smith, M Ulcickas-Yood, and K Chan. 2001. Multicenter epidemiologic and health services research on therapeutics in the HMO Research Network Center for Education and Research on Therapeutics. *Pharmacoepidemiology and Drug Safety* 10(5):373-377.

Quinn, V, V Stevens, J Hollis, N Rigotti, L Solberg, N Gordon, D Ritzwoller, K Smith, W Hu, and J Zapka. 2005. Tobacco-cessation services and patient satisfaction in nine nonprofit HMOs. *American Journal of Preventive Medicine* 29(2):77-84.

Raebel, M, E Lyons, S Andrade, K Chan, E Chester, R Davis, J Ellis, A Feldstein, M Gunter, J Lafata, C Long, D Magid, J Selby, S Simon, and R Platt. 2005. Laboratory monitoring of drugs at initiation of therapy in ambulatory care. *Journal of General Internal Medicine* 20(12):1120-1126.

Ritzwoller, D, K Kleinman, T Palen, A Abrams, J Kaferly, W Yih, and R Platt. 2005. Comparison of syndromic surveillance and a sentinel provider system in detecting an influenza outbreak—Denver, Colorado, 2003. *MMWR Morbidity and Mortality Weekly Report* 54(Suppl.):151-156.

Schaie, K. 1993. The Seattle Longitudinal Study: a thirty-five-year inquiry of adult intellectual development. *Zeitschrift fur Gerontologie* 26(3):129-137.

Simon, S, D Smith, A Feldstein, N Perrin, X Yang, Y Zhou, R Platt, and S Soumerai. 2006. Computerized prescribing alerts and group academic detailing to reduce the use of potentially inappropriate medications in older people. *Journal of the American Geriatrics Society* 54(6):963-968.

Smith, D, N Perrin, A Feldstein, X Yang, D Kuang, S Simon, D Sittig, R Platt, and S Soumerai. 2006. The impact of prescribing safety alerts for elderly persons in an electronic medical record: an interrupted time series evaluation. *Archives of Internal Medicine* 166(10):1098-1104.

Solberg, L, V Quinn, V Stevens, T Vogt, N Rigotti, J Zapka, D Ritzwoller, and K Smith. 2004. Tobacco control efforts in managed care: what do the doctors think? *American Journal of Managed Care* 10(3):193-198.

Somkin, C, A Altschuler, L Ackerson, A Geiger, S Greene, J Mouchawar, J Holup, L Fehrenbacher, A Nelson, A Glass, J Polikoff, S Tishler, C Schmidt, T Field, and E Wagner. 2005. Organizational barriers to physician participation in cancer clinical trials. *American Journal of Managed Care* 11(7):413-421.

Stevens, V, L Solberg, V Quinn, N Rigotti, J Hollis, K Smith, J Zapka, E France, T Vogt, N Gordon, P Fishman, and RG Boyle. 2005. Relationship between tobacco control policies and the delivery of smoking cessation services in nonprofit HMOs. *Journal of the National Cancer Institute Monographs* (35):75-80.

Taplin, S, L Ichikawa, M Yood, M Manos, A Geiger, S Weinmann, J Gilbert, J Mouchawar, W Leyden, R Altaras, R Beverly, D Casso, E Westbrook, K Bischoff, J Zapka,, and W Barlow. 2004. Reason for late-stage breast cancer: absence of screening or detection, or breakdown in follow-up? *Journal of the National Cancer Institute* 96(20):1518-1527.

Tunis, S, D Stryer, and C Clancy. 2003. Practical clinical trials: increasing the value of clinical research for decision making in clinical and health policy. *Journal of the American Medical Association* 290(12):1624-1632.

Wagner, E. 1998. Chronic disease management: what will it take to improve care for chronic illness? *Effective Clinical Practice* 1(1):2-4.

Wagner, E, S Greene, G Hart, T Field, S Fletcher, A Geiger, L Herrinton, M Hornbrook, C Johnson, J Mouchawar, S Rolnick, V Stevens, S Taplin, D Tolsma, and T Vogt. 2005. Building a research consortium of large health systems: the Cancer Research Network. *Journal of the National Cancer Institute Monographs* (35):3-11.

Yusuf, S, P Sleight, J Pogue, J Bosch, R Davies, and G Dagenais. 2000. Effects of an angiotensin-converting-enzyme inhibitor, ramipril, on cardiovascular events in high-risk patients. The Heart Outcomes Prevention Evaluation Study Investigators. *New England Journal of Medicine* 342(3):145-153.

6

The Patient as a Catalyst for Change

OVERVIEW

There is a growing appreciation for the centrality of patient involvement as a contributor to positive healthcare outcomes, and as a catalyst for change in healthcare delivery. This chapter presents the views of several individuals involved with programs that look to empower patients through improvements in access to health information as well as methods to make the patient an equal partner in health decision making. The era of the Internet and the personal health record greatly expands the types of information and evidence available to patients, but in a truly learning healthcare system, learning is bidirectional such that it works not only to better inform patients but also to ensure that patient preference is incorporated into "best care." These contributions only introduce the complexities and possibilities of a truly patient-centered healthcare system, but they represent important shifts towards a system that seeks to learn from patients and provide the means for their collaboration in the delivery of care. In the first essay, Janet Marchibroda reviews a number of recent public and private initiatives promoting the use of health information technology and health information exchange and widespread adoption of the electronic health record (EHR). These initiatives are aimed at improving the quality, efficiency, and value of care, in part by providing better information to consumers and patients. Also outlined by Marchibroda are results of a recent survey by eHealth Initiative and others to determine consumer perceptions and expectations for these technologies. While there is overestimation of the current use of health IT and of interoperability, there is also growing interest in using these tools to connect with providers and to manage care. Andrew Barbash then discusses possibilities to build on patient interests to connect with care and move toward true patient-provider collaboration. He notes that while the primary focus has been on building the tools that allow patients to take on new roles and responsibilities in managing personal health, equal effort should be put into thinking about new information models that can provide the types of information needed to appropriate users and into developing new rules of engagement for how accountability for the integrity of data, communication and response, and safeguarding privacy might be governed.

Understanding how to develop an evidence base that can incorporate patient preference is an important move toward a patient-centered system. James Weinstein's and Kate Clay's work at the Dartmouth-Hitchcock Medical Center has helped to develop the concepts of informed choice and shared decision making as a way to get the "right rates of treatment" and "catalyzing a patient-driven change of the healthcare system." This approach is particularly useful in cases where there is no clear "best" treatment option because such conditions are particularly value sensitive with a clear role for patient preference. Implicit in such an approach will be the use of high-quality decision aids and evidence-based information.

THE INTERNET, eHEALTH, AND PATIENT EMPOWERMENT

Janet M. Marchibroda
eHealth Initiative

Over the last five years, there has been a growing consensus among recognized experts, including many of the nation's leading providers, employers, health plans, and patient groups; members of both the House and the Senate; leaders in nearly every federal agency involved in health care; and state and local policy makers, that healthcare information technology, and specifically mobilizing health information exchange electronically, will contribute to significant improvements in the quality, safety, and efficiency of health care.

Because of the highly fragmented nature of the U.S. healthcare system, information about the patient is stored in a variety of locations, often in paper-based forms and is not easily accessed. As a result, clinicians often do not have comprehensive information about the patient when and where it is needed most—at the point of care—and those responsible for managing and improving the health of populations do not have the information they need to measure progress and facilitate improvement. In addition, those responsible for protecting the public's health don't have access to the information they need to identify threats and manage their response. Finally, those who are driving new research don't have effective access to the information they need to support the creation and monitoring of the effectiveness of both evidence-based guidelines and new, more effective therapies to improve health and health care for Americans.

Interoperable health information technology (HIT) and health information exchange—or the mobilization of clinical information electronically—facilitates access to and retrieval of clinical data, privately and securely, by different entities involved in the care delivery system, to provide safer, more timely, efficient, effective, equitable, patient-centered care.

There are several drivers for the use of HIT and health information exchange in health care, including concerns about quality and safety, driving various incentive or "pay for performance" programs as well as programs designed to drive public reporting or transparency of measures related to quality; concerns about rising healthcare costs, driving transparency in pricing; and consumerism. These drivers have led the federal government, Congress, state leaders, and many members of the private sector to take action to increase the use of HIT in health care.

This paper highlights environmental drivers, including those emerging at the national, state, and local levels, for the use of HIT in health care and explores the role of the patient as a catalyst for change for these efforts.

Rapidly Emerging Policy Advancements Related to the Use of HIT to Address Healthcare Challenges

In response to the fragmented healthcare system, and the quality and safety issues that result, reports from the Institute of Medicine (IOM), the Department of Health and Human Services (HHS), and several private sector groups have been pointing toward the need for an electronic, interoperable healthcare system to get information where it is needed, when it is needed, in an efficient manner. In addition to considerable leadership demonstrated in the private sector, a number of initiatives are now under way funded by HHS to address standards harmonization, application certification, prototype development, and privacy and confidentiality issues related to a nationwide health information network. On August 22, 2006, an Executive Order was issued calling for healthcare programs that are administered or sponsored by the federal government to promote quality and efficient delivery of health care through the use of HIT and to utilize HIT systems and products that meet recognized interoperability standards.

As recently as December 8, 2006, HHS announced its intent to advance a "nationwide health information network initiative," "bringing together the significant expertise and work achieved this year by the current efforts with state and local health information exchanges" to "begin to construct the network of networks that will form the basis of the NHIN." While details are currently under development with the announcement of a Request for Information (RFI) process in the spring of 2007, HHS appears to be interested in conducting "trial implementations of the NHIN [National Health Information Network]" that are likely to leverage its investments made to date, including those related to the development of an NHIN architecture prototype, which include, among other things, functional requirements, security approaches, and needed standards.

In addition to activities in the administration, Congress is also playing a considerable role. Over the last three years, much legislation has been introduced by Democrats and Republicans alike in both the House and the Senate, addressing the role of government in driving adoption of HIT, the need for standards, funding, and a host of other issues. On July 27, 2006, the U.S. House of Representatives passed the Health Information Technology Promotion Act (H.R. 4157), which was anticipated to be conferenced in the 109th Congress with the Senate version of the bill passed in November 2005. Despite considerable momentum, talks were suspended and this issue will be taken up in the 110th Congress as part of the Democratic agenda of economic, foreign policy, and healthcare reforms.

A number of states are also moving forward—in parallel with federal efforts—to develop and adopt policies for improving health and health care through HIT and electronic health information exchange. State legislators are increasingly recognizing the role of HIT in addressing healthcare challenges, with 121 bills introduced in 38 states since 2005—64 of which were introduced in the first seven months of 2006. Thirty-six of such bills in 24 states were passed in the legislature and signed into law (eHealth Initiative 2006). State legislatures are not the only policy makers driving change in states—U.S. governors are increasingly recognizing the value of HIT in addressing their healthcare goals. To date, 12 U.S. governors have issued an executive order designed to drive improvements in health and health care through the use of information technology (IT).

At the same time, the number of collaborative health information exchange initiatives at the state, regional, and community levels has grown considerably over the last three years. In September 2006, the eHealth Initiative (eHI) released the results of its Third Annual Survey of Health Information Exchange at the State, Regional and Community Levels, analyzing results from 165 responses from initiatives in 49 states, the District of Columbia, and Puerto Rico. Primarily nonprofit, multistakeholder organizations, these initiatives are beginning to mobilize health information electronically to support primarily services related to the delivery of care, such as those related to clinical results delivery, providing alerts, et cetera. About 20 percent of those surveyed reported that they were currently exchanging data types such as laboratory results, dictation or transcription data, inpatient and outpatient episodes, and enrollment and eligibility information.

Federal Efforts Toward Value-Based Health Care Are Also Likely to Have Impact

Concerns about cost and quality are also driving the federal government to take action on initiatives designed to drive value-based health care. In addition to requiring healthcare programs that are administered or sponsored by the federal government to utilize HIT systems and products that meet recognized interoperability standards, the August 22, 2006, Executive Order called for such programs to make available cost and quality information to their beneficiaries.

Secretary of Health and Human Services Leavitt has spoken frequently to public audiences, calling for action to drive better care and lower costs through four cornerstones, which are detailed in the HHS Prescription for a Value-Driven Health System (Leavitt 2006):

1. *Connecting the system:* Every medical provider has some system for health records. Increasingly, these systems are electronic. Standards need to be set so that all health information systems can quickly and securely communicate and exchange data.
2. *Measure and publish quality:* Every case, every procedure, has an outcome. Some are better than others. To measure quality, we must work with doctors and hospitals to define benchmarks for what constitutes quality care.
3. *Measure and publish price:* Price information is useless unless cost is calculated for identical services. Agreement is needed on what procedures and services are covered in each "episode of care."
4. *Create positive incentives:* All parties—providers, patients, insurance plans, and payers—should participate in arrangements that reward both those who offer and those who purchase high-quality, competitively priced health care.

Several large employer groups are exploring similar measures designed to drive value-based health care. The Business Roundtable and several other employer groups joined Secretary Leavitt on November 17, 2006, to discuss taking steps similar to that of the administration's Executive Order, utilizing an "employer toolkit" to drive implementation across markets in the United States.

In September 2006 the IOM released a report entitled *Rewarding Provider Performance: Aligning Incentives in Medicare*, which provided a series of recommendations related to pay for performance, recognizing that "existing (payment) systems do not reflect the relative value of healthcare services in important aspects of quality, such as clinical quality, patient-centeredness, and efficiency" (IOM 2006).

To add strength to fast-moving federal initiatives, on December 8, 2006, Congress passed the Tax Relief and Health Care Act of 2006 (H.R. 6408) as the 109th Congress came to a close. Among other things, the bill creates a quality reporting system for the voluntary reporting by eligible professionals of data on quality measures specified by the HHS secretary starting in July 2007. Beginning in 2008, quality measures used for data reporting will be measures adopted or endorsed by a consensus organization (such as the National Quality Forum or the AQA [Ambulatory Care Quality Alliance]), and it is specified that measures will include structural measures such as the use of electronic health records and electronic pre-scribing technology.

A majority of emerging policies and initiatives within both the public and the private sectors, related to what has most recently been termed "value-based health care" introduce the notion that the use of HIT and health information exchange can play an integral part in increasing the likelihood that improvements in quality and efficiency will result from these initiatives. Efforts are now under way to articulate specifically how HIT and health information exchange can play a critical role in rapidly emerging quality and efficiency-focused programs. Some value-based healthcare efforts incorporate structural measures designed to promote the adoption of interoperable EHRs. Nearly all such efforts currently require or plan to require the reporting of performance measures by clinicians, which will be difficult without the existence of a either a data warehouse or a health information exchange network.

Exploring the Role of the Consumer as a Catalyst for Change

Consumer activation can play a key role in driving improvements in quality and efficiency, as well as the use of HIT. This section explores consumer perceptions regarding the value of HIT and health information exchange, as well as their concerns.

According to research conducted by the Markle Foundation, there is a widespread overestimate of the current use of health IT and of interoper-ability: 40-65 percent of the public believes their doctor now has electronic health records, and 25 percent believes the emergency department can ac-cess their health record. Recent public opinion research sponsored by the eHealth Initiative Foundation further supports this overestimation, indicat-ing that of Gulf state citizens, 29 percent believe that their doctors keep their records electronically, and 54 percent believe that backup copies of their health information are kept in electronic form, which is simply not the case. In fact, according to a recent study conducted by David Blumenthal, only 17 to 25 percent of physician offices have EHRs, with 17 percent being the best estimate based on high-quality surveys (Blumenthal 2006).

According to research conducted by the eHealth Initiative Foundation in June 2006, 70 percent of Americans on the Gulf Coast favor the creation of secure, electronic health information (eHealth Initiative Foundation 2006). A similar survey by the Markle Foundation also found considerable support for the creation of a nationwide health information exchange network that has the following attributes: access to information controlled in secure online accounts; requirement for patient permission for medical information to be shared through a network; patient control of which information is made available to other physicians; and information held and maintained by individual physicians instead of a central database (Markle Foundation 2005). A survey by Public Opinion Strategies in September 2005, on the behalf of the Markle Foundation, found significant interest in using EHR-related tools: 65 percent of Americans are interested in accessing their records online, a service that could be enabled by a creation of the NHIN. While younger Americans are most likely to express interest, more than half of those 60 and older (53 percent) are interested in seeing their health information online (Markle Foundation 2005).

When asked about perceived benefits, the research indicates that for the most part, consumers believe a great deal of value emerges from the use of electronic health records, HIT, or health information exchange. For example, according to the Markle Foundation, 60 percent of Americans support the creation of a secure online "personal health record" service, and a substantial number of consumers would use this tool to check and refill prescriptions (68 percent); get results over the Internet (58 percent); check for mistakes in individual medical records (69 percent); and conduct secure and private e-mail communication with physicians (57 percent) (Markle Foundation 2005). A recent report released by the Markle Foundation offers similar insights. According to this report, the public feels that access to personal electronic health records would have the following benefits: ability to see what their doctors write down (91 percent); ability to check for mistakes (84 percent); and reduction in the number of repeated tests and procedures (88 percent) (Markle Foundation 2006).

Despite these benefits, there are some concerns about the use of HIT and health information exchange. According to the Markle Foundation (2006) report, while Americans see many benefits of electronic personal health information, they express concern that such information would be used for purposes other than their own care; some of the concern expressed include identity theft or fraud (80 percent) and marketing firms (77 percent), employers (56 percent), or health insurance companies (53 percent) gaining access to their records.

Opportunities for Consumer Engagement

Initiatives are beginning to emerge that engage the consumer, including personal health record services offered by private organizations such as WebMD, initiatives led by health plans such as that announced by America's Health Information Plans and the Blue Cross and Blue Shield Association, and those supported by some of the nation's largest employers—including Intel and Wal-Mart. Such initiatives—primarily national in nature—are designed to empower consumers, giving them the ability to access health information—that to date is primarily claims-based information—to help them navigate the health system.

At the same time, efforts to connect clinical data and information across disparate systems are beginning to take place at the state, regional, and community levels—where health care is delivered—in many parts of the country. The eHealth Initiative Foundation survey, however, indicates that only 6 percent of such efforts are currently interfacing with consumers or patients. Data services that support provision of information to clinicians—whether in their practices, in the emergency room, or in the hospital—are ordinarily the first step for these initiatives.

As efforts at the national, state, and local levels continue to mature and expand, there exists an enormous opportunity to engage consumers, who—according to research—are increasingly interested in accessing their information online. By connecting national efforts that are now beginning to interact directly with the consumer with claims-based information, to primarily state and local efforts that mobilize clinical information residing in laboratories, hospitals, and physician offices, the U.S. healthcare system has the opportunity to take a giant leap forward, bringing information not only to those who provide care and pay for care—but most importantly, to those receiving care.

JOINT PATIENT-PROVIDER MANAGEMENT OF THE ELECTRONIC HEALTH RECORD

Andrew Barbash, M.D.
Apractis Solutions

The increasing adoption of the electronic health record across a variety of settings will bring new roles and responsibilities to all those involved. As patients, family members, clinicians, and other caregivers begin to view, use, contribute to, and interact with information in the EHR, a new set of "rules of engagement" will evolve, in which accountability for integrity of data, for acting on reminders, for guardianship of privacy, and for responsible communication will require a new level of collaboration. The EHR is increasingly considered a tool that will allow for personal ownership of health information, which by necessity means that we will move away from the "institution" creating the data as a single system into a more collaborative environment that crosses the boundaries of a clinical practice, organizations, the individual patient, and the family. This paper outlines some pragmatic aspects of this for the present and future.

Considering patient-provider collaboration and the electronic health record opens a new paradigm for how to think about decision support. Medical decision making is a difficult process and is even more difficult to translate into something that is easily understood by patients in general. Many medical decisions are akin to complex statistical computations and factor in likelihood of risk and benefit, with the overall issue of our confidence in the data superimposed on these elements. Does the average consumer have any concept of how to make a risk-based decision? Looking at some of the considerations, does the healthcare decision-making equation mimic any other daily decision? For example, consider:

% risk of benefit
– % risk of adversity
× N (confidence in the data)
+ cost of making the choice
– chance of car accident on way to the test

As patients and family members gain ownership and control of more information, either through the EHR or through the vast resources now available to anyone with a computer and an Internet connection, they are asked to take a larger role in this complex process of medical decision making. Asking them to do this simply because they have the information at hand is not sufficient, and we need to think about ways to foster collaborative decision making.

There are large-scale efforts under way to achieve collaboration between consumers, patients, and doctors using online resources. In addition, there is a large and growing field that examines the decision-making behavior of consumers and the internal processes that drive these decisions. Many organizations are involved in getting consumers engaged through portals, products, software, and communication processes, such as the Veterans Health Administration, Kaiser Permanente, Regional Health Information Organizations, and the Centers for Medicare and Medicaid Services (CMS), as well as commercial vendors and small practices. The true goal of these initiatives is ultimately to move toward a consumer-centered world in terms of interaction with information. However most people in the healthcare sector don't consider collaboration tools that have been used in other industries as useful in health care because fundamentally, the healthcare system as it exists today lacks a culture of collaboration.

The opportunities to use EHRs as a basis for increased collaboration between patient and provider are immense. One major consideration in everyday health care is medication list management. This is a truly important area because we are caught in a paradigm where there is a disconnect between what a physician thinks a patient is taking and what the patient is taking in reality. In this case, patients have the opportunity to play a critical role in the translation of everyday information to their provider through the utility of tools such as EHRs. Currently, however, few patients think it is their responsibility to keep track of what they are actually taking. These new tools present an opportunity to change the culture that fosters this disconnect for both the patient and the provider.

Another opportunity centers around the ability to update conditions and status. There is a lot of work being done on interactive patient portals where patients can manage personal health records. This will require a better understanding of how patients view their own condition relative to how a health professional would characterize them, but nonetheless has significant opportunity to benefit the patient, make disease states more understandable to the provider, and provide a means to generate information for the healthcare system.

One of the key elements of EHRs is the ability to facilitate automatic alerts and reminders for physicians and patients. There are problems with assuming that this will be a great solution across the board though, because many busy providers will turn off these systems unless they are geared to be germane and timely. Alerts and reminders delivered to patients will perhaps have to have an even higher level of accuracy than they do for doctors. For example, at Mayo there only needed to be a couple of alerts sent out for an annual mammogram for patients who had had bilateral mastectomies to embarrass the whole system. There is a level of sophistication that needs to occur before something that seems so straightforward can be enacted in reality. On the other end of the spectrum, disease management and prevention are clearly areas where the role of the patient in receiving messages and the role of providers in receiving reminders to notify the patient create an important, and beneficial, communication interaction.

Health care, while often talked about as a data problem, is fundamentally just as much a communication problem. Communication, on an organizational level, is highly nonpersonalized and noncustomizable. The solutions emerging are the organization's view of how to communicate with patients, but this is very different from the patient's perspective of what level of communication is actually desired. On the organizational level, we view patient centeredness as one context for the EHR, but in reality for patients, this is just one piece of an otherwise large puzzle. From the patient perspective, there are many other components that are part of this picture, including legal documents and financial records. Thus, we must be cognizant of the real context of EHRs, which is the reality that health care and health records are only a fraction of the multitude of factors the consumer deals with each day.

Patients, families, clinicians, and care coordinators are all dealing with changing technologies, changing demographics, changing knowledge, and changing rules. We have to be highly cognizant that as patients and doctors are trying to collaborate around order management, results management, alerts management, and preventive reminders, the technology in many cases moves faster than the ability to keep up with it, which creates a very complex dynamic. Looking at patient-provider collaboration, we have key, common tasks that each entity shares at some time; they communicate, collaborate, decide, document, and validate or authenticate information. True patient-provider(s) collaboration is the same set of intersections, but with consumers playing a bigger role. For instance in MyHealtheVet, which is an interactive portal for Veterans Administration (VA) patients, patients will have access to their personal health information. If they see errors, what is their role, their responsibility, and who do they communicate with on these issues? Each entity also plays different roles at different times and the EHR needs to accommodate inquiries and searches, transforming information, ordering and requesting, communicating, documenting, and responding.

Different information models are also needed. What do different users need to know and how can we best convey this to them? Agreement that everyone plays a role in even something as simple as a common shared medication list might be reasonable, but what are the relative values of similar accuracy for other "shared information?" Understanding the role of the consumer is complex enough and will be compounded by issues related to EHRs.

Suppose that instead of thinking heath record collaboration specifically being oriented around the EHR, thinking shifts to collaboration in health care in general, about how consumers think about how they collaborate, and assigning tasks for different emerging "roles." For example, most doctors do not think of themselves as collaborators online. In addition, current focus is "web-centric" but perhaps becoming "communication-centric" will allow better leveraging of the web as a communication vehicle. Finally, consumers (patients and providers) need to be more educated about the changing tools they are being confronted with that could put them at the center of their own health management.

There is tremendous opportunity to begin to tackle these issues. Collaboration, occurring online, will provide insights into what new evidence is needed to move forward: what level of adoption or critical mass creates the transition point for stakeholders; how dependent "compliance" is on the "technology vehicles"; what the business models are that maximize productive participation; and what impact more "ambiguous" data have on an increasingly evidence-driven system.

EVIDENCE AND SHARED DECISION MAKING

James N. Weinstein, M.D.,[1] *and Kate Clay, M.A., B.S.N., R.N.*
Dartmouth-Hitchcock Medical Center

The challenges to the healthcare system are so formidable that patients must be central players in the decisions necessary. In 1935, Lawrence Henderson noted that "patients and doctors are part of the same system." Seventy years later, Alan Greenspan, the former chairman of the Federal Reserve Board, noted in effect that they must be directly engaged because of the potentially "abrupt and painful" choices when baby boomers reach retirement age unless Medicare and Social Security benefits are cut back so retirees are not expecting more than can be delivered. Increasing life expectancy, decreasing birth rates, and limits on the impact of productivity and economic growth all contribute to the impending crisis (Greenspan 2004).

Reduction in public programs is code for rationing health care in a society that has fostered the attitude that some of its members should have access to the latest, newest, and best without regard to cost. With a 7 percent annual increase in healthcare costs, and a $2 trillion annual bill, at this point in our history, the question seems to be: Should we do less (*ration* health care), or should we see this as an opportunity to do better (create a *rational* healthcare system that offers care that works, and make patients our partners in healthcare decision-making)?

Given the current opportunity and challenges, how do we move forward to implement best practices; narrow the currently observed practice variations that result in under-, over-, and inappropriate utilization of care; and provide rationalized best care for all? This crossroad calls for innovative strategies and the willingness to change. Focusing on the patient is our single best course of action and the source of partnership in catalyzing systemic change.

---

[1]Dr. Weinstein has in the past served as a consultant to the Foundation of Informed Medical Decision-Making which develops the content for the shared decision-making videos (proceeds directed to the Center for the Evaluative Clinical Sciences (CECS) and the Department of Orthopaedics); and to United Healthcare (proceeds directed to the Brie Fund, a fund for children with disabilities in the name of his daughter who passed away from leukemia).

The Informed Patient Model

We have limited resources, yet members of the public want health care to improve and they want their doctors to improve it. So, how do we partner with patients toward this goal? We can start by taking the best evidence from reliable sources (e.g., the Cochrane Collaboration (http://www.cochrane.org/) and altruistic clinical trials (Weinstein 2006)) and begin to apply evidence-based information to clinical practice. Today, health care is at a critical juncture, trying to implement a continuous stream of new treatments and *technologies* into a system that is already struggling with overuse of unproven and unnecessary care that increases utilization and cost without the necessary "best" evidence. The *"informed choice"* model being proposed here is one vehicle to inform patients of best evidence at the point of care—during their appointments with their doctors—the interface wherein medical decisions are being made.

The aim is to partner with our patients in the healthcare decisions that are "close calls," where clinicians are at equipoise with regard to treatment options (e.g., back pain, hypertension, benign prostate conditions, breast cancer, coronary artery disease, and end-of-life decisions). Technology (in this case, *shared decision making, as a means to informed choice*) needs to be brought into clinical practice to support close call decision making. Making the right choice for a given patient or population of patients lies with our patients, not with individual doctors, who either have no unbiased evidence-based treatment alternatives to offer their patients or, less often, have a conflict of interest that prevents them from doing so freely. The result of informing our patients in this way is to get the "right" rates of treatment options by catalyzing a patient-driven change of the healthcare system.

Well-informed patients making values-sensitive (close call) decisions in concert with their clinicians will utilize healthcare resources at the "right" rate: *the rate at which they prefer* to undertake more or less expensive and intensive care. In a Canadian study of patient preferences for knee replacement surgery (Hawker et al. 2001), only 15 percent of those who were eligible by clinical measures actually preferred to have surgery. Imagine the savings: if all candidates for elective medical treatments and surgery were asked to express their values and state their treatment preferences, we might save enough money to keep Alan Greenspan's worst fears at bay. More importantly, we could leverage these savings to provide evidence-based effective care for those in need.

Directing decision making toward patients activates a partnership that provides them with the latest information on what is known or not known about a condition, engages them in a shared decision-making conversation that elicits values and screening or treatment preferences, gathers data from them at the point of care for use in the clinical encounter, and reaches an *informed choice* that is agreed on by patient and clinician and acted upon.

Doing What Works: Evidence-Based Medicine

Archie Cochrane, whose contributions to epidemiology are best known through the Cochrane Collaboration, offered the challenge of evidence-based medicine. In particular, he advocated that "because resources would always be limited, they should be used to provide equitably those forms of health care which had been shown in properly designed evaluations to be effective" (The Cochrane Collaboration 2006). Today there are numerous Cochrane groups around the world synthesizing the literature on effective care. Most are attempted meta-analyses based on inadequate studies, and nearly all suggest that more studies are needed. This is not a criticism of investigations or investigators of the past; randomized trials are difficult at best, especially in the surgical disciplines (Carragee 2006; Flum 2006; Weinstein et al. 2006b; Weinstein et al. 2006c). Yet both patients and physicians would do well to understand that at this point, medicine, in many cases, is truly more art than science, and the struggle to keep up with unproven scientific innovations threatens to overwhelm patient care.

In the continuum of science and technology, the objective is to follow the trail of new evidence as it evolves and to act accordingly. Many beneficial treatments and processes in current practice are underutilized, as demonstrated by the tremendous variation in the use of such things as aspirin and beta blockers after myocardial infarction (MI), prophylactic antibiotics before surgery, and protection against deep vein thrombosis (DVT). Basing clinical practice on evidence will adjust underuse of beneficial care and overuse of preference-sensitive care that is recommended by clinicians but not preferred by patients.

The Learning Healthcare System

The United States is lagging behind in providing meaningful support for clinical excellence. The British National Health Service (NHS) has taken the lead in fostering a *learning healthcare system* by creating the National Institute for Health and Clinical Excellence (NICE). The essential components of such a system are multidisciplinary evidence-based clinical practice and a process for learning from errors (Sheaff and Pilgrim 2006). The institute is tasked with advising healthcare professionals on how to provide patients the highest standards of care. NICE is using a three-pronged approach: an appraisals program, a guidelines program, and an interventional procedures program (Rawlins 2004). It is charged with assessing clinical and cost-effectiveness of drugs, devices, and diagnostic tools. Based on these assessments, practice guidelines provide advice on whether and how these should be used.

To date, NICE has produced reports on nearly 250 products. As in the Cochrane model, its work is grounded in systematic reviews of randomized trials (*and* observational studies when appropriate) in order to estimate the true effect size more accurately. The guidelines are developed by independent, unpaid advisory boards drawn from the NHS, academia (including economics), professional societies, and patients and patient groups; the NHS has a legal obligation to provide the resources necessary for implementation. It is fully intended that physician pay will be linked to the quality of care. Paul Shekelle, M.D., described this as "an initiative . . . that is the boldest such proposal attempted anywhere in the world. . . . With one mighty leap, the NHS has vaulted over anything being attempted in the US, the previous leader in quality improvement initiatives" (Roland 2004).

Patient surveys are another new tool for the NHS. Physicians are rewarded, not for the scores, but for having surveyed the patients and then acted on the results by discussing them with patients. Physicians are now beginning to compare practices using these scores. This is a learning healthcare system in action. Rather than asking patients to learn from providers about healthcare options and recommendations, they are asked to let providers learn from them and to partner with providers in an exchange of information used to make an informed choice in real time during the clinical encounter.

The use of patient surveys in the United Kingdom is a strategy that has been in place within the Spine Center at the Dartmouth-Hitchcock Medical Center (DHMC) in Lebanon, New Hampshire, since 1997 (Weinstein et al. 2000), and in the Comprehensive Breast Program at DHMC since 2004. In the late 1990s, both the Spine Center (SC) and the first Center for Shared Decision-Making (CSDM) in the United States opened at DHMC. The Spine Center was designed to be a high-performing micro-system of care that incorporates a feed forward-feed back model at the point of care. The Spine Center Patient Summary Report uses patient self-reported data "commonly used for measurement of outcomes (feedback) to the clinician for use in clinical assessment (feed forward)"(Weinstein and Clay [submitted 2006]). This design was based in part on a trial done in the early 1990s, which found that after patients viewed a shared decision-making CD on treatment choices, procedure rates changed; patients chose lower rates of surgery for herniated disc and slightly higher rates for spinal stenosis (Ciol et al. 1996; Deyo et al. 1998). The face validity of this trial was consistent with the best evidence available at the time, which called for different rates of intervention than were being observed. It was this knowledge that inspired the pursuit of the "patient as a catalyst for change" using *shared decision making* as the vehicle. This has become the Spine Center Learning Microsystem.

Validated measurement tools are used at Dartmouth to give a snapshot of how each patient is doing in comparison to the last visit, so that care plans can be tailored by taking into account self-ratings and treatment preferences. Planning for DHMC institution-wide use of patient self-reported intake questionnaires for all patients at all points of care is well under way. This approach remains limited to pockets of excellence, because the U.S. healthcare system does not offer incentives for such patient-focused innovations, which is a significant barrier to their widespread use.

Doing What Works: Shared Decision Making

A minority of current healthcare practices are grounded in evidence-based information. As a profession and a system we have experienced some costly mistakes, such as recommending hormone replacement therapy to reduce cardiovascular risk in women. Millions of women were treated largely for the indication of cardiovascular health before a randomized trial demonstrated no benefit (Rossouw et al. 2002). Yet only a limited number of treatment recommendations are based on high-quality clinical trial evidence of efficacy. Decisions in health care do not, in general, have clear answers. The risk-benefit ratios are either scientifically uncertain or unknown, and their presentation to patients has not incorporated the role of values in weighing risks or benefits (Weinstein and Clay [submitted 2006]).

How do we approach healthcare decision making in cases where good evidence exists and also where it does not? There is a growing movement toward the concept of shared decision making as a process that can lead clinicians and patients to an informed choice based on a clear understanding of clinical evidence or lack thereof. Shared decision making is the collaboration between patients and clinicians to come to an agreement about a healthcare decision. The process is especially useful when there is no clear "best" treatment option. Clinicians and patients share information with each other in order to understand the likely outcomes of the options at hand, think about values as they relate to the risks and benefits of each option, and participate jointly in decisions about medical care.

Not all healthcare decisions are amenable to the shared decision-making process. In cases where there is strong evidence for the effectiveness of a treatment (e.g., treating a hip fracture or bacterial pneumonia), there is usually strong agreement among both clinicians and patients that these are valued interventions. However, many conditions, such as chronic low back pain, early-stage breast or prostate cancer, benign prostate enlargement, or abnormal uterine bleeding, are value sensitive. Reasons to consider higher-risk options in these cases are less clear and fall more under the purview of the patient. In such cases, the path of watchful waiting may be an option worth considering, and the valuing of risks and benefits becomes individual and personal (Weinstein et al. 2006b; Weinstein et al. 2006c).

In such decisions, the best choice should, in fact, depend on a patient's values with regard both to benefits and harms and to the scientific uncertainty associated with alternative treatment options. There is tremendous geographic variation in the use of value-sensitive options in our country. Low back pain treated with fusion is one example. Fusion surgery rates vary more than twentyfold and are dependent on where one lives and who one sees (Weinstein et al. 2006a). The rates of spine fusion rose more than 300 percent from 1992 to 2003, and the cost increased nearly 500 percent. In this example, lack of evidence-based medicine to support treatment decisions reveals significant scientific uncertainty expressed as increased regional variation and cost. Where there is significant regional variation, it is often the case that the proposed doctrine of informed choice is not considered. In such environments, the patient is the recipient of physician-based information rather than a partner in the decision-making process.

Another example is insurer-based limitation of information. Recently CMS, for the first time, made a decision not to pay for a new artificial disk technology, despite Food and Drug Administration (FDA) approval. Patients should know about this option; when they are engaged in informed choice and given a balanced presentation of *all* options and the evidence of efficacy (or lack thereof), patients tend to make the right decisions that set the benchmark for the right rates of surgeries and medical treatments (Ciol et al. 1996; Deyo et al. 1998; Deyo et al. 2000; O'Connor et al. 2004; Weinstein 2005).

Doing What Works: Patient Decision Aids

One good way to ensure the provision of balanced, evidence-based information is to integrate high-quality decision aids into the informed choice process whenever possible. Numerous randomized trials indicate that decision aids improve decision quality and prevent overuse of treatments that informed patients do not value (O'Connor et al. 2004).

Research has shown that the use of a patient decision aid (PtDA) as part of the process of making a treatment choice has unique value. Decision aids are defined as "interventions designed to help people make specific and deliberative choices among options (including the status quo) by providing (at the minimum) information on the options and outcomes relevant to a person's health status" (O'Connor et al. 2004). Thirty-four randomized trials have shown that decision aids improve decision-making by:

- Improving knowledge of the options, pros and cons;
- Creating more realistic expectations;

- Lowering decisional conflict;
- Reducing uncertainty about what to choose;
- Enhancing active participation in decision making;
- Decreasing the proportion of people who are undecided; and
- Improving agreement between values and choices (O'Connor et al. 2004).

Patients who use decision aids at DHMC rate them as having the right amount of information, being balanced in presenting information about the options, and being helpful in making their decisions, and say they would recommend the videos to others who are facing the same decision (see Table 6-1).

Doing What Works: Informed Choice

Focusing on patients changes the doctrine of informed consent, now antiquated and inadequate to meet the need of the current doctor-patient

TABLE 6-1 Treatment Intention Before and After Video Decision Aid for Spinal Stenosis, Herniated Disc, Knee, and Hip Osteoarthritis

Video Decision Aid	Before Video Intention	N	After Video Intention (N)		
			Unsure	Nonsurgical	Surgery
Spinal stenosis	Unsure	65	31	30	4
	Nonsurgical	91	8	80	3
	Surgery	42	4	1	37
	Total	198	43	111	44
Herniated disc	Unsure	38	21	12	5
	Nonsurgical	91	6	83	2
	Surgery	45	2	3	40
	Total	174	29	98	47
Knee osteoarthritis	Unsure	17	7	4	6
	Nonsurgical	14	0	12	2
	Surgery	93	4	2	87
	Total	124	11	18	95
Hip osteoarthritis	Unsure	8	5	0	3
	Nonsurgical	3	0	3	0
	Surgery	49	2	0	47
	Total	60	7	3	50

SOURCE: Author's summary of self-reported patient questionnaires.

relationship to share information in a partnership. The patient-based doctrine of *informed choice* transforms informed consent with the addition of shared decision-making and the use of decision aids as an impartial source of information. This process includes the following:

- Provision of balanced, evidence-based information on all options;
- Discussion of benefits and risks of each option and the likelihood that they will occur, using framing and language understandable to the patient;
- Elicitation of patient values and preferred role in decision making; and
- Arriving at a treatment decision through discussion between clinician and patient.

Using these steps in the clinical encounter has been shown to actively engage patients in decision making and to arrive at a treatment choice that is the right choice because it is based on good information and on the patient's values.

Barriers to Doing What Works

As with any intervention that is perceived to alter the usual doctor-patient relationship, recommendations for basing patient-focused care on evidence and fully engaging the patient in decision making can be threatening and become a barrier to implementation. The first hurdle to overcome is the resistance that comes with any change at the level of the clinician-patient encounter. In addition to resistance on the part of clinicians, there are barriers to implementing these strategies at other levels: health plans, health systems, even patients, some of whom just want the doctor to decide. Current practice incentives (e.g., fee-for-service model) are not aligned for the patient and are certainly not aligned to provide the best health care has to offer. The lack of appropriate incentives represents an important barrier to utilizing novel approaches to catalyze meaningful change.

Overcoming Barriers—
Value-Added Proposition for Clinicians and Patients

How do we incorporate informed choice into the flow of a busy physician's practice? How do we make decisions based on evidence and real knowledge, whether it comes from practical, pragmatic, observational, or randomized trials (Weinstein et al. 2000)? Remember, informed choice is by definition the process of interacting with patients and arriving at informed, values-based choices when options have features that patients value differently. We all value risks and benefits differently, so a one-size-fits-all approach will not work. Any new approach must be integrated easily into the normal workflow; it must improve clinical care and it must help the doctor or the doctor won't be an advocate for it.

The Spine Patient Outcomes Research Trial (SPORT) (Weinstein et al. 2006c; Weinstein et al. 2006b; Birkmeyer et al. 2002) is one example of how these barriers can be addressed in clinical practice (Weinstein et al. 2000). SPORT is a novel, practical clinical trial that utilized shared decision making as part of a generalizable, evidence-based enrollment strategy. It also took advantage of the computer as a technology partner in healthcare delivery (Birkmeyer et al. 2002; Arega et al. 2006). The SPORT multicenter trial enrolled patients at 13 centers in 11 states. It was not an add-on to the practice; it was usual care with systems already in place and shared decision making as part of the enrollment process. Patients who were eligible for SPORT viewed one of two shared decision-making videos: *Treatment Choices for Low Back Pain: Herniated Disc* or *Treatment Choices for Low Back Pain: Spinal Stenosis*. They were then offered trial enrollment and selected either the randomization cohort or the observational (preference) cohort, which allowed us to look at generalizability of the randomized arm versus the observational arm (Weinstein et al. 2006b; Weinstein et al. 2006c). The randomization cohort was randomly assigned surgical or medical management; the preference cohort chose surgery or the alternative. Using data from SPORT, we will be able to share probabilities with our patients so they have better information about their treatment options and the treatment outcomes. The issues of numeracy and patient understanding of risk-benefit information are well known and are not insignificant; thus we need to work on how we frame and transmit information to our patients and how patients interpret information so they can better understand it and make truly informed choices.

An added benefit may be that patient decision aids enhance minority enrollment in clinical studies. The SPORT protocol and its use of shared decision making may have facilitated enrollment across racial groups into SPORT (Arega et al. 2006). While previous studies have demonstrated low rates of minority participation in randomized trials, SPORT investigators discovered that this likely has more to do with treatment preference than with an unwillingness to randomize (Arega et al. 2006). Preference-based trials may be a mechanism to enhance enrollment of minority populations necessary for broader indications and use in clinical practice.

In a paper for *Health Affairs*, the principles of preference-sensitive care were applied to health economics (Weinstein et al. 2004). Data analysis showed that residents of Florida are much more likely to have surgical procedures if they live on the west coast rather than the east coast. In Florida, as in the United States in general, "geography is destiny." From a healthcare policy perspective, this speaks not only to the quality and costs of health care, but to the value of care delivered. Employing shared decision-making tools and the informed choice process on the west coast of Florida is an opportunity in waiting, to adjust surgery rates so they are driven by patient preference rather than zip code (Weinstein et al. 2006a; Weinstein et al. 2004).

In summary, resources must be redeployed utilizing best evidence and shared decision making. By allowing patients to be *active partners* in their healthcare decisions, there will be better prospects for resolving the economic crisis now faced. The patient as a *catalyst for change* is, in fact, where real change can be leveraged. Studies utilizing shared decision making for spine surgery showed a reduction in herniated disk surgery of about 30 percent (Deyo et al. 1998; Ciol et al. 1996). These tools work across the board; about 25 to 30 percent of our patients who have formed a "naïve" treatment preference actually change their preference when informed via shared decision making and tend to prefer the less aggressive procedure. Given the change in demand for procedures based on patient preferences, here is an opportunity to suggest that less is more (Fisher and Welch 2000, 1999). In a system wherein the evidence is mixed at best, why not respect patients and their values? If the evidence does not suggest a detrimental outcome, why not let our patients be the guide? Given that patients tend to be risk-averse, there is much to be gained by partnering with our patients: trust, better outcomes, better quality, and compliance. Of course, the cost of care also will be less. Now we can provide more of what really works to all of those truly in need.

What we are talking about is not new; patients and doctors have always been part of the same system. We need to shift from an independent doctor-patient relationship to a relationship where we are on the same team, shifting our roles so we are coaching each other and helping each other to improve health care for each individual patient. In this respect it is important to keep in mind a quote from a factory worker who said, "If we always do what we have always done, we will always get what we have always gotten."

It is time to adopt a doctrine of evidence-based *informed choice*, utilizing our patients as partners and catalysts to change health care. We must not ration health care but rationalize it based on best evidence. We must adopt and implement technologies that provide the evidence necessary for best clinical practice to help all at the expense of none.

REFERENCES

Arega, A, N Birkmeyer, J Lurie, T Tosteson, J Gibson, B Taylor, T Morgan, and J Weinstein. 2006. Racial variation in treatment preferences and willingness to randomize in the Spine Patient Outcomes Research Trial (SPORT). *Spine* 31(19):2263-2269.

Birkmeyer, N, J Weinstein, A Tosteson, T Tosteson, J Skinner, J Lurie, R Deyo, and J Wennberg. 2002. Design of the Spine Patient Outcomes Research Trial (SPORT). *Spine* 27(12):1361-1372.

Blumenthal, D. 2006 (September 12). Institute for Health Policy, Massachusetts General Hospital/Harvard Medical School, Presentation to the Department of Health and Human Services American Health Information Community. Washington, DC.

Carragee, E. 2006. Surgical treatment of lumbar disk disorders. *Journal of the American Medical Association* 296(20):2485-2487.

Ciol, M, R Deyo, E Howell, and S Kreif. 1996. An assessment of surgery for spinal stenosis: time trends, geographic variations, complications, and reoperations. *Journal of the American Geriatric Society* 44:285-290.

The Cochrane Collaboration. 2006. *The Name Behind the Cochrane Collaboration* (accessed November 30, 2006). Available from http://www.cochrane.org/docs/archieco.htm.

Deyo, R, E Phelan, M Ciol, D Cherkin, J Weinstein, and A Mulley. 1998. *Videodisc for Back Surgery Decisions: A Randomized Trial.* HS08079, Agency for Health Care Policy and Research, National Institutes of Health, Washington, DC.

Deyo, R, D Cherkin, J Weinstein, J Howe, M Ciol, and A Mulley Jr. 2000. Involving patients in clinical decisions: impact of an interactive video program on use of back surgery. *Medical Care* 38(9):959-969.

eHealth Initiative. 2006 (August). *States Getting Connected: State Policy Makers Drive Improvements in Healthcare Quality and Safety Through IT.* Washington, DC: eHealth Initiative.

eHealth Initiative Foundation. 2006 (October). *Gulf Coast Health Information Technology Services Project.* Funded by DHHS.

Fisher, E, and H Welch. 1999. Avoiding the unintended consequences of growth in medical care: how might more be worse? *Journal of the American Medical Association* 281(5):446-453.

———. 2000. Is this issue a mistake? *Effective Clinical Practice* 3(6):290-293.

Flum, D. 2006. Interpreting surgical trials with subjective outcomes: avoiding UnSPORTsmanlike conduct. *Journal of the American Medical Association* 296(20):2483-2485.

Greenspan, A. 2004 (August 27). *Remarks by Chairman Alan Greenspan* (accessed April 3, 2007). Available from http://www.federalreserve.gov/boarddocs/speeches/2004/20040827/default.htm.

Hawker, G, J Wright, P Coyte, J Williams, B Harvey, R Glazier, A Wilkins, and E Badley. 2001. Determining the need for hip and knee arthroplasty: the role of clinical severity and patients' preferences. *Medical Care* 39(3):206-216.

IOM (Institute of Medicine). 2006. *Rewarding Provider Performance: Aligning Incentives in Medicare.* Washington, DC: The National Academies Press.

Leavitt, M. 2006. *Better Care, Lower Cost: Prescription for a Value-Driven Health System.* Washington, DC: Department of Health and Human Services.

Markle Foundation. 2005 (October). *Attitudes of Americans Regarding Personal Health Records and Nationwide Electronic Health Information Exchange: Key Findings From Two Surveys of Americans.* Conducted by Public Opinion Strategies. Available from http://www.phrconference.org/assets/research_release_101105.pdf (accessed April 4, 2007).

———. 2006 (November). *National Survey on Electronic Personal Health Records.* Conducted by Lake Research Partners and American Viewpoint. Available from http://www.markle.org/downloadable_assets/research_doc_120706.pdf (accessed April 3, 2007).

O'Connor, A, D Stacey, V Entwistle, H Llewellyn-Thomas, D Royner, M Holmes-Royner, V Tait, V Fiset, M Barry, and J Jones. 2004. *Decision aids for people facing health treatment or screening decisions.* Cochrane Library. Available from http://decisionaid.ohri.ca/cochsystem.html (accessed October 17, 2006).

Rawlins, M. 2004. NICE work—providing guidance to the British National Health Service. *New England Journal of Medicine* 351(14):1383-1385.

Roland, M. 2004. Linking physicians' pay to the quality of care: a major experiment in the United Kingdom. *New England Journal of Medicine* 351(14):1448-1454.

Rossouw, J, G Anderson, R Prentice, A LaCroix, C Kooperberg, M Stefanick, R Jackson, S Beresford, B Howard, K Johnson, J Kotchen, and J Ockene. 2002. Risks and benefits of estrogen plus progestin in healthy postmenopausal women: principal results from the Women's Health Initiative randomized controlled trial. *Journal of the American Medical Association* 288(3):321-333.

Sheaff, R, and D Pilgrim. 2006. Can learning organizations survive in the newer NHS? *Implementation Science* 1:27.

Weinstein, J. 2005. Partnership: doctor and patient: advocacy for informed choice vs. informed consent. *Spine* 30(3):269-272.

———. 2006. An altruistic approach to clinical trials: the national clinical trials consortium (NCTC). *Spine* 31(1):1-3.

Weinstein, J, and K Clay. Submitted 2006. Informed patient choice: assessment of risk/benefit tradeoffs for surgical procedures and medical devices. *Health Affairs.*

Weinstein, J, P Brown, B Hanscom, T Walsh, and E Nelson. 2000. Designing an ambulatory clinical practice for outcomes improvement: from vision to reality: the Spine Center at Dartmouth-Hitchcock, year one. *Quality Management in Health Care* 8(2):1-20.

Weinstein, J, K Bronner, T Morgan, and J Wennberg. 2004. Trends and geographic variations in major surgery for degenerative diseases of the hip, knee, and spine. *Health Affairs (Millwood)* Supplemental Web Exclusive:VAR81-9.

Weinstein, J, J Lurie, P Olson, K Bronner, and E Fisher. 2006a. United States' trends and regional variations in lumbar spine surgery: 1992-2003. *Spine* 31(23):2707-2714.

Weinstein, J, J Lurie, T Tosteson, J Skinner, B Hanscom, A Tosteson, H Herkowitz, J Fischgrund, F Cammisa, T Albert, and R Deyo. 2006b. Surgical vs. nonoperative treatment for lumbar disk herniation: the Spine Patient Outcomes Research Trial (SPORT) observational cohort. *Journal of the American Medical Association* 296(20):2451-2459.

Weinstein, J, T Tosteson, J Lurie, A Tosteson, B Hanscom, J Skinner, W Abdu, A Hilibrand, S Boden, and R Deyo. 2006c. Surgical vs. nonoperative treatment for lumbar disk herniation: the Spine Patient Outcomes Research Trial (SPORT): a randomized trial. *Journal of the American Medical Association* 296(20):2441-2450.

7

Training the Learning Health Professional

OVERVIEW

In a system that increasingly learns from data collected at the point of care and applies the lessons for patient care improvement, healthcare professionals will continue to be the linchpin of the front lines, assessing the needs, directing the approaches, ensuring the integrity of the tracking and the quality of the outcomes, and leading innovation. However, what these practitioners will need to know and how they learn will dramatically change. Orienting practice around a continually evolving evidence base requires new ways of thinking about how we can create and sustain a healthcare workforce that recognizes the role of evidence in decision making and is attuned to lifelong learning. Presentations throughout the workshop revealed concern from many different sectors on how to best fill the pipeline with students dedicated to building and applying an expanded evidence base for health care and establish a culture that encourages collaboration across the spectrum of care delivery and health professions. This session explored three of the many conduits for educating health professionals: existing and emerging decision support, formal educational requirements, and continuing education programs. In addressing this broad topic, speakers raised a wide range of issues and emphasized the pressing need for culture change throughout the healthcare system.

In the first paper, William Stead discusses the challenges that confront the health professional in acquiring the knowledge relevant to providing individualized care to patients. With the expansion of genomics and proteomics, he predicts a one- to two-order-of-magnitude change in the amount of information needed for clinical decisions—far exceeding the capacity of the human mind. The electronic health record (EHR) will help health professionals accommodate this overload and deliver evidence-based, individualized care. In such a system, EHRs would change the practice eco-system by making learning continuous, with clinical practice augmented by "just-in-time" access to information and curricula. In addition, when paired with clinical informatics tools, EHRs can support a number of learning strategies ranging from identification of variation in care, to hypothesis generation, to phenotype-genotype hypothesis testing. Achieving this potential will require a completely new approach, entailing discontinuous changes in how we define the roles of health professionals and how we learn.

Mary Mundinger of the Columbia School of Nursing then outlines some of the challenges in health professions education with regard to orienting training around an evolving evidence base. Grounding the teaching approach in evidence and adopting translational research as a guiding principle can lead to a continuous cycle in which students and faculty engage in research, implementation, dissemination, and inquiry. Yet most institutions find considerable variance in the level of integration of evidence into education across health professions. While intellectual engagement with evidence-based practice is evident in faculty publications, it often has not yet found its way substantially into the curriculum as a framework for training. In part, educational efforts always lag behind academic practice, but changes in the culture of medical practice are needed to ensure that educating health professionals about the benefits and methods of bringing evidence to their daily practice actually produces a skill that is recognized and utilized in the healthcare setting.

In the chapter's final paper, Mark Williams discusses the shortfalls of current continuing medical education (CME) efforts and urges a shift to a knowledge translation approach that is integrated with practice and occurs on a daily basis. He notes that change is needed not only in the content and approach of CME but also in the culture of medical practice, advocating for a shift toward collaborative teamwork and increased cross-departmental collaboration, coupled with incentives for change and the provision of tools to facilitate such change.

CLINICIANS AND THE ELECTRONIC HEALTH RECORD AS A LEARNING TOOL

William W. Stead, M.D.
Vanderbilt University

The electronic health record is one key to a shift to systems approaches to evidence-based care that is nonetheless individualized. EHRs enable change in the practice ecosystem (Stead 2007). They change roles and responsibilities, what the clinician needs to know, and how the clinician learns, while providing a new source of information. These changes are discontinuous, not an incremental improvement in what we do today. Hence, conversations about using the EHR are not generally focused on issues of providing evidence to, or generating evidence from, our current practice processes. Yet let us consider nine ways the EHR and clinical informatics tools could potentially be used to generate and apply evidence: using billing data to identify variability in practice; EHR data to direct care; EHR data to relate outcomes back to practice; EHR data to monitor open-loop processes; decision support systems for alerts and reminders within clinical workflow; decision support systems for patient-specific alerts to change in practice; decision support systems for links to evidence within clinical workflow; de-identified EHR data to detect unexpected events; and de-identified EHR and Biobank data for phenotype-genotype hypothesis generation. Illustrative examples will be drawn from how Vanderbilt uses informatics, coupled with electronic health records, to support learning in clinical workflow and population management.

Call for a Discontinuous Change in How Clinicians Learn

Figure 7-1 depicts the current medical decision-making model. The clinician is an integrator, aggregating information from the patients and their records with biomedical knowledge, recognizing patterns, making decisions, and trying to translate those decisions into action. Cognitive research has shown that the human mind can handle about seven facts at a time in a decision-making process (Miller 1956; Cowan 2000). We are bumping up against that limit today. This cognitive overload is one of the

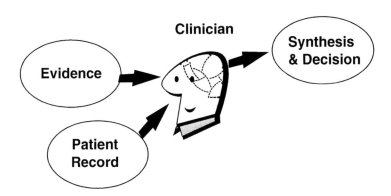

FIGURE 7-1 The decision model of the 1900s.

reasons we see the overuse, underuse, and misuse in health care that the Institute of Medicine (IOM) has highlighted in the Quality Chasm Series. This overload will get worse by one or two orders of magnitude as biomedical research turns functional genomics and proteomics into clinically useful information. We need a new decision-making model to deliver reproducible quality in the face of increasingly rich information sources.

Figure 7-2 depicts a possible alternative that emerged during Vanderbilt University Medical Center's strategic planning process (Vanderbilt Medical Center September 2005) and the visioning phase of the National Library of Medicine's long range planning process (NLM Board of Regents, National Institutes of Health 2006). Basically we envision a personal health knowledge base. This new resource would be much more than the personal health records emerging today. It would be a pre-computed intelligent integration of the individual's health information, together with the subset of biomedical evidence relevant to that individual, presented in a way that lets the clinician and the patient—with very different learning levels and learning styles—make the right decisions. Such a model changes what the clinician needs to know to perform. For example, factual recall becomes less important and coaching skills become more important.

We also envision a change in how we learn. In 1973, I was taught in medical school a defined body of biomedical information, "just in case" I needed it. I was also trained as a scientist so that I could discover and learn through reading and practice. I was tested on the body of knowledge and credentialed as "knowing enough" through my degree, my license, and my boards in internal medicine and nephrology. If you think about it, you will realize that we can not achieve acceptable healthcare quality with that ap-

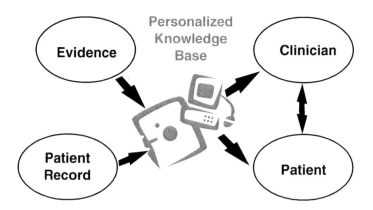

FIGURE 7-2 A possible model for the 2000s.

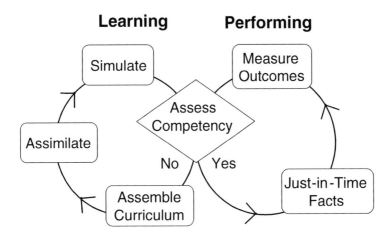

FIGURE 7-3 Continuous learning during performance.

proach to learning. It is not just that we have more biomedical information than anyone can learn or keep up with, even with ever-increasing specialization and a fifth year of medical school. The bigger problem is the variability in practice that comes from letting individuals learn, one by one, from their practice. Process reproducibility is a key to ensuring quality.

The clinician of tomorrow should be trained as a pilot to "fly" a system of care. In such a system, learning would be continuous and augmented with "just-in-time" access to information in clinical workflow. Credentials would be competency-based, reflecting current information about the individual's learning record and outcomes. Figure 7-3 depicts how a systems approach to learning might work. At its center is assessment. The system would decide if the clinician knows what she needs to know to do what she is going to do next. If the answer is yes, based on her learning and outcome records, she proceeds to perform the clinical task (right-hand circle). Her knowledge of how to use facts is assisted by computer recall of details, such as specific drug-drug interactions. Electronic records track the patient's progress and provide feedback regarding the effectiveness of the "system" and the clinician. After each cycle of clinical performance, her competency is reassessed. She flips into the learn cycle (left-hand circle) whenever additional knowledge or improvement is needed. The learn cycle begins by assembling a targeted curriculum using tools such as the Vanderbilt University School of Medicine's KnowledgeMap (Denny et al. 2003). Next she reads and assimilates the information. Finally, she uses simulation to test understanding and technical skill. The simulator pushes her past her limit of competency, ensuring individual understanding of that boundary. The simulator takes her back to the assessment point. If knowledge and skill are adequate, she flips back over into the performance mode. If not, she repeats the learn cycle.

Electronic Health Records as Learning Tools

Box 7-1 presents a framework of nine ways the EHR and clinical informatics tools can be used to support aspects of learning. It is a "splitter's" view to point out the many data sources available and the "niche" of various tools. Certain learning strategies can be supported by billing data, others take full EHR, others take decision support systems, others take de-identified EHR data or a combination of de-identified health record and a bio bank.

The easiest step is to use billing data to identify variability in practice. You can use the data for a practice group to help members identify where they have variability. At Vanderbilt, we started with a top-to-bottom sort of range in resource utilization by Diagnosis-Related Group (DRG) or procedure code. Since this measures intragroup variability, it avoids the comparable population challenge of external benchmarks. We then got the group around the table, helped members look at areas where they had high variability, and asked what they wanted to do most of the time. We reflected these decisions in collaborative care pathways. In many cases, we took out

---

BOX 7-1
A Splitters View of EHR Data and Tools to Support Learning

Billing Data
1. Data to identify variability in practice
Electronic Health Records
2. Data for direct care
3. Data to relate outcomes back to practice
4. Data to monitor open-loop processes
Decision Support Systems
5. Alerts and reminders within clinical workflow
6. Patient-specific alerts to change in practice
7. Links to evidence within clinical workflow
8. Detection of unexpected events
De-identified EHR and Biobank
9. Phenotype-genotype hypothesis generation

as much as 40 percent of the work, while decreasing morbidity and mortality (Koch, Seckin, and Smith 1995). So utilizing just billing data—which almost everyone has today —we have seen significant improvement.

Full EHRs are more complicated and more powerful. For the purposes of this discussion, uses of EHR data can be separated from uses of the clinical workflow software that is commonly bundled in the purchase of an electronic medical record system. EHRs provide ready access to data about the patient, freeing up the clinician's mind during direct care to focus on synthesis and pattern recognition. In addition, they provide a hypothesis generation resource as a "free" by-product of care. For example, the Duke Cardiovascular Databank (Rosati et al. 1975), begun in the mid-1970s, was probably the first large-scale case of using the computer as a time-lapse camera to tie clinical outcome back to the practice that produced it. Baseline data were captured for each patient admitted with cardiovascular disease, the results of their studies and procedures were entered, and a research team added outcome data with long-term follow-up. The Databank led to early ambulation post-myocardial infarction. Before the Databank, patients were put on prolonged bed rest. A query to the Databank showed a patient would not have complications if they did not occur in the first few hours. This "dry lab" hypothesis was then tested through a targeted controlled trial (McNeer et al. 1978). It is unlikely this finding would have been reached so quickly with conventional trails alone. Finally, data in the EHR can provide the feedback to trigger an external monitor of an open-loop process. Open-loop processes operate without internal feedback for real-time model adaptation. If an open-loop process makes frequent status reports, an external monitor can intervene if the status moves out of an acceptable range. Consider the requirement to administer antibiotics in a fixed time to patients presenting with pneumonia. One approach would be to force every clinician to use a programmed work process for every patient. This branching logic approach works at a microsystem level where a decision situation needs to be handled the same way over and over. By contrast, patients, who may ultimately turn out to have pneumonia, present in many ways and to all parts of the health system—a macrosystem problem. A better approach combines the open-loop process of the human clinician with a real-time event monitor. The clinician would be free to obtain data and recognize patterns. The monitor would check all records to see if recently arriving patients have been ruled in or out of the pneumonia population. If this event has not occurred within a specified period, the monitor could intervene to notify the clinician to make a decision whether or not the probability of pneumonia justified proceeding with administration of an initial dose of antibiotic.

Decision support systems, when informed by data from the EHR, permit alerts and reminders in clinical workflow as a helpful check on memory.

For example, the clinician is alerted to an allergy to a drug being ordered or reminded to order levels of aminoglycosides. Patient-specific alerts to information about a recommended change in practice can take the next step by supporting learning at a "teachable moment." For example, the pharmacy and therapeutics committee at Vanderbilt recommends use of cephepime instead of ceftazidime for antipseudomonal treatment. When a clinician begins to order ceftazidime, a web page comes up with the recommendation, radio buttons pre-computed as to how to apply the recommendations to the particular patient, and links to the evidence leading to the recommendation. This approach closes the gap between new information, learning, and translation into practice. The direct link to the evidence provides the hook for processes to keep the recommendation up-to-date as information changes.

As we look to the future, we expect to aggregate de-identified extracts of EHR data on large populations and to use pattern discovery algorithms to detect unexpected events, an approach the National Library of Medicine is funding a dataset to test (Miller 2006). Derivatives of the electronic patient chart are being constructed—for example, converting all dates to an offset to a random start time. This approach maintains the temporal relationships within the record while removing reference points that might result in re-identification. Such abstracts might be aggregated on a large scale to detect more quickly problems such as the complications of Vioxx. It might then be possible to decrease pre-market testing by assuring robust post-market surveillance with systematic translation of problem detection into practice. As a next step, Vanderbilt is going live with a project to bank de-identified DNA samples of all patients who do not opt out. A one-way hash will link these samples to the synthetic derivative of the electronic chart, permitting phenotype-genotype hypothesis testing.

Challenges to Achieving the Potential

The potential use of EHRs as a tool for learning has been clear for decades. I include a number of older citations to underscore the maturity of many of these ideas. Until recently, the underlying information technology did not scale up to handle the amount or complexity of biomedical information. Such technical limits are behind us. Google shows the ease with which information can be aggregated from across the globe and made accessible. A number of challenging problems remain to work through. Examples include how to authenticate a patient to his or her record without requiring yet another identifier; how to support both confidentiality and access; and how to achieve interoperability for core items such as allergies while enabling access to data that are too highly dimensional to be regularized;

and so forth. However, these informatics challenges are not the major rate-limiting steps at this juncture.

Our capacity to envision a new way of working and to manage the transition is the rate-limiting step. The changes to systems approaches to care and learning are discontinuous. By discontinuous, I mean that we cannot achieve the ultimate potential by fixing aspects of our current health non-system. The goal is a completely new approach. People's roles and responsibilities, the process, and the technology all need to change. These changes must be coordinated and take place in steps that can be accommodated within the current non-system while leading to another system. At the end of the journey we will see quite different professions, credentialing, decision-making strategies, et cetera.

The Institute of Medicine has taken a leadership role in highlighting the quality problems inherent in today's health non-system and in calling for systems approaches to care. To date its reports recommend how to cross the chasm through a set of targeted fixes such as adoption of information technology or addition of certain competencies to the health science curriculum. It is not likely that we can achieve the discontinuous change in how we provide care without equally discontinuous changes in our definitions of professional roles and how we learn. We need to develop pictures of alternative visions of various combinations of roles, processes, and infrastructure that scale up to translate our scientific breakthroughs into the quality we want, at a price we can afford. Next, we need an actionable road map that shows how we can implement key aspects of these visions in the context of current reality.

EMBEDDING AN EVIDENCE PERSPECTIVE IN HEALTH PROFESSIONS EDUCATION

Mary Mundinger, Dr.P.H., R.N.
Columbia University School of Nursing

With rapid advances in medical knowledge, teaching health professionals to evaluate and use evidence in clinical decision making becomes one of the most crucial aspects of future efficacy and patient safety. This paper discusses Columbia University School of Nursing's approach to teaching about evidence at the baccalaureate, masters, and clinical doctoral levels.

Fifty years ago in 1956, Sydney Burwell, dean of Harvard Medical School, said to his students, "Half of what you are taught as medical students will in ten years have been shown to be wrong. And the trouble is none of your teachers knows which half" (Sackett et al. 2001). What was once generally considered conventional care is no longer acceptable; many think of it as undisturbed ignorance. In 1985, Skolnick, in *Medicine and*

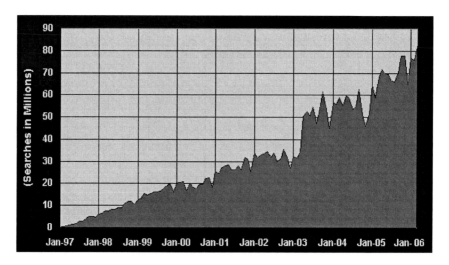

FIGURE 7-4 Medline searches.
SOURCE: NLM: www.nlm.nih.gov/bsd/medline_growth.html.

Law noted, "Failure to search the appropriate scientific literature is an obvious breach of the broader duty to perform at the level of knowledge and practice in a … clinical specialty" (Skolnick 1985). Searching the literature to guide practice is clearly a necessary first step, but only when sophisticated search and analysis skills are utilized. Evidence to direct practice is being sought more consistently as the most recent National Library of Medicine (2006a) graph on 10 years of database searches illustrates (Figure 7-4). But stronger educational efforts related to evidence assessment are needed to equip healthcare professionals with the tools and skills to continually bring the best evidence to bear on practice.

In thinking about teaching students to become evidence-based clinicians, there are three main questions. First is: Why teach it? This question has been quite cogently analyzed in this workshop; essentially, it is the best way to provide the best outcomes for our patients. The previous chapter addresses how it helps patients participate in treatment decisions and adopt best self-care practices. This is particularly important as we move beyond the era in which we expected passive patient compliance with physician-prescribed regimens. In addition, evidence-based practice is the way to achieve highest value with available resources. There isn't enough money to deliver the kind of care we are delivering now and still achieve the best possible outcomes. To improve the value of care we need to rely more on evidence.

The second question is: What do we do? It is not enough to give one course and expect the concept of evidence-based practice to take hold. At Columbia University School of Nursing, we found that we needed to examine the context and the core of how we engage in practice to get evidence-based practice fully integrated in our curricula. Our approach was to adopt a new guiding principle: translational research would inform everything we did. By this we do not mean the linear bench-to-bedside approach. Our school, in addition to having a program for college graduates to enter nursing through a second degree program, also has 12 master's programs in a number of clinical specialties and a doctoral research program, and we were considering instituting the first clinical doctoral program in the country. The doctor of nursing practice degree uses a teaching approach entirely grounded in evidence. Translational research is essentially a process that moves from conventional data collection, analysis, conclusions, and recommendations to actively incorporating the new evidence into practice (the hardest part), then to institutionalizing the change into policy (regulatory, reimbursement, liability), and then to ensuring that the new ways of doing things are taught to students. New research questions emanating from the new "state of the art" practice close the circle.

The beauty of this continuous circular process is that it does not stop after research changes practice. In our school, both research and clinical faculty actively engage in this process. Research doctoral students select studies emanating from faculty practice themes, and clinical doctoral students engage in the process of generating data for faculty research studies. Some examples follow. Dr. Suzanne Bakken's research on developing informatics-based approaches to patient care that enable data collection, secondary use of datasets, and building of evidence across evidence-based practice studies also includes teaching data collection to B.S. students using personal digital assistants. Doctoral research studies based on questions arising from faculty clinical practices include such topics as adult liver donation; testing acupressure for relief of AIDS-related nausea and vomiting; development of a fall and injury risk assessment instrument; diabetes treatment in the Hispanic population; and breast cancer screening practices. Changes in clinical practice guidelines resulting from faculty research include the cardiac effects of Parkinson's drugs and depression screening for children. Policy change as a result of clinical research and faculty practice includes a new hospital emergency room (ER) discharge policy for pregnant women. The interaction and active progression of translational research is a vibrant core of faculty scholarship.

Students are taught to understand different levels of evidence and to distinguish among good and bad studies and good studies with flawed conclusions or wrong recommendations. If practitioners cannot make these distinctions, the literature as an instrument of putting best evidence into practice will be insufficient. Although understanding the five levels of evidence is the first step in becoming an evidence-based clinician, students are also taught to focus on the critical relationship between design methods and conclusions and recommendations and to understand how the design of a trial might affect the ultimate strength of its recommendations. Simply having the gold standard of a randomized control trial is simply not enough. Strategies to analyzing and implementing evidence vary. Education of doctoral research students concentrates on analyzing evidence; training of clinical doctoral students focuses on implementing evidence.

The third and final question is: How will we get where we want to go? Clearly a main enabler is the electronic health record, which will be fundamental for data mining, evidence application, and evidence generation. Although the Institute of Medicine and some of the most sophisticated clinicians in the country have long advocated EHRs, we are still far from achieving broad utilization. We must help students become sophisticated readers of the literature and help them find systematic ways to phrase questions and collect data. We need to ensure that our advanced research courses teach the data-mining techniques that practitioners and the country will need to move forward.

Columbia's experience—as an academic health center that includes medical, public health, nursing, and dentistry—is illustrative. Collectively we have about 2,500 students, and the schools are highly integrated. More than half the public health faculty are physicians; many faculty members in each school have dual appointments; in nursing, 40 clinical faculty have joint appointments in medical school departments. Yet the curricula of these schools are quite disparate. We may be a collegial, academic campus, but we could not be more different in how we teach evidence-based practice. In medicine, evidence-based practice is incorporated into the curricula of three intensive courses that span one month in the fourth year of training. In this one month, students are introduced to the clinician scientist role, the practicing physician role, and biomedical informatics. Nationwide, physicians are clearly involved in evidence-based practice publications and research, but medical school curricula do not reflect this. In dentistry, evidence-based practice is introduced in the first semester, first year with courses in "Scientific Inquiry and Decision Making in Dentistry" and "Informatics, Epidemiology, Ethics, and General Dental Practice." Again while this school is cognizant of bringing discussion of evidence into its curricula, there isn't a strong evidence-based component that is identifiable. In public health, elements of evidence-based medicine are integrated into courses on "Informatics" and "Health Information Technology." Both the public health and the medical schools have National Institutes of Health (NIH) grants on evidence-based practice and clinical decision making. Columbia also has the best bioinformatics department in a medical school. The intellectual property for evidence-based practice certainly is present and is seen in faculty research publications, but it has not yet found its way into the curricula as a very specific way to train students. Education lags somewhat behind academic practice, and this may be true nationally as well.

In nursing, we have three separate curricula to train students for our different-level nursing programs. To educate college graduates to become nurses and earn a second B.S. degree we require a research utilization course. Master's degree students take a course titled "Assessing Clinical Evidence" (the ACE course). For our bachelor's nursing program we help nurses understand established evidence-based care, understand the science and how care protocols evolve, and how to know when to deviate from protocols because of patient responses. In the master's advanced practice nursing program, we are helping our students to learn, distinguish, and apply levels of evidence to literature analysis.

In the doctoral nursing program, students learn how to use evidence, how to assess literature using informatics, and how to collect data and generate evidence. They gain an understanding of research design and methods in relation to study outcomes and conclusions, the systematic use of data to adopt and generate evidence, and interdisciplinary and cross-site collaboration. In our research doctoral program we offer several biostatistics and research design and methods courses; our clinical doctoral students take some of these same courses and also "Synthesizing, Translating, and Integrating Clinical Evidence." The research doctoral graduates, training to be principal investigators, will ultimately be designing and conducting trials; the clinical doctoral graduates will need to know when and how to use evidence.

One particularly important point is that, although Columbia provides this kind of training, often it is not utilized because of restrictions on the nurse's role in providing patient care. If we allowed nurses the opportunity to employ evidence-based practice methods as part of their work, we might not have a nursing shortage. Nurses are trained to look at evidence, think critically and intelligently, and make decisions based on their knowledge, but they are not being allowed to do this in their jobs.

The three-tiered curricula progression (B.S.-M.S.-doctorate) at Columbia University Nursing School prepares graduates to distinguish and use evidence to guide practice. Applying the evidence, however, is very much limited by scope of practice. Hospital nurses, for example, are expected to abide by hospital policy, established nursing protocols, and physician orders. Professional responsibility requires the nurse to report any patient responses that could contraindicate following current protocols or orders. However actively initiating or changing regimens is not expected of nurses, and often not tolerated, even if the scientific evidence validates those actions. This kind of practice is deeply unsatifisfying to knowledgeable professionals. Shift work with its shared accountability, but without any authority for nurses, and a hierarchy that negates the nurse's decision making are all factors contributing to a broken system. In the 1970s, models with nursing accountability, M.D. partnerships, and flexibility in devising care regimens were developed. Hospitals found them too complex in the context of industrial organization, and physicians found giving up their total and easy determination of ordering care irksome. So the models disappeared (Mundinger 1973).

Nurses prepared as nurse practitioners with a master's degree in a specialty (adult primary care, for example) have more authority and can utilize their decision-making ability in a more independent way. This level of practice is again limited by regulation—this time at the state level rather than institutional level. Each state determines the level of independence (full, shared with a physician, or supervised by a physician) and prescriptive authority (full, only certain categories of drugs, or cosigned by a physician). Many qualified nurse practitioners shun opportunities in states where practice is limited.

Doctoral-level clinicians are those educated for more sophisticated practice and decision making, and regulatory bodies (hospitals for admitting privileges and states for prescribing and Medicaid reimbursement) have not yet made distinctions between them and M.S.-prepared practitioners. Regulation almost always lags behind practice. The Balanced Budget Act of 1997 was an exception in authorizing master's-prepared nurse practitioners for direct Medicare reimbursement in any site (United States Congress 1997), even though nurse practitioners are not educated for care of hospitalized patients. The doctor of nursing practice degree catches up with this regulation, educating nurses to care for patients across sites and over time—a true professional model of responsibility that, if the principles of educational philosophy are implemented, will be fully dedicated to advancing the application of evidence.

Several changes must occur in order to fully utilize the professional nursing workforce and ensure application of best evidence. Hospitals must adopt models of care that recognize nursing decision making. This is true for bedside nurses and for doctoral-level clinicians who admit and order care for their patients. Hospital medical boards must also change their by-laws and provide accessible consultations, as well as privileges for doctoral-level clinicians. Second, state regulations must be changed to standardize and authorize nurse decision making in outpatient settings, including increasing prescriptive authority, decreasing M.D. oversight, and nonrestrictive reimbursement from Medicaid. Third, private insurers and Medicare must recognize doctoral clinicians and grant them parity with physicians. Nurses have consistently demonstrated thoughtful responsibility for the care decisions they make, and a number of studies attest to this quality of care and outcomes (Mundinger et al. 2000). Nurses will be attracted to positions where their competency is operationalized, and the nursing "shortage" would disappear.

The changes enumerated above all relate to increasing the focus by nurses on generation and application of evidence. Especially important to optimizing evidence-based practice is to ensure that nurses can also develop evidence. Given the time, hospital nurses are particularly attuned to nuanced changes in a patient's condition and see themes of patient response to a variety of interventions. With a way to chart patient responses and to indicate their nursing-specific observations and treatment, they could be the frontline voice in guiding scientific evaluation of new or emerging evidence. The EHR can be developed to capture these data, but its utility depends on accurate input—a function that is often the responsibility of nurses.

Teaching baccalaureate nursing students how evidence is generated will spark their interest as graduates to play an important role. Master's-prepared nurse practitioners generate evidence through the more complete and comprehensive data they collect on their own primary care patients. Knowing how to collect data and publish their practice perspectives will add to the science of given clinical conditions or context of care. Doctoral clinicians will be the major source of identifying emerging patterns or new insights of care outcomes. Researchers will use these carefully collected data to carry out analytical outcomes leading to new evidence-based practice guidelines.

KNOWLEDGE TRANSLATION: REDEFINING CONTINUING EDUCATION AROUND EVOLVING EVIDENCE

Mark V. Williams, M.D.
Emory University School of Medicine

It's an incredibly simple idea and one that is blindingly obvious to most lay people. . . . Assess the existing evidence and concentrate on the reliable stuff.

Iain Chalmers, 1996

Dramatic increases in the generation of new medical knowledge practically overwhelm practicing clinicians; in fact, entire books have been published on how best to manage all the "evidence" available (Rennie and Guyatt 2001; Strauss et al. 2005). Each year, thousands of clinical trials are added to the already voluminous research literature in hundreds of journals. For example, to keep up with germane developments in the field of internal medicine, physicians now face the prospect of learning from thousands of relevant articles being published each month. Not surprisingly, numb resignation may supplant the desired eager and interactive approach to lifelong learning. Recognizing that learning all the evidence is impossible, some experts recommend that healthcare providers develop information management skills while allowing others to help identify, review, and summarize salient and valid clinical information (Slawson and Shaughnessy 2005). Even with successful transfer of this responsibility for knowledge organization, clinicians must still know how to access and deliver recommended advances in clinical care and systems of delivery. Unfortunately, physicians are doing a mediocre job of delivering recommended care to patients, with one well-designed study showing success about half the time (McGlynn et al. 2003); national reports confirm this though there are signs of improvement (AHRQ 2003).

To foster the dissemination of innovation and application of new evidence, clinicians must undertake efforts to ensure that clinical practice reflects the best current evidence. While the best evidence should always inform medical decisions and health choices, simply providing more bedside evidence may only worsen the informational plight of busy clinicians. Continuing education after initial training plays an essential role in allowing them to apply such new evidence effectively to patient care. The standard approach to postgraduate physician education, traveling to a continuing medical education course and listening to presentations in a classroom setting, is endorsed by medical societies, supported by pharmaceutical companies, and required by many state licensing boards. Yet, previous systematic reviews have documented for decades that standard CME is ineffective at changing physician behavior and translating proven interventions into practice (Haynes et al. 1984; Davis et al. 1995; Davis et al. 1999). While typical didactic sessions unsuccessfully influence practice, interactive workshops (e.g., role playing, case discussion, practicing skills) do seem to generate moderate changes in performance and offer hope (O'Brien et al. 2006). A variant of CME, continuous professional development, has been advocated by the American Board of Internal Medicine and attempts to incorporate adult learning principles and reflection (Baron 2005), but its economic value is yet to be determined (Brown et al. 2002). Additionally, it employs self-directed learning as a principal method, but physicians have limited ability to self-assess their own competency (Davis et al. 2006). All of these approaches to continuing education tend to focus on the physician to the exclusion of other members of the healthcare team.

Demands from patients, insurers, and regulatory agencies such as the Joint Commission on Accreditation of Healthcare Organizations (JCAHO) and the Centers for Medicare and Medicaid Services (CMS), combined with increased emphasis on pay for performance to improve overall quality of care, mandate changes in methods for CME (Rowe 2006). Popular magazines such as *Reader's Digest* suggest that hospitalization is equivalent to gambling with your life and portray patients as feeling suspended above a chasm between known medical evidence and the care actually provided (IOM 2001). Healthcare professionals do not have it any better; as a cover of *Time* magazine proclaimed in 2006, doctors also fear for the safety of their family members and themselves when they enter a hospital. The overarching message is to stay out of the hospitals if you value your life. Despite the lack of certainty regarding whether or not pay for performance will actually improve care (Petersen et al. 2006), healthcare insurers will increasingly use it to control costs, attempting to align payment incentives to promote better-quality care by rewarding providers who perform well (IOM 2007). For hospitals and healthcare systems to succeed in this new environment, involvement of the entire healthcare team will be necessary to utilize innovative approaches and take advantage of evolving evidence, including both scientific advances and learning how to deliver existing effective therapies more consistently. Of note, governmental healthcare leaders support the reinvention of CME and linking it to care delivery (Clancy 2004).

Knowledge translation may represent an approach that combines the right tools with involvement of the entire healthcare team to yield truly effective CME (Davis et al. 2003). This approach moves CME to where we deliver care, it targets all participants (patients, nurses, pharmacists, and doctors), and the content is based around initiatives to improve health care. Such a model marks an important shift toward translating evidence into practice and crossing the current perceived quality chasm, while also promoting an interdisciplinary approach. The theoretical underpinnings to this approach maintain not only that we make physicians and other healthcare providers aware of the evidence, but also that it is important that adoption occurs, and adherence is encouraged through thoughtful incentives as well as reminders to accomplish these goals. A review of the various components of knowledge translation with comparison to standard CME elucidates the advantages.

First, this approach moves CME out of the classroom into the actual setting of care delivery. By focusing on changing participants' behavior at the site of care (e.g., ordering and giving influenza vaccinations to eligible patients, measuring and treating pain post-operatively) and providing tools or toolkits to facilitate such changes, best evidence can be delivered where it is needed. The Society of Hospital Medicine, the medical society for hospitalists, now promotes the use of such tools on its web site (http://www.hospitalmedicine.org) to enhance patient safety and the quality of inpatient care, and examples of their use are being published (McKean et al. 2006). All that is lacking is the link to CME credits.

Knowledge translation also has a different target than the standard CME focus on physicians. This model can involve the entire healthcare team and group learning (Davis et al. 2003). It may even include patients in addition to nurses, pharmacists, and other healthcare providers. By centering the content on evidence that improves patient health care, instead of purely clinical or pathophysiologic material (e.g., the need and indications for administering an angiotensin-converting enzyme [ACE] inhibitor to a patient with heart failure vs. the mechanism by which the medications act on the renin-angiotensin pathway), there is a more direct impact on outcomes. Finally, knowledge translation pursues an interdisciplinary approach with inclusion of all relevant staff in the care process, instead of the teacher determining the goals of instruction, and employs a model that guides implementation and evaluation of interventions. This broadens expertise to include the fields of informatics, organizational learning, social marketing, and quality improvement (Davis et al. 2003). Although mainly still in the conceptual phase, the continuing education model of knowledge translation should be advanced by recent changes introduced by the Accreditation Council for Graduate Medical Education (ACGME) (Leach and Philibert 2006).

With the formation of a Committee on Innovation in the Learning Environment, the ACGME seeks to achieve implementation of the expectation that physicians be taught six general competencies: patient care, medical knowledge, practice-based learning and improvement, interpersonal communication skills, professionalism, and systems-based practice (Batalden et al. 2002). This forces a shift from residents' learning predominantly through clinical experiences to also include an emphasis on mastering and leading systems that deliver safe care (Leach and Philibert 2006). Fortunately, multiple quality improvement strategies, including some with robust research supporting their efficacy (e.g., audit and feedback), are available to be utilized in this effort (Stein 2006).

There are some anticipated challenges with the knowledge translation approach. We will need monitoring systems to support and document provider participation in these activities and evidence on specific mechanisms that promote learning and change. Yet, similar to healthcare delivery, the future of CME needs to function through collaborative teamwork in which we pull physicians out of their autonomous role and into collaboration with nurses, pharmacists, occupational and physical therapists, and dieticians. Achieving team-based, patient-centered, evidence-based care as the objective might occur at the local level and even nationally. The Institute for Healthcare Improvement attempted this with its 100,000 Lives Campaign and the newer 5 Million Lives Campaign (http://www.ihi.org/IHI/Programs/Campaign/). Collaborative projects by large organizations such as the Hospital Corporation of America (HCA; a large corporation with almost 200 hospitals) also have the potential to impact large numbers of patients profoundly. For example, HCA is partnering with expertise from an academic medical center (Vanderbilt) on a project funded by the Agency for Healthcare Research and Quality (AHRQ) to improve care and reduce errors in intensive care units (ICUs) across many of their hospitals. Yet, neither of these efforts includes official CME credits in its implementation. Forging this link might dramatically augment their success because physicians would have the added push from their state medical boards and accreditation agencies to become involved.

As mentioned earlier, impending pay for performance (P4P) initiatives should also facilitate adoption of the knowledge translation approach, even outside academic medical centers (Rowe 2006). The old model of healthcare reimbursement follows the simple principle that essentially the more you do, the more you make. A new model of pay for performance could help us move beyond this, and in an important sign, CMS is considering lowering payments for cases with medical errors and tying the National Quality Forum's "never events" to lower reimbursement. Tying knowledge translation to mandated CME seeking to accomplish this goal may powerfully drive healthcare systems both to apply evidence and to generate it through healthcare delivery. Instead of physicians traveling to a distant location (typically a vacation resort) for CME, healthcare delivery can become a learning experience as they experience practice-based learning with their colleagues. This will require consistent integration with care delivery occurring everyday. If data can be collected simultaneously with this implementation, we can also learn and have practice-based evidence to guide future practice improvements (Horn 2006). Not only would healthcare professionals be learning, but the entire system would also learn how to optimize care delivery.

REFERENCES

AHRQ (Agency for Healthcare Research and Quality). *National Healthcare Quality Report.* 2003. Available from http://www.ahrq.gov/qual/nhqr05/nhqr05.htm. (accessed December 19, 2006).

Baron, R. 2005. Personal metrics for practice: how'm I doing? *New England Journal of Medicine* 353:1992-1993.

Batalden, P, D Leach, S Swing, H Dreyfus, and S Dreyfus. 2002. General competencies a accreditation in graduate medical education. *Health Affairs (Milwood)* 21:103-111.

Brown, C, C Belfield, and S Field. 2002. Cost effectiveness of continuing professional development in health care: a critical review of the evidence. *British Medical Journal* 324:652-655.

Clancy, C. 2004. Commentary: Reinventing continuing medical education. *British Medical Journal* 4:181.

Cowan, N. 2000. The magical number 4 in short-term memory: a reconsideration of mental storage capacity. *Behavioral and Brain Sciences* 94:87-185.

Davis, D, M Thomson, A Oxman, and R Haynes. 1995. Changing physician performance: a systematic review of the effect of continuing medical education strategies. *Journal of the American Medical Association* 274:700-705.

Davis, D, M O'Brien, N Freemantle, F Wolf, P Mazmanian, and A Taylor-Vaisey. 1999. Impact of formal continuing medical education: do conferences, workshops, rounds, and other traditional continuing education activities change physician behavior or health care outcomes? *Journal of the American Medical Association* 282(9):867-874.

Davis, D, M Evans, A Jadad, L Perrier, D Rath, D Ryan, G Sibbald, S Strauss, S Rappolt, M Wowk, and M Zwarenstein. 2003. The case for knowledge translation: shortening the journey from evidence to effect. *British Medical Journal* 327:33-35.

Davis, D, P Mazmanian, M Fordis, R Van Harrison, K Thorpe, and L Perrier. 2006. Accuracy of physician self-assessment compared with observed measures of competence: a systematic review. *Journal of the American Medical Association* 296:1094-1102.

Denny, J, J Smithers, R Miller, and A Spickard 3rd. 2003. "Understanding" medical school curriculum content using KnowledgeMap. *Journal of the American Medical Informatics Association* 10(4):351-362.

Haynes, R, D Davis, A McKibbon, and P Tugwell. 1984. A critical appraisal of the efficacy of continuing medical education. *Journal of the American Medical Association* 251:61-64.

Horn, S. 2006. Performance measures and clinical outcomes. *Journal of the American Medical Association* 296:2731-2732.

IOM (Institute of Medicine). 2001. *Crossing the Quality Chasm. A New Health System for the 21st Century.* Washington, DC: National Academy Press.

———. 2007. *Rewarding Provider Performance: Aligning Incentives in Medicare, Pathways to Quality Health Care.* Washington, DC: The National Academies Press.

Koch, M, B Seckin, and J Smith Jr. 1995. Impact of a collaborative care approach to radical cystectomy and urinary reconstruction. *Journal of Urology* 154(3):996-1001.

Leach, D, and I Philibert. 2006. High-quality learning for high-quality health care: Getting it right. *Journal of the American Medical Association* 296:1132-1134.

McGlynn, E, S Asch, J Adams, J Keesey, J Hicks, A DeCristofaro, and E Kerr. 2003. The quality of health care delivered to adults in the United States. *New England Journal of Medicine* 348:2635-2645.

McKean, S, J Stein, G Maynard, T Budnitz, A Amin, S Johnson, and L Wellikson. 2006. Curriculum development: the venous thromboembolism quality improvement resource room. *Journal of Hospital Medicine* 1:124-132.

McNeer, J, G Wagner, P Ginsburg, A Wallace, C McCants, M Conley, and R Rosati. 1978. Hospital discharge one week after acute myocardial infarction. *New England Journal of Medicine* 298(5):229-232.

Miller, G. 1956. The magical number seven plus or minus two: some limits on our capacity for processing information. *Psychological Review* 63(2):81-97.

Miller, R. 2006. *TIME (Tools for Inpatient Monitoring using Evidence) for Safe & Appropriate Testing.* NLM Grant 5R01LM007995-03.

Mundinger, M. 1973. Primary nurse role evolution. *Nursing Outlook* 21(10):642-645.

Mundinger, M, R Kane, E Lenz, A Totten, W Tsai, P Cleary, W Friedewald, A Siu, and M Shelanski. 2000. Primary care outcomes in patients treated by nurse practitioners or physicians: a randomized trial. *Journal of the American Medical Association* 283(1):59-68.

NLM Board of Regents, National Institutes of Health. 2006. *Charting a Course for the 21st Century: NLM's Long Range Plan 2006-2016.* Available from http://www.nlm.nih.gov/pubs/plan/lrpdocs.html. (accessed April 4, 2007).

O'Brien, M, N Freemantle, A Oxman, F Wolf, D Davis, and J Herrin. 2006. Continuing education meetings and workshops: effects on professional practice and health care outcomes. *Cochrane Database of Systematic Reviews* 4.

Petersen, L, L Woodard, T Urech, C Daw, and S Sookanan. 2006. Does pay-for-performance improve the quality of healthy care? *Annals of Internal Medicine* 145:265-272.

Rennie, D, and G Guyatt. 2001. *Users' Guides: Manual for Evidence-Based Clinical Practice.* Chicago, IL: American Medical Association.

Rosati, R, J McNeer, C Starmer, B Mittler, J Morris Jr., and A Wallace. 1975. A new information system for medical practice. *Archives of Internal Medicine* 135(8):1017-1024.

Rowe, J. 2006. Pay-for-performance and accountability: related themes in improving health care. *Annals of Internal Medicine* 145:695-699.

Sackett, D, W Richardson, W Rosenberg, and R Haynes. 2001. *Evidence-Based Medicine: How to Practice and Teach EBM.* New York: Churchill Livingstone.

Skolnick, M. 1985. Expanding physician duties and patients rights in wrongful life: Harbeson v. Parke-Davis, Inc. *Medicine and Law* 4(3):283-298.

Slawson, D, and A Shaughnessy. 2005. Teaching evidence-based medicine: should we be teaching information management instead? *Academic Medicine* 80:685-689.

Society of Hospital Medicine. Ongoing. *Quality Improvement Tools.* Available from http://www.hospitalmedicine.org/Content/NavigationMenu/HQPS/QualityImprovementTools/Quality_Improvement_.htm. (accessed December 18, 2006).

Stead, W. 2007. Rethinking electronic health records to better achieve quality and safety goals. *Annual Review of Medicine* 58(14):1-14.

Stein, J. 2006. The language of quality improvement: therapy classes. *Journal of Hospital Medicine* 1:327-330.

Strauss, S, W Richardson, P Glasziou, and R Haynes. 2005. *Evidence Based Medicine.* London, UK: Churchill Livingstone.

United States Congress. 1997. *Balanced Budget Act of 1997.* Washington, DC: Government Printing Office.

Vanderbilt Medical Center. 2005 (September). *Strategic Plan for VUMC Informatics & Roadmap to 2010* September 2005. Available from http://www.mc.vanderbilt.edu/infocntr/IC_Strategic_Plan_05.pdf. (accessed April 4, 2007).

8

Structuring the Incentives for Change

OVERVIEW

A fundamental reality in the prospects for a learning healthcare system lies in the nature of the incentives for inducing the necessary changes. Echoed throughout this report are calls for incentives that are structured and coordinated to drive the system and culture changes, as well as to establish the collaborations and technological developments necessary to build learning into every healthcare encounter. Public and private insurers, standards organizations such as National Committee for Quality Assurance (NCQA) and the Joint Commission (formerly JCAHO), and manufacturers have the opportunity to shape policy and practice incentives to accelerate needed changes. In this chapter, representatives from private and public payer organizations, a manufacturer, and a standards organization give their perspectives on how the field might support specific and broad policy changes that provide incentives for systemwide progress. These perspectives engage only a sampling of the sorts of incentives to development of a learning healthcare system, but they represent important focal points for stakeholder alignment.

Alan Rosenberg of WellPoint offers a perspective from the health insurers industry on opportunities for encouraging both evidence development and application. For payers, incentives for change are structured around their three major functions: reimbursement, benefit plan design, and medical policy formation. Rosenberg gives several examples of past and current efforts by insurance providers to encourage evidence generation and application. Steven Phurrough discusses the Centers for Medicare and Medicaid

Services' (CMS's) opportunities for influencing change through regulatory and payment processes but also notes that its leadership in implementing policies that assist in developing evidence might encourage similar efforts throughout the healthcare system. A very powerful approach taken by CMS in this respect is Coverage with Evidence Development (CED), in which reimbursement is conditional on the creation or submission of additional data. Phurrough describes recent revisions of CED that define two CED components: Coverage with Appropriateness Determination and Coverage with Study Participation, as well as the range of gaps in the evidence base that such policies may help to fill.

Wayne A. Rosenkrans and colleagues discuss the importance of providing incentives for appropriate evidence creation and appropriate use of evidence. Establishing standards of evidence and processes for reimbursement decisions would help manufacturers design better studies and work to provide the evidence needed. In addition, flexibility to account for individual variation needs to be built into the system. Evidence generated must be put to good use through thoughtful structuring of guidelines, decision support, and outreach to providers and patients. New models for product development such as evidence-based drug development will accelerate the creation of a learning healthcare system by making clear breaks with outdated approaches. For example, embedding the creation of effectiveness data into the process of drug development or developing a continuous process of evidence creation in partnership with the regulators and payers might provide sufficient financial incentives to drive change.

Margaret E. O'Kane discusses the important role that standards organizations have played in improving the quality of health care by measuring performance and identifies the significant barriers to extending this across the healthcare system: the absence of evidence from basic science, to complex comorbidities, subpopulations, and comparative effectiveness; the lack of usable guidelines; difficulty in obtaining data; and lack of accountability throughout the system. All are significant impediments to improving quality and efficiency of care. O'Kane calls for payment reform, regulatory reform, and liability reform as the key instruments to confront these challenges. System-wide change requires new ways of thinking about gathering, managing, and deploying knowledge and an evolution in our approaches.

OPPORTUNITIES FOR PRIVATE INSURERS

Alan Rosenberg, M.D.
WellPoint Inc.

Private insurers have many opportunities to structure the incentives for change both in evidence development *and* in evidence-based application.

This paper addresses both the private insurance industry as a whole and gives specific examples from my own organization, WellPoint Inc., which provides health benefits through its affiliated companies for 34 million Americans. The area to be covered is very broad, but this overview provides a sense of the opportunities that the private insurers have for collaboration with others in health care to build a learning health-care system for evidence-based medicine.

Three major functions of private insurers provide such opportunities: reimbursement and financing methodologies, including reimbursement to physicians, other practitioners, and healthcare institutions, can be and are currently used to structure incentives; claims data through their analysis can be and are used to support this environment; benefit plan design (BPD) and, within BPD, medical policy formation also can be and are used.

This paper also discusses two initiatives—data integration for electronic health records (EHRs) and consumer-focused initiatives—along with the methods used, the importance of collaboration, and some of the hurdles from the private insurer perspective in achieving these goals.

Private insurers have and will continue to fund significant components of evidence development and evidence-based applications (Blumenthal 2006). Certain of these are still evolving but worthy of special note. Several health plans now provide benefit coverage for individuals in National Institutes of Health (NIH) sponsored trials. The Centers for Medicare and Medicaid Services has recently embarked on a model of coverage based on participation in registries such as the implantable cardioverter defibrillator registry. Several insurers, including WellPoint, helped provide funding for the development of this registry. WellPoint also recently announced its collaboration, including economic support, with the Society of Thoracic Surgeons (STS), for its cardiac surgery registry. Use of the data from these registries to support evidence development and evidence-based care remains a priority. WellPoint uses such data, including data from STS and Joint Commission on Accreditation of Healthcare Organizations (JCAHO) registries to determine variable reimbursement for facilities in a variety of its pay for performance (P4P) programs. Payers recognize that evidence for and analysis of the effectiveness of P4P programs are still under evaluation (Rosenthal et al. 2005). At the same time, payers continue to fund this important and significant modification in traditional insurance-based reimbursement methodology. Today, P4P programs include enhanced reimbursement for physicians who perform better on a wide array of evidence-based measures including mammography rates, immunization rates, diabetic retinal eye exam rates, and rates of measurement of hemoglobin A1c levels. WellPoint has already paid to physicians and medical facilities more than 100 million dollars through these programs.

The second area for review is how we can collaborate with others to advance evidence development through claim data analysis. WellPoint databases have claims history for 34 million Americans and integrated pharmacy claims data on 17 million of these. Through analysis of this dataset, and by other insurers as well, post-market surveillance can be undertaken. WellPoint, with its affiliate HealthCore, did submit information to the Food and Drug Administration (FDA) on cyclooxygenase-2 (COX-2) inhibitor complications based on analysis of this dataset. Health-Core is currently working with a variety of academic research centers and specialty societies on projects using this dataset to evaluate comparative effectiveness including projects on cardiac care, controller effectiveness in asthma, and an analysis of blood growth factors. Some of the individuals and organizations contributing to this workshop summary have worked for years and developed sophisticated models of data analysis. Ongoing efforts and collaborations will continue to tap these valuable resources for evidence development. In addition to WellPoint's initiatives, the Blue Cross Blue Shield Association (BCBSA) announced its plan to bring together an array of claims datasets that will eventually include claims data on more than 70 millions Americans. Unlike currently available CMS datasets, but similar to WellPoint's, these data will include integrated pharmacy and medical claims data.

Claims data are also an important component in evaluating evidence application. While having many limitations, efficiency is a real advantage of claims-based quality measures. The National Committee for Quality Assurance has catalyzed and significantly supported this effort by the development of standards for quality and preventive health initiatives through its Health Plan Employer Data and Information Set (HEDIS) measurement set. This is an example of a long-term collaboration involving practitioners, insurers, and employers that has significantly moved this field forward. Insurers continue to use this and other nationally developed measurement sets to provide feedback to the practitioner community participating in networks. However the defined datasets remain limited, and ongoing development of broader, nationally recognized, consistently defined, and efficient-to-gather standardized measurement sets needs to continue. In addition to NCQA's ongoing work, the majority of large insurers continue to actively engage in and support recent efforts by the AQA (previously known as the Ambulatory care Quality Alliance). Benefit plan design and, specifically, medical policy formation support evidence-based application. A key component of most health insurance benefit plans is that covered services are those that are medically necessary and services that are investigational are not covered. The benefit plans are legal contracts, and definitions of "medical necessity" and "investigational" vary, but they are routinely incorporated into these legal contracts. Therefore these definitions are at the core of insurers' benefit determinations. Based on the benefit plan language, insurers can and do develop evidence-based models for those things that may be considered medically necessary and those that may be considered investigational or not medically necessary. Insurers use inputs from a variety of evidentiary sources, including literature-based review, governmental review bodies, Cochrane reviews, and other technology assessment entities. (See publicly posted coverage or medical policies on numerous BCBSA-affiliated entities and Aetna web sites.) In addition, WellPoint uses specialty society and academic medical center input regarding medical policy and medical necessity determinations, working actively with more than 30 specialty societies. This process is an active effort at developing evidence-based evaluation that includes input from the practice community on when the evidence, in conjunction with national practice patterns, has developed to support benefit coverage. Collaboration in this regard is essential. However, litigation continues to be a significant mitigation in the insurers' ability to fully apply evidence-based medical necessity benefit determinations.

One significant initiative at WellPoint to better support the diffusion of claims information into practice is data integration for electronic health records. This is an effort to use our claim and pharmacy information datasets to support clinical practices. Through this initiative, WellPoint is making available claims-based data regarding diagnoses, procedures, and pharmaceutical information to emergency rooms on a real-time basis. This has already been undertaken in Missouri and is under way in California.

Insurers are actively involved in efforts to reengage their members through consumer-directed health plans. Initial evaluations regarding the effect of these programs have been published (Newhouse 2004). Some of the consumer-directed opportunities that these programs offer include disease management programs; web-based information, including films on conditions or procedures; mail-based information that is procedure and disease specific; web-based, paper, and personalized mailings with health information based on combinations of claim and pharmacy information; and safety information on drug recalls and new drug alerts.

Health insurers have excellent opportunities to support evidence development and evidence-based application. Private insurers also understand that we are only one part of the mosaic and that better value will be created through collaboration. This collaboration needs to occur across the industry and across the healthcare sector with manufacturers, with government, with academic and medical communities, and with our members to move healthcare delivery to a more evidence-based approach. Examples of collective opportunities include the following:

- With *government:* develop national registries, support and conduct research, educate, develop national standards;

- With the *academic medical community:* provide evidence-based care, conduct research, establish evidence-based guidelines, educate practitioners and patients;
- With *members and patients:* strengthen demand for evidence-based along with preference-based care;
- With *manufacturers:* conduct research, support full publication of data, innovate and bring to market health-enhancing products; and
- With *employers and insurers:* enhance individual and physician decision support, integrate data sources, educate, develop performance-based reimbursement plans, and provide evidence-based coverage determinations.

There are also significant hurdles faced by insurers. One of the most significant is the litigation environment and the large dollar court settlements that do not align with evidence-based practices. For a bit of context, AHRQ's budget is approximately $330 million dollars a year, but insurers have had and continue to have $50 million to $100 million dollar settlement costs for failing to provide benefit coverage for an intervention that has inadequate evidentiary support. The most broadly described has been autologous bone marrow transplantation for breast cancer, but new examples occur each and every year. Insurers recognize that we are not viewed favorably in terms of court cases and have very significant risk—this continues to make it difficult for us to maintain strong evidence-based decision making. The opportunity here is to develop some safe harbors built around a national evidence-based process similar to Britain's National Institute for Clinical Excellence (NICE) (Rawlins 2004). Second, insurers recognize that we are not the healthcare sector that most people come to as a trusted partner for getting health information. These ongoing trust issues with the consumer and medical community make communications by us less effective. We are working hard to transform this perception through continued collaborations, but we recognize we have a way to go.

The last significant hurdle that must be addressed is cost. One important example of this is the discussion of conversion from the Ninth Revision of the International Classification of Diseases (ICD-9) to the Tenth Revision (ICD-10). Healthcare researchers generally agree that this will increase the availability of useful clinical information in claim databases. However the cost to systems for conversions is enormous. The ICD-9 to ICD-10 conversion cost to the health insurance industry alone (not including cost to physician practices or hospitals) is estimated to be between $432 million and $913 million, according to a Robert E. Nolan company report and subsequently by independent IBM reports. Therefore careful evaluation of the true value of these changes versus the total cost remains an ongoing imperative—each dollar spent on this is a dollar that cannot be spent on one of the other initiatives outlined.

OPPORTUNITIES FOR CMS

Steve Phurrough, M.D., M.P.A.
Centers for Medicare and Medicaid Services

What opportunities does CMS have to develop policies that can provide incentives for the developments necessary to build learning—evidence development and application—into every healthcare encounter? Issues around trial design, rapid technology advancement, and healthcare culture are crucial and of concern to CMS, and have been discussed in earlier chapters. This discussion focuses on options that CMS has to influence these changes.

CMS influences changes either through its regulatory and payment processes or through its leadership role in the healthcare system. Over the last few years, CMS has attempted to use the latter more broadly, with its emphasis on public health and not just paying claims. This role is very important in itself but with better prospects when accompanied with payment or regulatory changes.

Prerequisites

There are certain prerequisites to these policy changes. For all healthcare experiences to become learning experiences will require some technologies not currently in place. This global population-level learning requires information technology (IT) changes that allow simpler, faster, and more complete data collection and exchanges. Telephonic and paper surveys, multiple data entries, chart reviews for data, and extensive data validations are all impediments to this learning experience. Solutions are complex, but the technology exists. A national standard for the operational architecture for electronic health records is an essential first step. Many facilities, clinics, and offices are hesitant to enter into EHRs, fearful that standards may change and expensive systems become obsolete. While CMS does not have responsibility for this, it is interested in being part of that conversation.

Standard definitions for medical terminology are also necessary. Clinical trials, registries, FDA post-market approval studies, and payers do not have consistent definitions of basic medical terms necessary to simplify data collection. An industry-sponsored registry for a particular device may pay for data on a particular patient that also has a requirement to have the same data submitted to a payer. The definitions of the data elements may differ, and hospitals spend significant time sorting out the differences. However, although the time issue is significant, comparing results from the two data collections may not be useful because of this.

The Department of Health and Human Services (HHS) has contracted with the American National Standards Institute (ANSI) in cooperation with the Healthcare Information and Management Systems Society, the Advanced Technology Institute, and Booz Allen Hamilton to develop a widely accepted and useful set of standards specifically to enable and support widespread interoperability among healthcare software applications. ANSI created a Healthcare IT Standards Panel (American National Standards Institute 2006) to assist in the development of the U.S. Nationwide Health Information Network (NHIN) by addressing issues such as privacy and security within a shared healthcare information system. This panel recently presented its first set of 30 harmonized standards to the American Health Information Community in October 2006. A number of officials from both the public and the private sectors voiced concerns about the standards. This initial effort demonstrates the difficulty of this task.

Much of the learning discussed in this Institute of Medicine (IOM) workshop requires collecting data in ways that may not have the same scientific base as the typical clinical trial methodological sciences. Healthcare research has a fairly well thought out and well designed research methodology, but the research methodology for collecting, analyzing, and utilizing data in other manners—data from claims databases, registries, emerging death data—is much less clear. Increasing the opportunities to collect more information without a good scientific basis for how it will be used—and without broad acceptance in the healthcare community that it is valid evidence—is a fruitless endeavor. Good science behind the use of these types of data is needed.

Policies

Moving from prerequisites to policy options, CMS has several opportunities that could increase learning. Improving the information included with claims data could rapidly advance knowledge, particularly around safety and adverse events. Moving from ICD-9 to ICD-10 adds a greater level of detail for diagnoses and procedures than we currently have. The success of this option will require providers and coders to accurately select the more definitive diagnoses found in ICD-10.

Significant concerns have been raised about the ability of the healthcare industry to track adverse events from medical devices and to notify patients when those events occur or when a recall is initiated. If a particular implantable device is recalled, providers and hospitals have tremendous difficulties in identifying patients who have those devices. Payers, such as Medicare, have significant interest in ensuring that their beneficiaries are notified of the recall. That information is not available to payers. The FDA has begun discussions on an initiative to add unique product identifiers to medical devices, identifiable through bar coding, radio frequency, or other automated techniques. While this would allow easier recording of this information in hospital records, it still does not simplify notification of patients. Having data fields in the claims system that could be populated through the systems required by the FDA would allow payers to notify their beneficiaries when recalls or adverse events occur. In addition, device specific information on claims forms has the potential, when matched with subsequent claims data from patients' interactions with the healthcare system, to identify other events not recognizable through the current reporting systems.

Using claims data is not without problems. Claims forms are payment instruments and are completed with the goal of maximizing payments. In some instances, this may result in a lack of clarity as to the major diagnoses or procedures involved in the care of the patient. Using claims data also makes risk stratification difficult and results in outcomes that do not reflect true practices.

Another opportunity that CMS has already employed is to create requirements that condition payment on the submission of additional data. The CMS quality programs are representative of this. Hospitals currently participate in several quality initiatives that were required as a condition of the annual inpatient rate increase. In other instances, CMS has provided additional payment for information—the oncology demonstration is an example of that. CMS is currently working with the public to develop appropriate quality measures for ambulatory services as well. While the collection of this type of information has become de rigueur for CMS and most health plans, it is still challenging to present this information in manner that is beneficial to the public. In early 2005, CMS released a draft guidance document on Coverage with Evidence Development that outlined a policy on requiring additional evidence as a condition of payment. Several National Coverage Determinations (NCDs) over the previous two years had used this option, and the 2005 guidance document outlined how this process would be used in the future. Following extensive public comments and public forums, CMS issued a revised document in the summer of 2006. This revised document answered many of the concerns addressed by the public. In essence, the guidance document outlined two CED components: Coverage with Appropriateness Determination (CAD) and Coverage with Study Participation (CSP).

CAD requires additional data collection to ensure that the item or service is being provided in a manner consistent with the guidelines outlined in the CMS reasonable and necessary determination. CAD will be required when CMS is concerned that the data collected on a claims form are insufficient to determine that the item or service was appropriately provided as outlined in the NCD. The following are some concerns that may lead to a coverage decision that requires CAD as a condition of coverage:

- If the newly covered item or service should be restricted to patients with specific conditions and criteria;
- If the newly covered item or service should be restricted for use by providers with specific training or credentials;
- If there is concern among clinical thought leaders that there are substantial opportunities for misuse of the item or service; and
- If the coverage determination significantly changes how providers manage patients utilizing this newly covered item or service.

CSP may be an option in a national coverage determination when CMS does not find sufficient evidence to determine that the item or service is reasonable and necessary under section 1862(a)(1)(A). This option would condition payment on participation of the beneficiary in a clinical research study outlined in the NCD. The following list includes some of the evidentiary findings that might result in CSP:

- Available evidence may be a product of otherwise methodologically rigorous evaluations but may not have evaluated outcomes that are relevant to Medicare beneficiaries.
- The available clinical research may have failed to address adequately the risks and benefits to Medicare beneficiaries of off-label or other unanticipated uses of a drug, biologic, service, or device.
- Available clinical research studies may not have included specific patient subgroups or patients with disease characteristics that are highly prevalent in the Medicare population.
- New applications may exist for diagnostic services and devices that are already on the market, but there is little or no published research that supports a determination of reasonable and necessary for Medicare coverage at the time of the request for an NCD.
- Sufficient evidence about the health benefits of a given item or service to support a reasonable and necessary determination is available only for a subgroup of Medicare patients with specific clinical criteria and/or for providers with certain experience or other qualifications. Other patient subgroups or providers require additional evidence to determine if the item or service is reasonable and necessary.
- CSP research conducted may include a broader range of studies than randomized clinical trials to include observational research. However, all studies must conform to the standards that will be developed by the Clinical Research Policy.

In rare instances, for some items or services, CMS may determine that the evidence is very preliminary and not reasonable and necessary for Medicare coverage, but, if the following criteria are met, CSP might be appropriate:

- The evidence includes assurance of basic safety;
- The item or service has a high potential to provide significant benefit to Medicare beneficiaries; and
- There are significant barriers to conducting clinical trials.

The implantable cardioverter defibrillator (ICD) registry is one instance where payment for some beneficiaries was conditional on data submission to a registry. Hospitals implanting ICDs for primary prevention are required to submit several data elements to a national registry. This registry was initially managed by one of CMS' Quality Improvement Organizations. However, this has now been transferred to the National Cardiovascular Data Registry managed by the American College of Cardiology and the Heart Rhythm Society. The first year of the registry resulted in data on almost 45,000 ICD implantations with a compliance rate greater than 95 percent. The initial review of these data produced results not seen in the large trials for these devices. In those trials, no deaths were recorded during the initial hospitalization for the implantation. In the registry, a number of deaths were recorded. This provides a cautionary warning to both patients and providers that ICD implantation is not without risk.

The current CED concept limits its use to those few instances in which we believe that the evidence does not support coverage but is suggestive of a benefit and some additional data collection supported by CMS might provide that additional evidence. While yet to be clearly delineated, there is the potential for this concept to be broadened to the extent that new technologies receive CMS coverage at an earlier time in return for continuous data collection over the life cycle of the technology and a more streamlined process for technologies to enter and leave the CMS coverage toolbox. This concept, somewhat similar to ongoing discussions at FDA, will require significant public discussion and potential legislative action.

CMS does have limits in its abilities to influence learning behavior. Its policy options are essentially payment options. We do think there is a leadership role for government; as we implement on a small scale a particular policy that we think will assist in developing more evidence, we think that particular leadership role will trickle down into other settings. In our current healthcare system, physician learning typically comes from training and experience. Patient learning comes from physicians or the Internet—a fairly inaccurate database. Movement toward a system in which both providers and patients are basing decision about their health care on good, reliable information is a challenge. It is a challenge that CMS and HHS are engaged in and we look forward to engaging the rest of the community in making this work.

OPPORTUNITIES FOR PHARMACEUTICAL COMPANIES

Wayne A. Rosenkrans, Jr., Ph.D., Catherine Bonuccelli, M.D., and Nancy Featherstone, M.B.A.
AstraZeneca Pharmaceuticals

From the point of view of a pharmaceutical firm, the opportunities and challenges in moving toward a learning healthcare system fall into three categories: appropriate evidence creation, appropriate use of evidence, and evidence-based drug development.

Appropriate Evidence Creation

In evidence creation, policies should be pursued that encourage asking the right questions or, rather, avoiding asking the wrong questions. Specifically, for a question worth asking, we need to ensure that the methodology for answering that question is matched to the need and that we are applying the right level or standard of evidence to the question. The right question will depend on the severity of the health condition and the nature of the intervention. For serious life-threatening health conditions, there is a greater willingness to accept less than perfect information because critical decisions must be made by doctors and patients in a short time. In asymptomatic populations at risk for developing an illness, there is a greater desire for certainty before widespread use. Transparency in the question generation process between all stakeholders in health care is essential to the process.

Thus there is a dichotomy in the questions being asked and in the evidentiary standards used to answer each. Who defines what that standard is? Randomized trials frequently fail to find differences when there indeed are some. On the other hand, decision-modeling approaches frequently identify differences where there are none. How should this conundrum be engaged—what is the tie-breaker? When assessing the comparative effectiveness of therapeutic options, all of the evidence needed to fully assess the options is rarely available to decision makers; in fact it may never be available. At some level a decision must be made despite the lack of evidence. From the perspective of pharmaceutical companies, to generate the desired evidence we need to know what standards are going to be required. We have a long-standing set of standards with the FDA for demonstrating safety and efficacy, but lack standards of evidence for demonstrating effectiveness.

Clarification of the standards to be used to evaluate evidence is an area in need of development. For example, the overall size and scope of some

Health Technology Assessment (HTA) guidelines reach so far beyond that of the Academy of Managed Care Pharmacy (AMCP) dossier requirements as to be virtually impossible to meet as an evidentiary standard, even if we were to spend substantial amounts of time and money. Not only that, but there is little consistency between the various HTA requirements. We also know that most health plans don't conduct a thorough review of the AMCP dossier, the only standard we have today. What is the expectation here? We need a set of standards defining which evidence will be used for what purposes, transparency in the process of how evidence is used to make those decisions, and how that evidence translates into treatment guidelines and reimbursement policy.

Also, evidence by its nature is population based, but each individual patient responds differently to a given therapy. As we begin to recognize clinical differences in response to therapy, we need to work to identify the needs of patient subpopulations and individuals and tailor the delivery of care appropriately. There must be a process for exceptions or appeals of coverage rules that are established on population-based evidence, and this appeals process must be efficient and easy to navigate. We need to grapple with the challenge of tailoring population-based evidence to individualization of therapy. Physicians need to estimate the individual patient's response when initiating therapy and to make adjustments based on actual patient response. Evolving knowledge around the molecular nature of disease leading to personalized, or stratified, medicine may provide an answer here. Utilizing sophisticated diagnostic technology to identify therapeutic responders offers the promise of bridging the evidence gap from populations to the individual.

Appropriate Use of Evidence

Most of the current dialogue is around creating new evidence, rather than how we use the evidence we already have or how we embed it into practice. However, if we did nothing more than consistently use the evidence that already exists, we could significantly improve patient care. Appropriate use of evidence can be addressed in two areas of focus: the individuals involved, namely the patient and the provider, and the tools available, namely decision support tools and reimbursement incentives. There are clear benefits to educating patients with evidence-based health communications. Educated patients are believed to be more likely to strive toward effectively managing their own health—if they are provided meaningful and relevant information. Several obstacles hinder both the effective communication of good evidence to patients and the patients' subsequent action to embed that evidence into creating better health. The sheer volume and sometimes questionable quality of the information can work against us. In translating complex scientific material into usable content for patients, the patient's own medical literacy affects how he or she receives and responds to information, and failure to take cultural or ethnic differences into account may also interfere with effective communication. Finally, people being people, there are behavioral issues related to different beliefs, attitudes, and social milieus. We need to better understand how patient behavior impacts response to evidence-based therapy recommendations in order to create more effective communication paradigms.

As the primary treatment decision makers, physicians are in the best position to embed evidence into clinical practice. The physician-patient dyad is the most important component of the healthcare continuum. While formal physician training provides doctors with a baseline education in effectively treating patients, the evidence base is constantly evolving, and "best practices" can change at an unbelievable pace. As with patients, the sheer volume of information is working against us, as are cultural and behavioral issues. We need to understand how to support continuous, efficient physician learning and how physicians respond to a variety of media. New strategies for how to communicate evidence to the practicing physician are required.

Health information technology (HIT) can enable healthcare professionals to access real-time patient records and compare them to thousands of other patients with similar profiles to determine treatment options with the greatest probability of producing the desired results. Adoption of computerized decision-support systems paired with electronic health records has been shown to improve patient compliance with clinical guidelines. Personal health records may provide a vehicle for patients to own—and understand—their own health status and data. However we need to be cognizant of several issues here as well. The use of HIT to the degree of sophistication at Cleveland Clinic, Intermountain Health, and the Veterans Administration (VA) is not yet widespread. The cost hurdles to embedding the kind of sophistication seen at the major medical centers in small-practice offices and hospitals are significant, and there continue to be issues with standards and vocabularies for information exchange. We also need to be careful about what is embedded in these decision support systems. We need to avoid embedding financially based decision criteria that are counterproductive to good care. The emphasis needs to be on improving the quality of care by gaining intelligence from data gathered from those for whom services and treatments have been delivered.

Probably the most effective way of driving evidence into the system today is to follow the money. Payers have as much if not more power to embed evidence than the physician does. Reimbursement decisions by payers can effectively embed evidence-based practice patterns into clinical practice through decisions to cover or not to cover a product, device, procedure, or service. A payer is often seen as a trusted authority on evidence assessment and thus able to influence physicians' beliefs about best clinical practices. Payers have more resources than individuals and physicians to analyze large volumes of complex and sometimes conflicting information. Yet are the right questions being asked? Are the questions designed to assess treatment impact on health outcome or are they geared toward cost savings only? Were the correct methodologies used? There are both challenges and drawbacks to embedding evidence through reimbursement including provider incentives based on process efficiency rather than outcome of therapy.

Evidence-Based Drug Development

Pharmaceutical manufacturers spend most of their resources developing drugs to help people—an expensive undertaking. One estimate (DiMasi et al. 2003) found that it took an average of $802 million to develop a drug—with another $95 million in post-launch costs. Surveying a group of leaders in research and development (R&D) recently suggested that this number may have increased to $1.4 billion. Adding the costs of doing effectiveness research on top of doing research on efficacy and safety (estimated from internal costs for outcomes and epidemiological trials) may lead to a total between $2 billion and $2.3 billion to develop a new drug. The additive costs of comparative outcomes research extend beyond economics. The larger patient populations required to adequately power these studies significantly increase the resources needed, including logistical and manufacturing issues. The sterile environment of the traditional clinical trial is needed to reduce bias and other confounding elements, but the traditional clinical trial doesn't reflect real-world clinical use. These costs are unsustainable and we are coming to a tipping point rapidly in being able to afford innovation.

One of the things that could change is the way that we develop new medicines: we need new models, and one possibility is a concept of evidence-based drug development—embedding the creation of effectiveness data in addition to efficacy and safety data into the process of drug development rather than as an afterthought. We do drug development episodically today—Phase I, II, III, regulatory approval, and launch. Generating evidence of effectiveness largely occurs in Phase IV if at all. Could we think about changing this episodic process to something that looks very different, a more continuous process of evidence creation generating an ever-increasing databank of safety, efficacy, and effectiveness in partnership with not only the regulators but the payers as well? FDA's critical path, the NIH Roadmap, and CMS's Quality Roadmap are all beginning to align along this need for change, but much remains to be done in the regulatory and reimbursement arenas to generate sufficient financial incentive and drive the change.

Technologically, the development process should leverage information from qualified biomarkers, surrogate markers, and development simulations, in concert with regulatory authorities, prior to first patient exposure. Once available to some patients, use of the evolving EHR systems at major payer and academic medical centers can begin a process of continuous data capture and simulation confirmation in broadening patient numbers. At a point agreed between the innovator, regulator, and possibly the payer there is an initial release where the innovator can begin to recoup investment cost in a proscribed patient base while additional data accumulate until there is a full release of the new therapy. This is a very different way of doing drug development, a concept that drug development never stops, or maybe the learning development system.

It is not possible for any one stakeholder to solve these issues, and if we are going to make evidence-based medicine work for our healthcare system we all need to work together. This includes the pharmaceutical and biotech industry, provider organizations, government agencies, the diagnostic and device companies, payers, and technology providers. As we work through this new world for health care we need to keep the patient in the middle of our dialogue, which must be about putting patient health first.

OPPORTUNITIES FOR STANDARDS ORGANIZATIONS

Margaret E. O'Kane
National Committee for Quality Assurance

Foundational to any exploration of evidence development in health care is a restatement of the central mission of health care: to improve health. In many ways we have moved too far away from this mission and pursued a series of tangential goals that, while important, have led us to lose sight of where we are going. If we are to achieve the mission, healthcare regulators, accreditors, purchasers, consumers, and providers must build their efforts around this larger goal.

Today, the healthcare quality movement is being held hostage to ever-rising costs and the failure to manage evidence effectively. Our current payment system is irrational, wasteful, and inequitable by any measure; as a result, healthcare costs are being driven to the boundaries of society's ability and willingness to pay. Over the last six years, the average cost of health insurance for a family of four Americans has jumped 87 percent, a larger increase than any other sector of our economy (Kaiser Family Foundation 2006). Healthcare costs have eaten into corporate profits and family incomes. Even in 2005, when insurance inflation dropped to 7.7 percent, that increase and the accompanying shift of costs to employees ate up much of the average 3.8 percent rise in Americans' wages (Kaiser Family Foundation 2006). Until we deal with costs, our efforts to improve quality will always take a back seat. Yet we know that these two issues are intricately entwined. Poor-quality care can cost more than high-quality care. If a patient gets the right care at the right time for the conditions that ail her, there will often be less need for more expensive, high-cost treatment of complications in the future. High-quality care also leads to greater productivity on the job and healthier and happier families at home.

Addressing the Evidence Gaps

We need to think in terms of populations. If we really think clearly about how health care affects populations, we will all be better off. In their impressive book *Epidemic of Care*, George Halvorson and George Isham presented us with a visual representation of population-based health that offers a way of thinking about the health of the American public. It reflects the continuum of health of the population of the United States, of a state, of a city, of a community, or even of a health plan. As time goes by, however, some of those people move into "at-risk" or "high-risk" or "early-symptom" categories. This representation has been adapted in Figure 8-1 to illustrate how we need to keep healthy people healthy, and to identify those who are at risk and move them back to the healthy stage through treat-

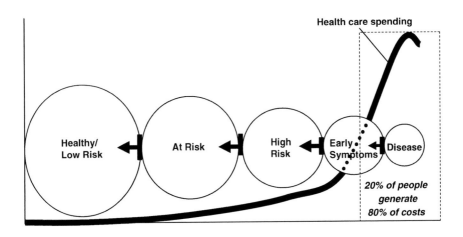

FIGURE 8-1 A value-based healthcare system moves people to the left—and keeps them there.
SOURCE: Essential Guide to Health Care Quality, NCQA 2007.

ment and behavioral modification. As a population moves further toward high risk and active illness, we must give people the appropriate care and support to keep them as healthy as possible. Finally, when people are living with active disease or are at the end of life, we need to help them manage their illness, coordinate their complex care, alleviate their pain, and assist them in dying with dignity. We also know that 80 percent of healthcare dollars are spent on the 20 percent of the population who are in this last stage of health. Sadly, much of that care is of poor quality or unnecessary and neither prolongs nor improves life. If we can reduce the amount of money we spend there—through improved quality in earlier stages and a more rational use of care in the latter stages—not only could we help address our overall cost problems but we could redirect some of that money toward the earlier stages of the continuum that provide a better payback in health for the healthcare dollar.

NCQA has adopted this framework to guide our efforts to accredit health plans and measure the performance of healthcare providers. We have developed a paradigm that holds the plan accountable for the quality of care and service provided to its members. The plans, in turn, often hold providers accountable for delivering care that is evidence-based and of high quality. In the health plan accreditation process, NCQA assesses the performance of health plans in three ways. First, we establish standards for structural and procedural activities meant to ensure patients' rights, appropriate utilization management, quality improvement, customer service, and access to care. Second, we require plans to measure and report on their performance through HEDIS, a set of standardized, evidence-based measures. This unique approach allows us to evaluate how often patients receive the right care at the right time. Finally, we ask patients about their experiences with their health plans and providers. The Consumer Assessment of Health Plans and Providers (CAHPS) examines both a plan's direct administrative performance and members' experience with the delivery system. Together, these three parts combine to form an accreditation program that has become a model for public and private oversight of health care. It is the only accreditation program in health care where performance measurement drives a substantial proportion of the scoring.

Clearly, when one considers the list of HEDIS measures (Table 8-1), there are many important aspects of care that are being measured. It is important to note that for what we measure, there have been notable gains for patients, purchasers, and the health plans that report. NCQA has documented enormous improvements on the issues that it does measure. For example, the use of beta-blockers has increased substantially over the last decade. Health plans are now reporting 95 percent of patients being discharged from the hospital after a heart attack or major cardiac procedure on a beta-blocker, up from 69 percent in 1996 when NCQA began measur-

TABLE 8-1 HEDIS Effectiveness of Care Measures

- Prevention
  - Cancer Screening
    - Breast cancer
    - Cervical cancer
    - Colon cancer
  - Immunizations (Children & Adolescents)
  - Chlamydia screen
  - Antibiotic prescribing
  - Elderly Care
    - Pneumonia vaccination
    - Influenza vaccination
    - Urinary incontinence
    - Vision Screening
    - Advice for physical activity

- Chronic Care Conditions
  - Hypertension
  - Diabetes (6)
  - Cardiovascular Disease
    - Cholesterol test & results
    - Betablocker after AMI
    - Betablocker long-term compliance
  - Smoking cessation
  - Osteoporosis
  - Arthritis
  - Asthma
  - COPD
  - Depression (3)
  - Substance Use (3)
  - Coordination of care psychiatry
  - ADHD
  - Low back pain
  - Safe Medication Management
    - Never medications
    - Appropriate testing

NOTE: ADHD = attention deficit hyperactivity disorder; AMI = acute myocardial infarction; COPD = chronic obstructive pulmonary disease.

ing this (National Committee for Quality Assurance 2006). Children are nearly three times as likely to have had all their recommended immunizations as they were in 1997. Diabetics are twice as likely to have their cholesterol controlled (< 130 mg/dL) as in 1998. These are just a few examples. We are extremely proud of the ground that we broke here because we know that there are people alive and healthier today because of this improvement (Figure 8-2). This transparency and accountability for quality is something really worth promoting—because we know it works. However, there are also many aspects of care that are not being measured, and this is where we need to focus as we move forward.

Despite our progress on accountability, significant barriers remain to robust measurement of performance across the healthcare system. These include the following:

- *The absence of evidence.* Despite tremendous growth in funding of biomedical research in the United States and abroad, there are significant gaps in our evidence base. The process of managing the evidence base toward a return on investment in health can

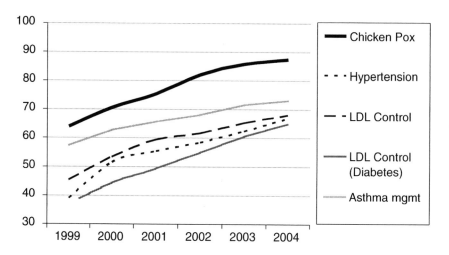

FIGURE 8-2 Selected HEDIS improvements: 1999-2004.

only be described as haphazard. Often research is conducted in areas that are already well understood, while areas that may be clinically important remain uncharted. As a result, in many areas, we simply do not know what constitutes effective care. There are many examples, such as the basic science behind effective treatment for esophageal cancer and the appropriate care for patients with multiple conditions. We lack clinical trial data for the elderly. We do not know about the comparative effectiveness of many treatments so that we cannot evaluate how treatment "A" compares to treatments "B" or "C" in terms of risks, outcomes, and costs. David Eddy has mapped the areas of what we know in diabetes and heart care, and he uses the metaphor "islands of knowledge." We have some islands of knowledge, supported by repetitive and redundant trials, while there remains a vast sea of ignorance that is unexplored. There is a tremendous need to proactively manage the evidence base. The funders of research must make sure that we are being strategic on where we need to develop more evidence. So it isn't just turning research into practice, it is figuring out where there are basic research gaps. The best way to identify priorities would be to look at issues that affect large numbers of patients with a high cost of disease burden and expense and where practice is not solidly evidence based. Issues could be prioritized using quality-adjusted life years per dollar spent. Finally, evidence-based guidelines for patients with a combination of conditions are needed, but randomized clinical trials rarely address more complex patients.

- *The absence of care guidelines.* Even where the evidence exists, there is often a failure to convert it into usable guidelines because we have a significant failure to develop consensus about the evidence. Medical specialty societies develop their own guidelines, often producing conflicting guidelines for the same patients, and this creates a lot of confusion. The model of specialty societies developing their own guidelines without some kind of overall organizing structure needs rethinking. For example, orthopedists, neurosurgeons, and internists disagree on when to do surgery for back pain. As a result, there is no cohesion in approaches or agreement on what is appropriate. We also have some guidelines that do not go far enough. For example, the guidelines for screening for depression or cholesterol levels in the general population do not specify the appropriate intervals. Here again, however, the evidence base that could determine the appropriate guideline has not been adequately marshaled to do so.

- *The lack of or difficulty in obtaining data.* There are also important barriers to getting the data to assess performance. NCQA had to abandon an otitis media measure because health plans were unable to find the data in patients' medical charts. This is true in many other areas.

- *The lack of accountability.* Appearances to the contrary, only a small part of the current healthcare system is being held accountable through quality measurement and reporting. Among health plans, only health maintenance organizations (HMOs) and point of service (POS) plans are called on to report HEDIS. Yet those plans account for only a third of all Americans enrolled in private health plans. Only a handful of preferred provider organizations (PPOs), which cover 64 percent of privately insured Americans, collect and report HEDIS (National Committee for Quality Assurance 2006).

Another significant barrier is the relative absence of performance measurement at the provider level. Some progress has been made in recent years in developing and implementing hospital focused measures. The Joint Commission on Accreditation of Healthcare Organizations, the Leapfrog Group, and the Hospital Quality Alliance have each developed measures that are now in broad use. There has been less progress on the physician side of the ledger. NCQA, working with the American Medical Association and its Physician Consortium for Performance Improvement, has developed physician-level HEDIS measures for certain conditions and has been working in partnership with CMS) to develop additional measures at the specialty level. Much more work needs to be done before we are even close to a system of physician-level accountability.

NCQA has developed a set of programs designed to recognize high-performing physicians in diabetes and heart or stroke care, as well as practices that utilize clinical information systems to improve care across the board. These recognition programs also form the basis for several pay for performance initiatives operating around the United States, including the Bridges to Excellence program sponsored by large employers and the Integrated Healthcare Association program in California that works with large medical groups. NCQA also has been working with a variety of partners to develop a new CAHPS survey for clinician groups.

Measuring at the physician level presents other challenges as well. When it comes to individual doctors, we have a limited, insufficient sample size to assess performance. Yet more than half of American doctors practice in one- or two-member practices. Except for some proceduralists, individual physicians simply do not treat enough patients with a particular condition to draw valid conclusions. We need to recognize these limitations and factor them into our planning and implementation in order to safeguard the integrity of the measurement process.

The advent of electronic health records will help decrease the burden and expense of data collection—but only if we get the right kind of EHRs. The current generation of EHRs leaves much to be desired in terms of their usefulness to improve quality. Partly, this is because processes in health care are often unique to the practice microenvironment and, to some extent, standardized software requires standardized process. Perhaps the biggest potential for EHRs is their theoretical ability to provide customized reminders and warnings for each patient based on specific medical history, diagnoses, and situations. Comprehensive EHRs can also support appropriate decision making, but the current generation of products generally does not have these capabilities. In fact, many current EHRs don't even have the capability of producing performance data after the fact.

How Can We Advance?

If we are to achieve a system that is truly accountable for quality, we must overcome the politics, the warring measures, resource use-cost measures, and political opposition that stand in the way of comprehensive quality assessment. We also need to address issues of appropriateness. Another problem that must be addressed is unclear accountabilities. There needs to be some entity or organization larger than the individual provider that is ultimately responsible for coordinating care across boundaries and practice settings and taking responsibility for at-risk patients after discharge. Once again, the sickest 20 percent of patients account for 80 percent of medical

---

BOX 8-1
Comprehensive evidence management will do the following:

- Identify the gaps
- Encourage priority research areas
- Promote paradigms of continuous learning and evidence development
- Gather patient reported impact/outcomes
- Consider patient preferences

---

costs and there are important opportunities to improve quality and reduce costs with this group.

As we attempt to move practice toward a stronger evidence base, it is crucial that we chart an approach to comprehensive evidence management in order to exercise responsible stewardship for scarce healthcare resources. This will require cooperation across stakeholder groups and specialty and disease organizations, as well as substantial public funding. We need a comprehensive function of evidence management (Box 8-1). This enterprise would identify the gaps, encourage priority research areas, and promote paradigms of continuous learning and evidence development.

In order to have the greatest impact, consider the establishment of an evidence stewardship board to do three things: (1) evaluate the current medical evidence and publish guidelines; (2) identify priority areas for new evidence development; and (3) consider ways to move beyond clinical trials in an era when much more real-time information can be gleaned from practice and used to study what works. Such a board would be analogous to the U.S. Preventive Services Task Force, but covering the broad scope of medical practice.

There are four basic policy enablers and each must play a role to drive systematic improvements in health care (Box 8-2).

First, we must change the way that we pay for health care in this country. Payment reforms such as pay for performance, and other current models, are a good beginning, but they are generally based on fee-for-service payment. With new technology we all know that the old models of care, even some team-based care, are hopelessly inefficient. We must stop providing financial rewards for what we know is inefficient and ineffective medicine. The move to Diagnosis-Related Groups (DRGs) in the early 1980s and the Resource-Based Relative Value Scale (RBRVS) in the early 1990s were significant advances, moving us away from true fee-for-service toward a system that is based more on the average cost of performing a group of

---

BOX 8-2
Policy Enablers Needed:

- Payment reform
- Regulatory reform
- Liability reform
- Patient Activation

---

services. It is time for a new generation of payment reform that utilizes bundled payments with strong incentives for efficient delivery of high-quality care. This kind of payment demands true quality transparency at the same time.

Second, we need regulatory reform. The role of policy makers is to encourage promising new models of care; figure out which ones are taking us toward higher-quality, affordable health care; and then push relentlessly to make the whole delivery system move in that direction. Old and outmoded regulatory requirements need to be dropped as new and more powerful techniques are adopted.

Third, liability reform is also part of the change management process. The current litigious environment is an impediment to good medicine, which requires a special partnership between patients and their healthcare providers. We need to make a new deal with society. We need to modify our practices going forward, and in return, we ask that we have some protection as we seek to improve the delivery system.

Finally, we need real patient activation. It is critical that we recognize that patient-centered health care requires that we do more than make data available or even provide it to patients and expect them to do the right thing. A very important area that needs to be more fully explored is determining the best ways to motivate patients. We need to take a comprehensive look at how both providers and the health system as a whole can help people make healthier choices, without creating dependency or increasing costs. We need to address issues such as health literacy and the need for culturally and linguistically appropriate services in order to communicate with patients in a manner that they understand and that motivates them to make lifestyle changes to improve their health and play an active role in managing their conditions.

At the end of the day, our purpose in quality measurement is not to derive knowledge in order to deliver it back into the same process. We will only maximize the benefits of performance measurement by addressing the structural elements that must be in place for systemic improvement.

We need to find different ways to gather information in the first place; then transformation becomes not only desirable but almost unavoidable. As we explore new models for knowledge development, there are important considerations for how to effectively use them. Also very importantly, regulators, accreditors, and certifiers must work hard to evolve their approaches to accountability to support and encourage and not stifle knowledge development. Old paradigms based on assumed relationships between structure and outcomes need to be either justified or replaced with more evidence-based constructs if regulators, accreditors, and certifiers are to be drivers and enablers of progress rather than impediments to it.

REFERENCES

American National Standards Institute. 2006. *Healthcare IT Standards Panel.* Available from http://www.ansi.org/standards_activities/standards_boards_panels/hisb/hitsp. aspx?menuid=3. (accessed April 4, 2007).

Blumenthal, D. 2006. Employer-sponsored insurance—riding the health care tiger. *New England Journal of Medicine* 355(2):195-202.

DiMasi, J, R Hansen, and H Grabowski. 2003. The price of innovation: new estimates of drug development costs. *Journal of Health Economics* 22(2):151-185.

Kaiser Family Foundation. 2006. *Employer Health Benefits Annual Survey.*

NCQA (National Committee for Quality Assurance). 2006. *State of Health Care Quality Report.*

———. 2007. *Essential Guide to Health Care Quality.*

Newhouse, J. 2004. Consumer-directed health plans and the RAND Health Insurance Experiment. *Health Affairs* 23(6):107-113.

Rawlins, M. 2004. NICE work—providing guidance to the British National Health Service. *New England Journal of Medicine* 351(14):1383-1385.

Rosenthal, M, R Frank, Z Li, and A Epstein. 2005. Early experience with pay-for-performance: from concept to practice. *Journal of the American Medical Association* 294(14):1788-1793.

Appendix
A

Workshop Agenda

THE LEARNING HEALTHCARE SYSTEM

A WORKSHOP OF THE IOM ROUNDTABLE ON EVIDENCE-BASED MEDICINE
THE KECK CENTER OF THE NATIONAL ACADEMIES
WASHINGTON, DC 20001

JULY 20-21, 2006
MEETING AGENDA

OBJECTIVE: To characterize the key features of the Learning Healthcare System, to identify the most important hindrances to its evolution, and to posit some remedies.

DAY 1: THE LEARNING HEALTHCARE SYSTEM

8:30   WELCOME AND OPENING REMARKS

Harvey Fineberg, Institute of Medicine

Darrell Kirch, Association of American Medical Colleges
What would be the features of a healthcare system designed not to learn—how might it be corrected?

9:00   SESSION 1: HINTS OF A DIFFERENT WAY—LEARNING FROM EXPERIENCE
CASE STUDIES IN PRACTICE-BASED EVIDENCE DEVELOPMENT

CHAIR: Carolyn Clancy, Agency for Healthcare Research and Quality (AHRQ) and EBM Roundtable Member
What "best practices" might be spotlighted to illustrate ways to use the health care experience as a practical means of both generating and applying evidence for health care? Are there lessons from certain examples that can help identify the most promising approaches?

15-minute presentations followed by discussion session

    Peter Bach, Centers for Medicare & Medicaid Services (CMS)
        Coverage with evidence development: Lung volume
        reduction surgery

    Jed Weissberg, Permanente Federation
        Use of large system databases: Cyclooxygenase-2 (COX-2)
        inhibitors

    Stephen Soumerai, Harvard Pilgrim Health Care
        Potential of quasi-experimental designs for evaluating
        health policy

    Sean Tunis, Health Technology Center
        Practical clinical trials

    Alan Morris, Latter Day Saints Hospital and University of Utah
        Computerized protocols to assist clinical research*

10:30   SESSION 2: THE EVOLVING EVIDENCE BASE—METHODOLOGIC AND POLICY CHALLENGES

CHAIR: Don Steinwachs, Johns Hopkins University and EBM Roundtable Member
What challenges confront methodologically rigorous learning from experience? How can alternatives to randomized controlled trials (RCTs) and innovative approaches to generating evidence be used to confront emerging challenges: broader post-marketing surveillance; linking Phase III and coverage requirements; increasingly complex patterns of comorbidity; subgroup analysis, and heterogeneity in treatment outcomes? How might learning that is more nimble also foster innovation and discovery?
15-minute presentations followed by discussion session

    Robert Califf, Duke Clinical Research Institute
        Alternatives to large RCTs

    David Goldstein, Duke Institute for Genome Sciences and Policy
        Engaging the implications of subgroup heterogeneity—
        prospects for pharmacogenetics

    Harlan Weisman, Johnson & Johnson
        Broader post-marketing surveillance for insights on risk and
        effectiveness

    Telba Irony, Food and Drug Administration (FDA)
        Evaluating interventions in a rapid state of flux

    David Eddy, Archimedes Inc.
        Mathematical models to fill the gaps in evidence*

Sheldon Greenfield, University of California at Irvine
    Heterogeneity of treatment effects: subgroup analysis*
Steve Teutsch, Merck & Co. Inc.
    Adjusting evidence generation to the scale of effects*
Janlori Goldman, Health Privacy Project
    Protecting privacy while linking patient records*

12:00   Lunch

1:00   SESSION 3: NARROWING THE RESEARCH-PRACTICE DIVIDE—SYSTEM
        CONSIDERATIONS

        CHAIR: Cato Laurencin, University of Virginia and EBM
        Roundtable Member
        What system changes are needed for the healthcare delivery
        environment to facilitate the generation and application of better
        evidence? What are the needs and implications for structuring
        "built-in" study designs, managing the data burden, and defining
        appropriate levels of evidence needed? What is needed to turn
        clinical data into an "epidemiologic utility," a public good?
        15-minute presentations followed by discussion session
            Brent James, Intermountain Healthcare
                Feedback loops to expedite study timeliness and relevance
            Walter Stewart, Geisinger Health System
                Clinical data system structure and management for better
                learning
            Steven Pearson, America's Health Insurance Plans
                Implications for standards of evidence
            Robert Galvin, General Electric
                Implications for innovation acceleration

2:30   SESSION 4: PANEL DISCUSSION—KEY BARRIERS AND PRIORITIES FOR
        ACTION
        CHAIR: Denis Cortese, Mayo Clinic and EBM Roundtable
        Member
        Members of the Roundtable on Evidence-Based Medicine

DAY 2: ACCELERATING THE PROGRESS

8:30   OPENING REMARKS

Denis Cortese, Mayo Clinic and EBM Roundtable Chair
What are some of the key challenges and opportunities if the
development of a sustainable capacity for real-time learning is to
be accelerated?

9:00   SESSION 5: HINTS OF A DIFFERENT WAY—LEARNING SYSTEMS IN
PROGRESS

CHAIR: Jonathan Perlin, Department of Veterans Affairs and
EBM Roundtable Member
What experiences of healthcare systems highlight the
opportunities and challenges in integrating the generation and
application of evidence for improved care? What's needed to take
to scale?
15-minute presentations followed by discussion session
  Joel Kupersmith, Veterans Health Administration
    Implementation of evidence-based practice in the Veterans
    Administration
  George Isham, HealthPartners
    AQA (Ambulatory Care Quality Alliance)
  Robert Phillips, Robert Graham Center
    Practice-Based Research Networks
  Lynn Etheredge, George Washington University
    A rapid learning health system

10:30   SESSION 6: DEVELOPING THE TEST BED: LINKING INTEGRATED DELIVERY
SYSTEMS

CHAIR: Helen Darling, National Business Group on Health and
EBM Roundtable Member
How can integrated healthcare delivery systems be better engaged
for structured real-time learning? How can the organizational,
logistical, data system, reimbursement and regulatory issues be
addressed?
15-minute presentations followed by discussion session
  Stephen Katz, National Institutes of Health (NIH)
    NIH Roadmap initiatives use of integrated delivery systems
  Cynthia Palmer, Agency for Healthcare Research and Quality
    Turning research to ACTION through delivery systems

       Eric Larson, Group Health Cooperative
          Health Maintenance Organization Research Network
          (HMORN)
       Michael Mustille, Permanente Federation
          Council of Accountable Physician Practices

12:00   LUNCH

12:30   SESSION 7: THE PATIENT AS A CATALYST FOR CHANGE

       CHAIR: **Andrew Stern, Service Employees International Union and EBM Roundtable Member**
       What is the changing role of the patient in an age of the Internet and the personal health record? Reengineering a system focused on patient needs and built around best care requires improved communication of evidence. How does patient preference fit into evidence development?
       15-minute presentations followed by discussion session
          Janet Marchibroda, eHealth Initiative
             The Internet, eHealth, and patient empowerment
          Andrew Barbash, Apractis Solutions
             Joint patient-provider management of the electronic health record (EHR)
          James Weinstein, Dartmouth-Hitchcock Medical Center
             Evidence and shared decision making

1:35   SESSION 8: TRAINING THE LEARNING HEALTH PROFESSIONAL

       CHAIR: **Nancy Nielsen, American Medical Association and EBM Roundtable Member**
       What are the educational needs for the health professional in the Learning Healthcare System? How must qualification exams and continuing education be adjusted? What approaches can bring the processes of learning and application into seamless alignment?
       15-minute presentations followed by discussion session
          Mary Mundinger, Columbia University School of Nursing
             Health professions education and teaching about evidence
          William Stead, Vanderbilt University
             Providers and the electronic health record as a learning tool
          Mark Williams, Emory University School of Medicine
             Redefining continuing education around evolving evidence

2:40   SESSION 9: STRUCTURING THE INCENTIVES FOR CHANGE

CHAIR: **John Rother, AARP and EBM Roundtable Member**
What policies can provide the incentives for the developments
necessary to build learning—evidence development *and*
application—into every healthcare encounter?
15-minute presentations followed by discussion session
    Alan Rosenberg, WellPoint
       Opportunities for private insurers
    Steve Phurrough, Centers for Medicare and Medicaid Services
       Opportunities for CMS
    Wayne Rosencrans, Jr., AstraZeneca
       Opportunities for manufacturers
    Margaret O'Kane, National Care Quality Alliance
       Opportunities for standards organizations

4:00   CONCLUDING SUMMARY REMARKS

Denis Cortese, Mayo Clinic and EBM Roundtable Chair
J. Michael McGinnis, Institute of Medicine

4:30   ADJOURN

*Presentation included in workshop materials, but not delivered.

Appendix
B

Biographical Sketches of Participants

Peter B. Bach, M.D., M.A.P.P., joined the Centers for Medicare and Medicaid Services (CMS) as a senior adviser to the administrator in February 2005. Dr. Bach's work at CMS focuses on improving evidence about the effect of therapies and devices, and revising payment to enhance care quality. He also is the agency lead on cancer policy. Dr. Bach is board certified in internal medicine, pulmonary medicine, and critical care medicine and is an associate attending physician at Memorial Sloan-Kettering Cancer Center in New York. He is a National Institutes of Health (NIH) funded researcher with expertise in quality of care and epidemiologic research methods. His research on health disparities, variations in healthcare quality, and lung cancer epidemiology has appeared in the *New England Journal of Medicine*, the *Journal of the American Medical Association*, and the *Journal of the National Cancer Institute*. During the Rwandan Civil War, he was a camp physician in Goma, Zaire, caring for refugees. Dr. Bach received his bachelor's degree in English and American literature from Harvard College, his M.D. from the University of Minnesota, and his master of arts degree in public policy from the University of Chicago, where he was also a Robert Wood Johnson clinical scholar. He completed his clinical training in internal medicine and pulmonary and critical care at the Johns Hopkins Hospital.

Andrew Barbash, M.D., is the chief executive officer (CEO) of Apractis Solutions, LLC, Collaboration Partners. He is also a practicing neurologist and the medical director of the Holy Cross Hospital Stroke Care Program in Maryland. He was a vice president and member of the senior management of the Medical Group for Kaiser Permanente of the Mid-Atlantic states until 2001, where he managed the development and deployment of the electronic medical record for that region. He has been very active in the e-health, mobile health, and personal health records arena and has served on national-level workgroups related to consumer information empowerment and e-health. He was a member of the Task Force on Information Capture in 2001 and is also leading the Personal Medication Records project in the SOS Rx initiative, sponsored by the National Consumers League. In 2003-2004 he was actively engaged with the Medical Records Institute relative to mobile computing and the TEPR (Towards the Electronic Patient Record) awards. He is also very active in Health Tech Net, a Washington area consortium of health technology participants. He completed his B.A. at Bowdoin College, his M.D. at Northwestern University, and his neurology residency at the Mayo Clinic.

Marc L. Berger, M.D., is vice president for Outcomes Research and Management in the U.S. Human Health Division at Merck & Co., Inc While at Merck, Dr. Berger has held various positions of responsibility for Phase II to Phase IV clinical trials, outcomes research studies, and disease management programs. His current research interests include health-related productivity, cost-effectiveness analysis, and the value of pharmaceutical innovation. He was recently invited to serve on the CMS Medicare Coverage Advisory Committee. He also serves on advisory boards for the Health Industry Forum and the Program on the Economic Evaluation of Medical Technology (PEEMT) at the Harvard Center for Risk Analysis, as well as for the journal *Value in Health*. He holds appointments as adjunct senior fellow at the Leonard David Institute of Health Economics at the University of Pennsylvania and adjunct professor in the Department of Health Policy and Administration at the University of North Carolina at Chapel Hill School of Public Health. Prior to joining Merck, he was on the faculty of the University of Cincinnati School of Medicine. Dr. Berger obtained his M.D. from Johns Hopkins University School of Medicine. He completed an internal medicine residency at New York University-Bellevue Hospital and a Liver Research Fellowship at the University of Texas Southwestern Medical School.

Robert M. Califf, M.D., is vice chancellor for clinical research, director of the Duke Clinical Research Institute (DCRI), and professor of medicine in the division of cardiology at Duke University Medical Center. He is board certified in internal medicine and cardiology and is a fellow of the American College of Cardiology. Author or coauthor of more than 600 peer-reviewed journal articles, as well as major textbooks on cardiovascular disease, Dr. Califf has also served on the Cardiorenal Advisory Panel of the U.S. Food and Drug Administration (FDA) and the Pharmaceutical Roundtable of the Institute of Medicine (IOM). He is director of the coordinating center for the Centers for Education and Research on Therapeutics (CERTs), a public-private partnership among the Agency for Healthcare Research and Quality, the DCRI, academia, the medical products industry, and consumer groups focused on research and education that strives to advance the best use of medical products. Dr. Califf graduated from Duke University in 1973 summa cum laude and Phi Beta Kappa and from Duke University Medical School in 1978, where he was selected for Alpha Omega Alpha. He completed his internship and residency at the University of California at San Francisco and his fellowship in cardiology at Duke University.

Carolyn M. Clancy, M.D., is director of the Agency for Healthcare Research and Quality (AHRQ). Prior to 2002 she was director of AHRQ's Center for Outcomes and Effectiveness Research (COER). Her major research interests include various dimensions of healthcare quality and patients', including women's health, primary care, access to care services, and the impact of financial incentives on physicians' decisions. Prior to joining AHRQ in 1990, she was an assistant professor in the Department of Internal Medicine at the Medical College of Virginia in Richmond. Dr. Clancy holds an academic appointment at George Washington University School of Medicine (clinical associate professor, Department of Medicine), is the senior associate editor of *Health Services Research,* and serves on multiple editorial boards. Dr. Clancy has published widely in peer-reviewed journals and has edited or contributed to seven books. She is a member of the Institute of Medicine and was elected a master of the American College of Physicians in 2004. Dr. Clancy, a general internist and health services researcher, is a graduate of Boston College and the University of Massachusetts Medical School. Following clinical training in internal medicine, Dr. Clancy was a Henry J. Kaiser Family Foundation fellow at the University of Pennsylvania.

Denis A. Cortese, M.D., is president and CEO at Mayo Clinic and chair of the Executive Committee. He is a member of the Board of Trustees and is a professor of medicine at Mayo Clinic College of Medicine. He is a director and former president of the International Photodynamic Association and has been involved in the bronchoscopic detection, localization, and treatment of early-stage lung cancer. He is a member of the Healthcare Leadership Council and the Harvard-Kennedy School Healthcare Policy Group, and a former member of the Center for Corporate Innovation. He also is a charter member of the Advisory Board of World Community Grid and a founding member of the American Medical Group Association Chairs-Presidents-CEOs Council. Following service in the U.S. Naval Corps, he joined the staff of Mayo Clinic in Rochester, Minnesota, as a specialist in pulmonary medicine. He was a member of the Board of Governors in Rochester before moving to Mayo Clinic in Jacksonville, Florida. He has served as chair of the Board of Governors at Mayo Clinic and chair of the Board of Directors at St. Luke's Hospital in Jacksonville, Florida. He also served on the Steering Committee for the RAND Ix Project, "Using Information Technology to Create a New Future in Healthcare," and the Principals Committee of the National Innovation Initiative. Dr. Cortese is a graduate of Temple University and completed his residency at the Mayo Graduate School of Medicine. Dr. Cortese is a member of the IOM, a Fellow of the Royal College of Physicians in England, and an honorary member of the Academia Nacional de Mexicana (Mexico).

Helen Darling is president of the National Business Group on Health (formerly Washington Business Group on Health). Ms. Darling also currently serves as co-chair of the Committee on Performance Measurement of the National Committee for Quality Assurance. She is a member of the Medical Advisory Panel, Technology Evaluation Center, run by the Blue Cross Blue Shield Association; the IOM Board on Health Promotion and Disease Prevention; the Cancer Care Measures Steering Committee of the National Quality Forum; the Board of the VHA (Veterans Health Administration) Health Foundation, along with a number of other advisory and editorial boards. From 1992 through 1998, Ms. Darling directed the purchasing of health benefits and disability for Xerox Corporation and was previously a principal at William W. Mercer. Earlier in her career, Ms. Darling was an adviser to Senator David Durenberger, the ranking Republican on the Health Subcommittee of the Senate Finance Committee. Ms. Darling received a master's degree in demography-sociology and a bachelor of science degree in history-English, cum laude, from the University of Memphis.

David M. Eddy, M.D., Ph.D., is the director of Archimedes and is responsible for the medical development of the model. David started his career as a professor of engineering and medicine at Stanford, and the J. Alexander McMahon Professor of Health Policy and Management at Duke University. David received his M.D. from the University of Virginia and his Ph.D. in engineering-economic systems (applied mathematics) from Stanford. More than 25 years ago, David wrote the seminal paper on the role of guidelines in medical decision making, the first Markov model applied to clinical problems, and the original criteria for coverage decisions; he was the first to use and publish the term *evidence-based*. David is the author of five books, more than 100 first-authored articles, and a series of essays for the *Journal of the American Medical Association*. His writings range from technical mathematical theories to broad health policy topics. David has received top national and international awards in fields including applied mathematics, health technology assessment, healthcare quality, and outcomes research. He has been elected or appointed to more than 40 national and international boards and commissions, including Consumers Union, the National Board of Mathematics, the World Health Organization Panel of Experts, the Blue Cross Blue Shield Medical Advisory Panel, and the National Committee for Quality Assurance, and is a member of the Institute of Medicine of the National Academy of Sciences.

Lynn Etheredge is an independent consultant working on health care and social policy issues. His career started at the White House Office of Management and Budget (OMB). During the Nixon and Ford administrations, he was OMB's principal analyst for Medicare and Medicaid and led its staff work on national health insurance proposals. He returned to OMB as a senior career executive and headed its professional health staff in the Carter and Reagan administrations. He was a coauthor of the Jackson Hole Group's proposals for healthcare reform and a founding member of the National Academy of Social Insurance. During the last several years, Lynn has authored policy studies about Medicaid's future, Medicare reforms, evidence-based health care, and expanding health insurance coverage. His current projects include a "Medicaid + tax credits" model for expanding coverage and a national rapid learning system for evidence-based health care. He is author of more than 70 publications and is a graduate of Swarthmore College.

Harvey Fineberg, M.D., Ph.D., is president of the Institute of Medicine. He served as provost of Harvard University from 1997 to 2001, following 13 years as dean of the Harvard School of Public Health. He has devoted most of his academic career to the fields of health policy and medical decision making. His past research has focused on the process of policy development and implementation, assessment of medical technology, evaluation and use of vaccines, and dissemination of medical innovations. Dr. Fineberg helped found and served as president of the Society for Medical Decision Making and also served as consultant to the World Health Organization. At IOM he has chaired and served on a number of panels dealing with health policy issues, ranging from AIDS to new medical technology. He also served as a member of the Public Health Council of Massachusetts (1976-1979), chairman of the Health Care Technology Study Section of the National Center for Health Services Research (1982-1985), and president of the Association of Schools of Public Health (1995-1996). Dr. Fineberg is coauthor of the books *Clinical Decision Analysis, Innovators in Physician Education,* and *The Epidemic That Never Was,* an analysis of the controversial federal immunization program against swine flu in 1976. He has coedited several books on such diverse topics as AIDS prevention, vaccine safety, and understanding risk in society. He has also authored numerous articles published in professional journals. In 1988, he received the Joseph W. Mountain Prize from the Centers for Disease Control and Prevention (CDC) and the Wade Hampton Frost Prize from the Epidemiology Section of the American Public Health Association (APHA). Dr. Fineberg earned his bachelor's and doctoral degrees from Harvard University.

Robert Galvin, M.D., is director of global health care for General Electric (GE). He oversees the design and performance of GE's health programs, which total more than $3 billion annually, and is responsible for GE's medical services, encompassing over 220 medical clinics in more than 20 countries. In his current role, he focuses on issues of market-based health policy and financing, with a special interest in quality measurement and improvement. He has been a leader in pushing for public release of performance information and reform of the payment system. He was a member of the Strategic Framework Board of the National Quality Forum and is on the board of NCQA. He is a founder of both the Leapfrog Group and Bridges to Excellence. He is also a member of the Advisory Board of the Council of Health Care Economics and the IOM Committee on Redesigning Health Insurance Benefits, Payments and Performance Improvement Programs. Adjunct professor of medicine and health policy at Yale, he is also a fellow of the American College of Physicians and has published in various journals, including the *New England Journal of Medicine* and *Health Affairs.* Dr. Galvin completed his undergraduate work at the University of Pennsylvania, where he graduated magna cum laude and Phi Beta Kappa. He received his M.D. from the University of Pennsylvania and was elected to Alpha Omega Alpha. He received an M.B.A. in healthcare management from Boston University School of Management.

Janlori Goldman, J.D., is director of the Health Privacy Project and research faculty at the Center on Medicine as a Profession at Columbia University. She specializes in privacy and confidentiality issues within the physician-patient relationship, and her areas of expertise include the Health Insurance Portability and Accountability Act (HIPAA) privacy regulation, public health and bioterrorism, and e-health initiatives. She also directs the Health Privacy Project, based in Washington, D.C., which she founded after a year as a visiting scholar at Georgetown University Law Center. Ms. Goldman co-founded the Center for Democracy and Technology, a nonprofit civil liberties organization committed to preserving free speech and privacy on the Internet. She was the staff attorney and director of the Privacy and Technology Project of the American Civil Liberties Union (ACLU). Her efforts at the ACLU led to the enactment of the Video Privacy Protection Act, and she also led initiatives to protect people's health, credit, financial, and personal information held by the government. Her publications include "Bioterrorism, Public Health and Privacy," included in the publication *Lost Liberties: Ashcroft and the Assault on Personal Freedom*; two articles in *Health Affairs:* "Virtually Exposed: Privacy and E-Health," coauthored with Zoe Hudson, and "Protecting Privacy to Improve Health Care"; and "A Federal Right of Information Privacy," coauthored with Jerry Berman and included as a chapter in *Computers, Ethics, and Social Values.*

David Goldstein, Ph.D., is visiting professor of molecular genetics and microbiology and has been director of the Institute for Genome Sciences and Policy (IGSP) Center for Population Genomics and Pharmacogenetics since June 2005. Dr. Goldstein's principal interests include human genetic diversity, the genetics of neurological disease, and pharmacogenetics. He is the author of more than 75 scholarly publications in the areas of population and medical genetics. He is on the editorial boards of *Current Biology*, *Annals of Human Genetics*, *Molecular Biology and Evolution*, and *Human Genomics*. He is the recipient of one of the first seven nationally awarded Royal Society-Wolfson Research Merit Awards in the United Kingdom for his work in human population genetics. Dr. Goldstein received his Ph.D. in biological sciences from Stanford University in 1994, and from 1999 to 2005 was Wolfson Professor of Genetics at University College London.

Sheldon Greenfield, M.D., is director of the Center for Health Policy Research and professor in the Department of Medicine at the University of California (UCLA), Irvine College of Medicine. Previously, Dr. Greenfield was director of the Primary Care Outcomes Research Institute at New England Medical Center and Tufts University School of Medicine. Dr. Greenfield was associated with the UCLA Schools of Medicine and Public Health and the Rand Corporation in California, including the position of co-director of the Joint RAND-UCLA Center for Health Policy Study. He has pioneered research in increasing patients' participation in care and using outcomes to determine the value of that participation. Beginning in 1984, Dr. Greenfield served as the medical director of the Medical Outcomes Study, which sought to compare systems of care, specialties, various aspects of interpersonal care, and resource use to outcome. Dr. Greenfield was principal investigator (PI) of the Type 2 Diabetes Patient Outcome Research Team, and is chairman of the Diabetes Quality Improvement Program, a joint venture of the Health Care Financing Administration (HCFA), NCQA, and the American Diabetes Association (ADA). He is currently serving as chair of the National Diabetes Quality Alliance. He is also former president of the Society of General Internal Medicine and was chairman of the Health Care Technology Study Section for the Agency for Health Care Policy and Research (now AHRQ). Dr. Greenfield earned an A.B. from Harvard College and an

M.D. from the University of Cincinnati College of Medicine. He completed his residency and a fellowship in infectious disease at Beth Israel Hospital, Boston, Massachusetts.

Telba Irony, Ph.D., is chief of the General and Surgical Devices Branch in the Division of Biostatistics at the Center for Devices and Radiological Health (CDRH) of the FDA. She received her Ph.D. from the University of California at Berkeley in 1990 where she worked with applications of Bayesian Statistics. She was on the faculty of the George Washington University, Engineering School, from 1990 to 1998, when she joined the CDRH in order to help implement the use of Bayesian methodology in medical device clinical trials. She worked in several projects of applications of Bayesian statistics sponsored by the National Science Foundation (NSF) and produced more than 30 articles that were published in statistical journals.

George Isham, M.D., M.S., is medical director and chief health officer for HealthPartners. He is responsible for quality, utilization management, health promotion and disease prevention, research, and health professionals' education at HealthPartners, a consumer-governed Minnesota health plan representing nearly 800,000 members. Before his current position, Dr. Isham was medical director of MedCenters Health Plan in Minneapolis. In the late 1980s, he was executive director of University Health Care, an organization affiliated with the University of Wisconsin, Madison. Dr. Isham received his master of science in preventive medicine and administrative medicine at the University of Wisconsin, Madison; he received his M.D. from the University of Illinois; and he completed his internship and residency in internal medicine at the University of Wisconsin Hospital and Clinics in Madison. His practice experience as a primary care physician included eight years at the Freeport Clinic in Freeport, Illinois, and three and one-half years as clinical assistant professor in medicine at the University of Wisconsin.

Brent C. James, M.D., M.Stat., is executive director of the Institute for Health Care Delivery Research and vice president of Medical Research and Continuing Medical Education at Intermountain Healthcare. Based in Salt Lake City, Utah, Intermountain Healthcare is an integrated system of 23 hospitals, almost 100 clinics, a 450+ member physician group, and an HMO-PPO (health maintenance organization-preferred provider organization) insurance plan jointly responsible for more than 450,000 covered lives. Brent James is known internationally for his work in clinical quality improvement, patient safety, and the infrastructure that underlies successful improvement efforts, such as culture change, data systems, payment methods, and management roles. Before coming to Intermountain, he was an assistant professor in the Department of Biostatistics at the Harvard

School of Public Health, providing statistical support for the Eastern Cooperative Oncology Group, and staffed the American College of Surgeons' Commission on Cancer. He holds faculty appointments at the University of Utah School of Medicine, Harvard School of Public Health, Tulane University School of Public Health and Tropical Medicine, and University of Sydney, Australia, School of Public Health. He is also a member of the Institute of Medicine of the National Academy of Sciences.. Dr. James holds bachelor of science degrees in computer science (electrical engineering) and medical biology, an M.D., and a master of statistics degree from the University of Utah; he completed residency training in general surgery and oncology.

Stephen I. Katz, M.D., Ph.D., has been director of the National Institute of Arthritis and Musculoskeletal and Skin Diseases (NIAMSD) since August 1995 and is also a senior investigator in the Dermatology Branch of the National Cancer Institute (NCI). Dr. Katz has focused his studies on immunology and the skin. His research has demonstrated that skin is an important component of the immune system both in its normal function and as a target in immunologically mediated disease. In addition to studying Langerhans cells and epidermally derived cytokines, Dr. Katz and his colleagues have added considerable new knowledge about inherited and acquired blistering skin diseases. He also has served many professional societies, including as a member of the Board of Directors and president of the Society for Investigative Dermatology, on the Board of the Association of Professors of Dermatology, as secretary-general of the 18th World Congress of Dermatology in New York in 1992, as secretary-treasurer of the Clinical Immunology Society, and as president of both the International League of Dermatological Societies and the International Committee of Dermatology. Dr. Katz has twice received the Meritorious Rank Award and has also received the Distinguished Executive Presidential Rank Award, the highest honor that can be bestowed upon a civil servant. He earned a B.A. in history from the University of Maryland, an M.D. from Tulane University Medical School, and a Ph.D. in immunology from the University of London, England. He completed a medical internship at Los Angeles County Hospital and a residency in dermatology at the University of Miami School of Medicine, Florida.

Darrell G. Kirch, M.D., is president and chief executive officer of the Association of American Medical Colleges (AAMC), a position he assumed on July 1, 2006. Dr. Kirch's career spans all aspects of academic medicine and includes leadership positions at two medical schools and teaching hospitals, as well as at the National Institutes of Health. Before becoming the AAMC's fourth president, Dr. Kirch was selected to be chair-elect of the association, and served as co-chair of the Liaison Committee on Medical

Education and as a member-at-large of the National Board of Medical Examiners. He also has served as chair of the AAMC's Council of Deans Administrative Board and as chair of the American Medical Association (AMA) Section on Medical Schools. Dr. Kirch comes to the AAMC after six years as senior vice president for health affairs, dean of the College of Medicine, and CEO of the Milton S. Hershey Medical Center at the Pennsylvania State University, where he and his leadership team are credited with revitalizing the institution and guiding it through a period of major expansion. Dr. Kirch held a number of leadership positions at the Medical College of Georgia, including dean of the medical school, senior vice president for clinical activities, and dean of the School of Graduate Studies. As a psychiatrist and clinical neuroscientist, Dr. Kirch is a leading expert on the biological basis of and treatments for severe neuropsychiatric disorders. Following the completion of his residency training at the University of Colorado Health Sciences Center, he joined the National Institute of Mental Health, in Bethesda, Maryland, where he was named acting scientific director in 1993. Dr. Kirch is an active member of several professional societies, including the American College of Psychiatrists, the AMA, and the American Psychiatric Association. Dr. Kirch received both his B.A. and his M.D. from the University of Colorado.

Joel Kupersmith, M.D., is chief research and development officer of the Veterans Health Administration. He has completed projects and published papers on a number of health and research policy areas including how to fund, oversee, and promote effectiveness research; how academic medical centers should be accountable; quality of care in teaching hospitals; regional institutional review boards (IRBs); medical manpower; and other issues. Following his early research on cardiac rhythm abnormalities and implantable cardiac defibrillators, he published in the area of cost-effectiveness of heart disease treatments and outcomes following heart attacks. He is widely published, with at least 150 publications and two books, and has been on the editorial boards of numerous journals, including the *American Journal of Medicine*. Prior to joining the VHA, Dr. Kupersmith held faculty positions at the Mt. Sinai School of Medicine, University of Louisville, and the College of Human Medicine at Michigan State University. He served as dean of the School of Medicine and Graduate School of Biomedical Sciences and vice president for clinical affairs at Texas Tech University. He was a scholar-in-residence at both the IOM and the AAMC and a visiting scholar at the Hastings Center for Ethics and is a member of numerous professional organizations. Dr. Kupersmith is a winner of an Affirmative Action Award from the University of Louisville and an Alumni Association distinguished achievement award from New York Medical College. Dr. Kupersmith was elected to the Governing Council, Medical School Section of the AMA, is a member of the AAMC Task Force on Fraud and Abuse, and has been a site visit chair for the Liaison Committee on Medical Education. Dr. Kupersmith earned his M.D. from New York Medical College, where he also completed residency in internal medicine, and completed a cardiology fellowship at Beth Israel Medical Center-Harvard Medical School.

Eric B. Larson, M.D., M.P.H., M.A.C.P., is director of Group Health Co-operative's Center for Health Studies. His research spans a range of general medicine topics and has focused on aging and dementia topics, including a long running study of aging and cognitive change set in Group Health Cooperative: the UW-Group Health Alzheimer's Disease Patient Registry-Adult Changes in Thought Study. He has served as president of the Society of General Internal Medicine, chair of the Office of Technology Assessment-Department of Health and Human Services (HHS) Advisory Panel on Alzheimer's Disease and Related Disorders and was chair of the Board of Regents (2004-2005), American College of Physicians. He is currently PI on an NIH Roadmap project to expand existing clinical research networks: The Coordinated Clinical Studies Network of the HMO Research Network (HMORN). He also served as medical director of University of Washington Medical Center and associate dean for clinical affairs from 1989 to 2002. A graduate of Harvard Medical School, he trained in internal medicine at Beth Israel Hospital, completed a Robert Wood Johnson Clinical Scholars and M.P.H. program at the University of Washington, and then served as chief resident of University Hospital in Seattle.

Cato T. Laurencin, M.D., Ph.D., is the Lillian T. Pratt Professor and Chair of Orthopaedic Surgery, university professor, and professor of biomedical engineering and chemical engineering at the University of Virginia and an IOM member. The focus of Dr. Laurencin's research is novel methods for bone and musculoskeletal tissue engineering and polymeric systems for drug delivery. Prior to his appointment at Virginia University's Department of Biomedical Engineering, he was at Drexel University as the Helen I. Moorehead Professor of Chemical Engineering, and clinical associate professor of orthopaedic surgery at the Medical College of Pennsylvania and Hahnemann University School of Medicine, working with the team physicians for the New York Mets and St. John's University. Dr. Laurencin earned his B.S.E. in chemical engineering from Princeton University and went on to a Ph.D. in biochemical engineering-biotechnology from the Massachusetts Institute of Technology (MIT). In parallel with his research training, Dr. Laurencin attended the Harvard Medical School, graduating magna cum laude. While directing his laboratory at MIT, Dr. Laurencin undertook clinical residency training in orthopaedic surgery at Harvard and served as chief resident in orthopaedic surgery at Beth Israel Hospital,

Harvard Medical School; he subsequently completed fellowship training in shoulder surgery and sports medicine at the Hospital for Special Surgery in New York, Cornell University.

Janet M. Marchibroda is the CEO of the eHealth Initiative, a Washington, D.C.-based national multistakeholder nonprofit organization whose mission is to improve the quality, safety, and cost-effectiveness of health care through information technology. Ms. Marchibroda has a particular interest in issues related to the improvement of quality in health care. Prior to the eHealth Initiative, Ms. Marchibroda co-founded and served as a senior executive for two healthcare information companies, one that focuses on providing patient safety and compliance information to physicians and the other—a Bertelsmann AG subsidiary—that focuses on providing electronic publishing services to the managed care industry to better meet member information needs. Ms. Marchibroda has also served as the CEO of the NCQA, where she was responsible for accreditation, certification, education, the national HEDIS (Health Plan Employer data and Information Set) database, report cards and electronic information products, and other publications. She holds a B.S. in commerce from the University of Virginia and an M.B.A. with a concentration in organization development from George Washington University.

J. Michael McGinnis, M.D., M.P.P., is senior scholar at the Institute of Medicine. From 1999 to 2005, he served as senior vice president and founding director of the Health Group, and as counselor to the president, at the Robert Wood Johnson Foundation (RWJF), and from 1977 to 1995, he held continuous appointment as assistant surgeon general, deputy assistant secretary for health, and founding director, Disease Prevention and Health Promotion, through the Carter, Reagan, Bush, and Clinton administrations. Programs and policies launched at his initiative include the Healthy People process on national health objectives, now in its third decade; the U.S. Preventive Services Task Force; the *Dietary Guidelines for Americans* (with the U.S. Department of Agriculture [USDA]), now in its sixth edition; the RWJF Health and Society Scholars Program; the RWJF Young Epidemiology Scholars Program; and the RWJF Active Living family of programs. International service includes appointments as chair of the World Bank-European Commission Task Force reconstruction of the health sector in Bosnia (1995-1996); and state coordinator for the World Health Organization smallpox eradication program in Uttar Pradesh, India (1974-1975). He is an elected member of the IOM, fellow of the American College of Epidemiology, and fellow of the American College of Preventive Medicine. Recent board memberships include the Nemours Foundation Board of Directors, the IOM Committee on Children's Food Marketing (chair); the NIH State-of-the-Science Panel on Multivitamins in Chronic Disease Prevention (chair); the Health Professionals Roundtable on Preventive Services (chair); the FDA Food Advisory Committee, Subcommittee on Nutrition; and the Board of the United Way of the National Capital Area (chair, resource development).

Alan H. Morris, M.D., is professor of medicine and adjunct professor of medical informatics at the University of Utah, and director of research and associate medical director of the Pulmonary Function and Blood Gas Laboratories at the LDS Hospital. He has experience in the conduct of acute respiratory distress syndrome (ARDS) multicenter randomized clinical trials of treatments, including innovative therapies, for ARDS patients. He is PI of the 4-Hospital Utah Critical Care Treatment Group (CCTG) of the NIH-NHLBI (National Heart, Lung, and Blood Institute) ARDS Network for clinical trials and has directed this group since 1994. This 4-Hospital group includes the LDS, Cottonwood, McKay Dee, and Utah Valley Regional Medical Center Hospitals. He is also PI for the NIH-NHLBI Reengineering Clinical Research in Critical Care contract.

Mary O'Neil Mundinger, Dr.P.H., R.N., is the Centennial Professor in Health Policy and dean of the Columbia University School of Nursing. A noted health policy expert, primarily known for her work on workforce issues and primary care and author of *Home Care Controversy: Too Little, Too Late, Too Costly* (1983) and *Autonomy in Nursing* (1980), she has led Columbia's nursing school since 1986. Dr. Mundinger served as a member of the Commonwealth Fund Commission on Women's Health from 1993 to 1998 and was a founder and the first president of Friends of the National Institute for Nursing Research. In 1993 President Clinton appointed her to the Health Professionals Review Group, which analyzed the President's plan to reform the health care system before he presented it to Congress. In 1984-1985 she received a Robert Wood Johnson Health Policy Fellowship and worked as a staff member for Senator Kennedy on the Senate Labor and Human Resources Committee. Dr. Mundinger is the founder of Columbia Advanced Practice Nurse Associates (CAPNA), and recently established at Columbia the doctor of nursing practice degree, the first clinical nursing doctorate in the nation. In 1998 she was named Nurse Practitioner of the Year by the *Nurse Practitioner: The American Journal of Primary Health Care*. Dr. Mundinger holds a B.S. cum laude from the University of Michigan and a doctorate in public health from Columbia University School of Public Health. In 1996 she was awarded a doctor of humane letters (honorary) from Hamilton College. In 1995 she was the first nurse to be honored and profiled by the University of Michigan as a distinguished alumna. She is an elected member of the IOM and the

American Academy of Nursing. Dr. Mundinger currently sits on the board of directors of UnitedHealth Group, Gentiva Health Services, Welch Allyn, Inc., and Cell Therapeutics, Inc.

Michael A. Mustille, M.D., an occupational medicine physician and physician executive for 33 years with the Permanente Medical Group in Northern California, is currently associate executive director for external relations with the Permanente Federation, a national organization of physicians who practice in the Kaiser Permanente Medical Care Program. Dr. Mustille is also a senior adviser to the Council of Accountable Physician Practices (CAPP), a joint undertaking by 34 member groups of the nation's largest and most prominent physician practices. CAPP's mission is to foster the development of the accountable physician group model as a step toward the transformation of the American healthcare system. Before assuming his current role in 1997, Dr. Mustille served as assistant physician-in-chief of the Kaiser Permanente Medical Center in South San Francisco, California. He started with Kaiser Permanente at the Walnut Creek, California, Medical Center in 1973 as a staff physician, then moved to South San Francisco as assistant chief of medicine, and was later chief of occupational medicine at the South San Francisco and San Francisco facilities. While there, he developed a prototype occupational medicine specialty clinic that was adopted as the model for Kaiser Permanente medical centers throughout the state. Dr. Mustille received his undergraduate degree from Williams College in Massachusetts and his M.D. from Cornell University in New York. He completed a medical internship at the University of California's Moffitt Hospital in San Francisco as well as a residency in occupational medicine at the University of California, San Francisco. He is a member of the Phi Beta Kappa and Alpha Omega Alpha honor societies.

Nancy H. Nielsen, M.D., Ph.D., an internist from Buffalo, New York., was elected speaker of the American Medical Association House of Delegates in June 2003 and reelected in 2005. She is a delegate from New York and previously served two terms on the AMA Council on Scientific Affairs. She is clinical professor of medicine and senior associate dean for medical education at the State University of New York (SUNY) School of Medicine and Biomedical Sciences in Buffalo. Dr. Nielsen has also served as a member on the National Patient Safety Foundation Board of Directors, the Commission for the Prevention of Youth Violence, the Task Force on Quality and Patient Safety, and the HHS Secretary's Advisory Committee on Regulatory Reform and as the AMA representative to the National Quality Forum, Physicians Consortium for Performance Improvement, the Hospital Quality Alliance (HQA), and the Ambulatory Care Quality Alliance (AQA). She has served as a trustee of SUNY and as a member of the Board of Directors of Kaleida Health—a five-hospital system in western New York. She is currently associate medical director for quality and interim chief medical officer at Independent Health Association, a major health insurer in New York. Dr. Nielsen holds a doctorate in microbiology and received her M.D. from SUNY School of Medicine and Biomedical Sciences in Buffalo.

Margaret E. O'Kane is the president and founder of the National Committee for Quality Assurance, an independent, nonprofit organization whose mission is to improve healthcare quality. Under Ms. O'Kane's leadership, NCQA has developed broad support among the employer and health plan communities; most Fortune 500 companies will only do business with NCQA-accredited health plans and nearly all use HEDIS data to evaluate the plans that serve their employees. Ms. O'Kane was named Health Person of the Year in 1996 by *Medicine & Health;* in 1997 she received a Founder's Award from the American College of Medical Quality, and she is an elected member of the Institute of Medicine. In 2000, Ms. O'Kane received the Centers for Disease Control and Prevention's (CDC's) Champion of Prevention Award, the agency's highest honor. In 2005, Ms. O'Kane was named one of Modern Healthcare's Top 25 Women in Health Care, and she has previously been voted one of the nation's "100 Most Powerful People in Health Care." Under her leadership, in 2005 NCQA received awards from the National Coalition for Cancer Survivorship, the American Diabetes Association, and the American Pharmacists' Association. Ms. O'Kane is a sought-after public speaker, regularly addressing audiences across the country on topics such as pay-for-performance, the value of accountability, and the need to expand measurement in health care. She grants about 75 media interviews a year; has been a guest on the Today show, CNN, NBC, ABC, and NPR; and is regularly quoted in the *Wall Street Journal, New York Times,* and other major daily papers.

Steve E. Phurrough, M.D., M.P.A., is the director of the Coverage and Analysis Group at the Center for Medicare and Medicaid Services. Using evidence-based medicine principles, Dr. Phurrough assists in developing national policy on the appropriate devices, diagnostics, and procedures that should be provided by the Medicare program. Dr. Phurrough joined CMS in 2001 as the director of the Division of Medical and Surgical Services in the Coverage and Analysis Group after completing a long and distinguished career in the United States Army. In addition to being a practicing family practitioner, his military career also included managing Department of Defense regional healthcare delivery systems, creating national and international healthcare policy for the Army, and developing practice guidelines. Dr. Phurrough received his M.D. from the University of Alabama in

Birmingham and a master's in public administration from the University of Colorado in Colorado Springs. He is board certified by the American Board of Family Practice and is a certified physician executive by the American College of Physician Executives.

Cynthia Palmer, M.Sc., is the program officer for AHRQ's Integrated Delivery System Research Network (IDSRN) and its successor program, Accelerating Change and Transformation in Organizations and Networks (ACTION). ACTION includes 15 partners and approximately 150 collaborating organizations that link the nation's top researchers with some of the largest healthcare systems to conduct rapid cycle, demand-driven, applied research on issues important to healthcare delivery systems. Ms. Palmer is also the co-lead of the AHRQ team involved in a National Health Plan Collaborative to reduce racial and ethnic disparities. She has more than 20 years of experience in health services research and clinical epidemiology. She joined AHRQ in December 2001 from MEDTAP International, Inc., Bethesda, Maryland, where she served as a research scientist and deputy director of the Health Economics Group.

Steven D. Pearson, M.D., M.Sc., F.R.C.P., is a general internist and associate professor of ambulatory care and prevention at Harvard Medical School, and senior fellow at America's Health Insurance Plans (AHIP). Dr. Pearson's work examines the scientific and ethical foundations of evidence-based policy making in health care, and at AHIP, he performs research and policy analysis on issues related to evidence-based medicine. In addition, he is working to support the Institute for Clinical and Economic Review (ICER). ICER is a new initiative, created to integrate appraisals of the clinical effectiveness and cost-effectiveness of medical innovations, with the goal of providing new information to decision makers intent on improving the value of healthcare services His published work includes the book *No Margin, No Mission: Health Care Organizations and the Quest for Ethical Excellence*. Dr. Pearson serves on the management committee of the International Society for Priority Setting in Health Care, and in 2004 he was awarded an Atlantic Fellowship to pursue policy studies at the National Institute for Clinical Excellence in London, England. He returned to the United States to serve from 2005 to 2006 as special adviser, Technology and Coverage Policy, at the CMS. Dr. Pearson received his B.A. from Stanford University and his M.D. from the University of California at San Francisco. He was a medical intern and resident at Brigham and Women's Hospital in Boston, following which he completed a fellowship in health services research and received a master of science in health policy and management from the Harvard School of Public Health.

Jonathan B. Perlin, M.D., Ph.D., M.S.H.A., F.A.C.P., is under secretary for health in the Department of Veterans Affairs (VA). As the chief executive officer of the Veterans Health Administration, Dr. Perlin leads the nation's largest integrated health system. As VHA's chief quality and performance officer from 1999 to 2002, he was responsible for supporting quality improvement and performance management. He is also commissioner to the American Health Information Community (chartered to help realize the president's goal of making electronic health records available to most Americans within 10 years), president of the Association of Military Surgeons of the United States, and government liaison member to the Board of Directors of the National Quality Forum. Prior to joining VHA, Dr. Perlin served as medical director for quality improvement at the Medical College of Virginia Hospitals—Virginia Commonwealth University (VCU) Health System—where he is adjunct associate professor of medicine and professor of health administration at Virginia Commonwealth University. A fellow of the American College of Physicians, Dr. Perlin has a master of science in health administration. He received his Ph.D. in pharmacology and toxicology and an M.D. as part of the Medical Scientist Training Program at Virginia Commonwealth University's Medical College of Virginia campus.

Robert L. Phillips, Jr., M.D., M.S.P.H., is a family physician and director of the Robert Graham Center: Policy Studies in Family Practice and Primary Care, a research center sponsored by the American Academy of Family Physicians. His research interests include primary care safety and quality, healthcare geography, and collaborative care processes. He has been a co-investigator on several studies of errors reported in primary care settings and contributed to a resulting taxonomy. He has faculty appointments at Georgetown University and George Washington University, and he sees patients in Fairfax, Virginia. Dr. Phillips graduated from the University of Florida College of Medicine in Gainesville, Florida, and did residency training in family medicine at the University of Missouri-Columbia in Columbia, Missouri. He remained in Columbia for a two-year National Research Service Award (NRSA) research fellowship, during which he completed a master of science in public health and did clinical practice in a community health center in a federal housing authority. He has served on the AMA's Council on Medical Education and as the president of the National Residency Matching Program.

Alan B. Rosenberg, M.D., is the vice president of Medical Policy, Technology Assessment, and Credentialing Programs for WellPoint, Inc., and president of Anthem Utilization Management Services Inc. Among his responsibilities, Dr. Rosenberg leads WellPoint's programs (across all of its affiliated brands) for medical policy, technology assessment, credentialing, and utilization management. Prior to his current position, he served as chief medical officer for Rush Prudential Health Plans; director in Healthcare Business Consulting for Arthur Andersen; and vice president of medical affairs and medical director for Aetna US Healthcare of the Midwest, Inc. Dr. Rosenberg received his undergraduate training from Columbia University and received his medical degree from New York University Medical School. He completed his residency in internal medicine at the University of Chicago, Michael Reese Hospital. Dr. Rosenberg is a fellow of the Institute of Medicine of Chicago, serves as a board member of American Association of Preferred Provider Organizations (AAPPO), a member of the Blue Cross Association Medical Policy Panel, and several AHIP committees.

Wayne A. Rosenkrans, Jr., is business strategy director for external scientific affairs at AstraZeneca Pharmaceuticals. In that role he has responsibility for long-range strategy development supporting AstraZeneca's external scientific influencing policy through U.S. regulatory affairs and U.S. medical affairs. He is a recipient of the Society of Competitive Intelligence Professionals (SCIP) Fellows Award and a former president of the society. Previous positions include global director, intelligence affairs, at AstraZeneca; director, U.S. intelligence, at AstraZeneca; Competitive Technical Intelligence Group leader and research planning analyst at Zeneca Pharmaceuticals; director of Strategic Intelligence Systems for Windhover Information; director of Drug Intelligence Systems Sales and Marketing for Adis International; and associate director and head of strategic intelligence for SmithKline Beecham Pharmaceuticals R&D. He holds an S.B. in biology from MIT and a Ph.D. in cell and molecular biology from Boston University; he received postdoctoral training in cancer and radiation biology at the University of Rochester.

John C. Rother, J.D., M.A., is the group executive officer of policy and strategy for AARP. He is responsible for the federal and state public policies of the association, for international initiatives, and for formulating AARP's overall strategic direction. He is an authority on Medicare, managed care, long-term care, Social Security, pensions, and the challenges facing the boomer generation. Prior to coming to AARP in 1984, Mr. Rother served eight years with the U.S. Senate as special counsel for labor and health to former Senator Jacob Javits (R-NY), then as staff director and chief counsel for the Special Committee on Aging under its chairman Senator John Heinz (R-PA). He serves on several boards and commissions, including the National Health Care Quality Forum and the American Board of Internal Medicine Foundation. John Rother is graduated with honors from Oberlin College and the University of Pennsylvania Law School.

Stephen B. Soumerai, Sc.D., is professor of ambulatory care and prevention at Harvard Medical School and Harvard Pilgrim Health Care, where he directs the Drug Policy Research Group, a research program focused on pharmaceutical outcomes and quality of health care that is also a World Health Organization Collaborating Center in Pharmaceutical Policy. Dr. Soumerai is well-known for his research on the effectiveness of educational, administrative, and regulatory interventions to improve drug prescribing; economic access to medications; and the effects of pharmaceutical cost containment and coverage policies among vulnerable populations. He co-chairs the statistics and evaluative sciences concentration of Harvard University's Ph.D. program in health policy, and has served on numerous federal scientific review committees.

William W. Stead, M.D., is associate vice chancellor for health affairs and director of the Informatics Center at Vanderbilt University. In this role, he functions as chief information officer of the Vanderbilt Medical Center and chief information architect for the university. He was involved in early development of the Cardiology Databank, one of the first clinical epidemiology projects to change practice by linking outcomes to process and the Medical Record (TMR), one of the first practical computer-based patient record systems. He has led two prominent academic health centers through both planning and implementation phases of large-scale, Integrated Advanced Information Management System (IAIMS) projects. Dr. Stead is McKesson Foundation Professor of Biomedical Informatics and Professor of Medicine. He is a founding fellow of both the American College of Medical Informatics and the American Institute for Engineering in Biology and Medicine, and an elected member of both the IOM and the American Clinical and Climatological Association. He was the founding editor-in-chief of the *Journal of the American Medical Informatics Association* and served as president of the American Association for Medical Systems and Informatics and the American College of Medical Informatics. He serves on the Computer Science and Telecommunications Board of the National Research Council. He served as chairman of the Board of Regents of the National Library of Medicine and as a presidential appointee to the Commission on Systemic Interoperability. In addition to his academic and advisory responsibilities, Dr. Stead is a director of HealthStream and director of NetSilica. Dr. Stead received his B.A. and M.D. from Duke University, where he also completed specialty and subspecialty training in internal medicine and nephrology.

Donald M. Steinwachs, Ph.D., is the chair of the Department of Health Policy and Management at Johns Hopkins University. He also holds the Fred and Julie Soper Professorship of Health Policy and Management.

Dr. Steinwachs's current research includes (1) studies of medical effectiveness and patient outcomes for individuals with specific medical, surgical, and psychiatric conditions; (2) studies of the impact of managed care and other organizational and financial arrangements on access to care, quality, utilization, and cost; and (3) studies to develop better methods to measure the effectiveness of systems of care, including case mix (e.g., ambulatory care groups), quality profiling, and indicators of outcome. He has a particular interest in the role of routine management information systems (MIS) as source of data for evaluating the effectiveness and cost of health care. This includes work on the integration of outcomes management systems with existing MIS in managed care settings.

Andrew L. Stern is president of the Service Employees International Union (SEIU). Mr. Stern began his union career in 1973 as a state social service worker and rank-and-file member of SEIU Local 668. He become the first elected full-time president of the local when he was 27, and two years later in 1980 was named to the union's International Executive Board. In 1984 he began overseeing the organizing and field services programs, and in 1996 he was elected SEIU's international president. Stern serves on the board of directors of the Aspen Institute, Rock the Vote, and the Broad Foundation.

Walter "Buzz" Stewart, Ph.D., M.P.H., is an associate chief research officer at Geisinger Health System (Danville, Pennsylvania) and director of the Center for Health Research and Rural Advocacy. The center is involved in expanding clinical and population-based research, genomics research, and the use of information technology and new healthcare models to translate knowledge to clinical practice. An expert in neuroepidemiology, Dr. Stewart has spent his career understanding the debilitating effects of chronic episodic conditions such as migraine headaches and other pain conditions (among other topics) and exploring healthcare models to improve outcomes. Dr. Stewart has authored more than 220 journal articles and book chapters. Earlier in his career, Dr. Stewart founded IMR, a clinical trials and survey research company. In 1998 IMR was acquired by AdvancePCS, where Stewart served as vice-president of clinical research and development. Dr. Stewart also started the AdvancePCS Center for Work and Health, focusing on measuring the impact of illnesses on work productivity. Prior to his tenure with AdvancePCS, he was a full-time faculty member at the Johns Hopkins Bloomberg School of Public Health and he maintains an adjunct professor position at Johns Hopkins. He earned his bachelor's degree in the neurosciences from the University of California, Riverside; his M.P.H. from the University of California, Los Angeles; and his Ph.D. in epidemiology from Johns Hopkins School of Hygiene and Public Health.

Sean Tunis, M.D., M.Sc., is a senior fellow at the Health Technology Center in San Francisco, where he works with healthcare decision makers to design and implement "real-world" studies of new healthcare technologies. Through September 2005, Dr. Tunis was the chief medical officer at the Centers for Medicare and Medicaid Services. Before joining CMS, Dr. Tunis served as director of the health program at the congressional Office of Technology Assessment and as a health policy adviser to the U.S. Senate. He received his M.D. from Stanford University and did his residency training at UCLA and the University of Maryland in emergency medicine and internal medicine.

James N. Weinstein, D.O., M.S., is professor and chair of the Department of Orthopaedic Surgery and professor of community and family medicine at Dartmouth Medical School. He is the principal investigator of the Spine Patient Outcomes Research Trial (SPORT), the largest study ever funded by the NIAMSD. He founded the Spine Center at Dartmouth-Hitchcock Medical Center (DHMC), as well as the Center for Shared Decision-Making at DHMC. Dr. Weinstein is center director of the newly established NIH-sponsored, Multidisciplinary Clinical Research Center (MCRC) in Musculoskeletal Health Care at Dartmouth, in addition to directing other programs and centers at the Dartmouth Medical School: co-director of the Clinical Trials Center and senior member of the Center for the Evaluative Clinical Sciences. He is editor-in-chief of *Spine* and an award-winning scholar (e.g., Bristol-Myers Career Research Award in pain research and the prestigious Kappa Delta Award), Dr. Weinstein is a member of the American Academy of Orthopaedic Surgeons Board of Directors. He is also a director of the American Board of Orthopaedic Surgery. Dr. Weinstein was presented with the ISSLS Wiltse Lifetime Achievement Award in 2006.

Harlan F. Weisman, M.D., is the chief science and technology officer, medical devices and diagnostics, Johnson & Johnson (J&J). He supports the J&J Medical Devices & Diagnostics Group Operating Committee in steering the group's scientific and technical agenda, leading investments in group-level technologies, and sponsoring the group's research and development (R&D) talent agenda. Prior to this, he was company group chairman, research and development, pharmaceuticals, for Johnson & Johnson, where he had executive oversight of the ALZA Corporation, Johnson & Johnson Pharmaceutical Research & Development (J&JPRD), and TransForm Pharmaceuticals, Inc. Previously, Dr. Weisman was president of J&JPRD. Prior to this, he was president, research and development, at Centocor, another member of the Johnson & Johnson family of R&D companies. Before joining Centocor in 1990, Dr. Weisman was assistant professor of medicine at Johns Hopkins University School of Medicine; consultant cardiologist,

Johns Hopkins Hospital; and director of the Experimental Cardiac Pathology Laboratory there. He is a graduate of the University of Maryland and the University of Maryland School of Medicine. After his residency in internal medicine at Mount Sinai Hospital in New York, he did his postgraduate fellowship training in cardiovascular disease at Johns Hopkins Hospital. Dr. Weisman is a fellow of the American College of Cardiology, the American College of Chest Physicians, and the Councils on Clinical Cardiology and Arteriosclerosis, Thrombosis, and Vascular Biology of the American Heart Association. He is also a member of the American College of Physicians, the American Federation for Clinical Research, the American Medical Association, and the New Jersey Medical Society. Dr. Weisman is an author of more than 90 journal articles and book chapters in the fields of cardiovascular disease and medical product development.

Jed Weissberg, M.D., is associate executive director for quality and performance improvement at the Permanente Foundation. Jed chairs the board of the Care Management Institute, New Technology Committee, the Garfield Memorial Research Fund, and the Medical Director's Quality Committee. After joining the Permanente Medical Group in 1984, Jed became chief of GI and then became the physician-in-chief at the Fremont Medical Center. After six years, Jed joined the Permanente Federation, the governance umbrella organization for the eight Permanente Medical Groups across the country. Dr. Weissberg was educated at the University of Pennsylvania and Albert Einstein College of Medicine and completed an internal medicine residency at Boston City Hospital. This was followed by a gastroenterology fellowship at Stanford and an alcoholism and substance abuse fellowship at the Palo Alto VA Hospital.

Mark V. Williams, M.D., F.A.C.P., is a professor of medicine at Emory University School of Medicine and director of the Hospital Medicine Unit for Emory Healthcare. He is also executive medical director for the Emory HCA Medical Centers. Dr. Williams established the first hospitalist program at a public hospital and now supervises the largest academic hospitalist program in the United States. A past president of the Society of Hospital Medicine and editor-in-chief of the *Journal of Hospital Medicine*, he actively promotes the role of hospitalists as leaders in the delivery of health care to hospitalized patients. Dr. Williams' teaching activities center on promoting the use of evidence-based medicine (EBM) in patient care and a systems approach to patient safety. He developed the initial curriculum used to teach EBM to internal medicine residents at Emory. A strong advocate of EBM, he has participated as a tutor in the McMaster "How to Teach EBM" course and served as a member of the EBM Task Force for the Society of General Internal Medicine. With more than 50 publications,

Dr. Williams' research focuses on the role of health literacy in the delivery of health care and quality improvement, and he currently is studying the role of teamwork in the delivery of hospital care and the discharge process. Dr. Williams graduated from Emory University School of Medicine and completed residency in internal medicine at Massachusetts General Hospital. Board certified in internal medicine and emergency medicine, he also completed a Faculty Development Fellowship in general medicine at the University of North Carolina-Chapel Hill and the Woodruff Leadership Academy at Emory.

Appendix
C

Workshop Attendee List

Patricia Adams
NPC (National Pharmaceutical
    Council)

Kate Ahlport
Health Research Alliance

Dara Aisner
Institute of Medicine (IOM)

David Aron
Department of Veteran Affairs

David Atkins
Agency for Healthcare Research
    and Quality (AHRQ)

Peter Bach
Centers for Medicare and Medicaid
    Services (CMS)

Lynn Bale
Premier, Inc

Andrew Barbash
Apractis Solutions

Bart Barefoot
GlaxoSmithKline

Sinan Batman
Kodak

Martina Bebin
Robert Wood Johnson (RWJ)
    Foundation

Marc Berger
Merck

Cliff Binder
AARP

Gregg Bloche
Georgetown

Carmella Bocchino
America's Health Insurance Plans
    (AHIP)

Cathy Bonuccelli
AstraZeneca

Rosemary Botchway
Primary Care Coalition

Dianne Bricker
Medical Society of the District of
    Columbia

Jennifer Bright
National Mental Health
    Association

Sharon Brigner
Pharmaceutical Research and
    Manufacturers of America
    (PhRMA)

Lynda Bryant-Comstock
GlaxoSmithKline

Randy Burkholder
PhRMA

Robert Califf
Duke University

Daniel Campion
AcademyHealth

Tanisha Carino
Avalere Health

Shenan Carroll
IOM

Linda Carter
Johnson & Johnson

Samantha Chao
IOM

Carolyn Clancy
AHRQ

John Clarke
Drexel University

Steve Cole
Kaiser Permanente

Garen Corbett
Health Industry Forum

Denis Cortese
Mayo Clinic

John Courtney
Clinical Research Forum

Helen Darling
National Business Group on
    Health

Liza Dawson
National Institutes of Health (NIH)

Shoshana Derrow
AARP

Elise Desjardins
Grantmakers in Health

Emily DeVoto
Health Care Consultant

Carol Diamond
Markle Foundation

Andrea Douglas
PhRMA

Alison Drone
Aspen Institute

Joyce Dubow
AARP

Jill Eden
IOM

Sarah England
RWJ Foundation/Senate

Lynn Etheredge
George Washington University

Christina Farup
Johnson & Johnson

Nancy Featherstone
AstraZeneca

Reuven Ferziger
Ortho-McNeil Janssen Scientific
    Affairs

Shelley Fichtner
PhRMA

Harvey Fineberg
IOM

Diane Flickinger
Eli Lilly and Company

Irene Fraser
AHRQ

Deborah Fritz
GlaxoSmithKline

Richard Fry
Foundation for Managed Care
    Pharmacy

Robert Galvin
General Electric

Andrea Gelzer
CIGNA

Janice Genevro
AHRQ

Sharon Gershon
FDA, Center for Devices and
    Radiological Health (CDER)

Daniel Gesser
Overture

David Goldstein
Duke University

Stuart Guterman
Commonwealth Fund

Douglas Hadley
CIGNA

Bruce Hamory
Geisinger Health System

Catherine Harrison
Avalere Health

Robin Hemphill
Office of Senator Jeff Bingaman

Giselle Hicks
National Breast Cancer Coalition
    Fund

Peter Highnam
NIH

Telba Irony
FDA, CDRH

George Isham
HealthPartners, Inc.

Jeannie Jacobs
Virginia Hospital Center

Dawn Marie Jacobson
U.S. Department of Health and
    Human Services (HHS)

Brent James
Intermountain Healthcare

Roger Johns
Office of Senator Orrin Hatch

Maya Johnson-Nimo
HHS, Health Resources and
    Services Administration
    (HRSA)

Peter Juhn
Johnson & Johnson

Michael Kafrissen
Ortho-McNeil Janssen Scientific
    Affairs, LLC

Ming-Chih Kao
University of Michigan Medical
    School

Stephen Katz
NIH

Jessica Kidwell
Veterans Health Administration
    (VHA)

Darrell Kirch
Association of American Medical
    Colleges (AAMC)

Joel Kupersmith
VHA

Eric Larson
Group Health Cooperative

Cato Laurencin
University of Virginia

Paul Lee
IOM

Craig Lefebvre
Lefebvre Consulting Group

Sandy Leonard
AstraZeneca

Jeffrey Lerner
ECRI

Patricia MacTaggart
EDS

Janet Marchibroda
eHealth

J. Michael McGinnis
IOM

Robert Mechanic
Brandeis University

Erik Mettler
FDA

Marie Michnich
IOM

Lisa Minich
Robert Graham Center

Hazel Moran
National Mental Health
    Association

Tom Mowbray
Freelance Member of the National
    Press Club

Mary O'Neil Mundinger
Columbia University

Horacio Murillo
AAAS

Michael Mustille
Permanente Federation

Nicole Newburg-Rinn
Johns Hopkins University

Nancy Nielsen
American Medical Association

Margaret O'Kane
National Committee for Quality
    Assurance (NCQA)

LeighAnne Olsen
IOM

Ann Page
IOM

Cynthia Palmer
AHRQ

Steven Pearson
AHIP

Eleanor Perfetto
Pfizer Inc.

Jonathan Perlin
Department of Veterans Affairs

Anuradha Phadke
Consumers Union

Robert Phillips
American Academy of Family
    Physicians (AAFP)

Steve Phurrough
CMS

William Pilkington
Cabarrus Health Alliance

Sarah Pitluck
Genentech, Inc.

Leonard Pogach
Veteran Affairs

G. Gregory Raab
Raab & Associates, Inc.

Nancy Ray
MedPAC

Joseph Reblando
PhRMA

John Ring
IOM

Alan Rosenberg
WellPoint

Wayne Rosenkrans
AstraZeneca Pharmaceuticals

John Rother
AARP

Forough Saadatmand
Howard University

Lindsay Sabik
Harvard University

Khaled Saleh
University of Virginia

Karen Sanders
American Psychiatric Association

Adam Scheffler
Health Policy Analyst

Karen Schoelles
ECRI

David Schulke
American Health Quality
    Association

Nirav Shah
Geisinger Health System

Katherine Shear
Columbia University

Gail Shearer
Consumers Union

Kirsten Sloan
AARP

Stephen Soumerai
Harvard Pilgrim

Fran Spigai
Lincoln County Community Health
    Improvement Partnership
    (CHIP)

William Stead
Vanderbilt University

Ben Steffen
Maryland Health Care
    Commission

Donald Steinwachs
Johns Hopkins University

Andrew Stern
Service Employees International
    Union (SEIU)

Walter Stewart
Geisinger Health System

Nancy Sung
Burroughs Wellcome Fund

Meghan Taira
Arnold and Porter LLP

Patrick Terry
Genomic Health, Inc.

Steven Teutsch
Merck

Paul Tibbits, Jr.
American Diabetes Association

Tricia Trinité
AHRQ

Anne Trontell
AHRQ

Sean Tunis
Health Technology Center

I. Steven Udvarhelyi
Independence Blue Cross

Craig Umscheid
Center for Evidence-Based Practice

Jill Wechsler
Managed Healthcare Executive

Richard Weil
Kodak

James Weinstein
Dartmouth University

Kathleen Weis
Pfizer, Inc.

Harlan Weisman
Johnson & Johnson

Jed Weissberg
Permanente Federation

Karen Williams
NPC

Kendal Williams
University of Pennsylvania Health
    System

Mark Williams
Emory University

Reggie Williams
Avalere Health

Appendix
D

IOM Roundtable on
Evidence-Based Medicine

The Institute of Medicine's Roundtable on Evidence-Based Medicine provides a neutral venue for key stakeholders—patients, health providers, payers, employers, manufacturers, health information technology, researchers, and policy makers—to work cooperatively on innovative approaches to generating and applying evidence to drive improvements in the effectiveness and efficiency of medical care in the United States. Participants seek the development of a *learning healthcare system* that is designed to generate and apply the best evidence for the collaborative health care choices of each patient and provider; to drive the process of discovery as a natural outgrowth of patient care; and to ensure innovation, quality, safety, and value in health care. They have set a goal that, by the year 2020, ninety percent of clinical decisions will be supported by accurate, timely, and up-to-date clinical information, and will reflect the best available evidence.

This is not currently the case. Today, far too often care that is important is not delivered, and care that is delivered is not important. Despite per capita health expenditures much higher than any other nation—now more than $2 trillion—the United States ranks far down the list on international comparisons on many basic measures of health status. As leaders in their fields, Roundtable members work with their colleagues to identify issues not being adequately addressed, the nature of the barriers and possible solutions, and the priorities for action. They marshal the energy and resources of the sectors represented on the Roundtable to work for sustained public-private cooperation for change. Anchoring this work is a focus on three dimensions of the challenge:

1. Accelerating progress toward the *long-term vision* of a learning healthcare system, in which evidence is both applied and developed as a natural product of the care process.
2. Expanding the *capacity* to meet the acute need for evidence to support medical care that is maximally effective and produces the greatest value.
3. Improving *public understanding* of the nature of evidence, the dynamic character of evidence development, and the importance of insisting on medical care that reflects the best evidence.

For the purpose of the Roundtable activities, we define evidence-based medicine broadly to mean that, to the greatest extent possible, the decisions that shape the health and health care of Americans—by patients, providers, payers and policymakers alike—will be grounded on a reliable evidence base, will account appropriately for individual variation in patient needs, and will support the generation of new insights on clinical effectiveness. Evidence is generally considered to be information from clinical experience that has met some established test of validity, and the appropriate standard is determined according to the requirements of the intervention and clinical circumstance. Processes that involve the development and use of evidence should be accessible and transparent to all stakeholders.

A common commitment to certain principles and priorities guides the activities of the Roundtable and its members, including the commitment to: the right health care for each person; putting the best evidence into practice; establishing the effectiveness, efficiency and safety of medical care delivered; building constant measurement into our health care investments; the establishment of health care data as a public good; shared responsibility distributed equitably across stakeholders, both public and private; collaborative stakeholder involvement in priority setting; transparency in the execution of activities and reporting of results; and subjugation of individual political or stakeholder perspectives in favor of the common good.

Roundtable Sponsors

Agency for Healthcare Research and Quality
America's Health Insurance Plans
AstraZeneca
Blue Shield of California Foundation
Burroughs Wellcome Fund
California Healthcare Foundation

Centers for Medicare & Medicaid Services
Food and Drug Administration
Johnson & Johnson
sanofi-aventis
Stryker
Veterans Health Administration